Praise for *Food Sanity*

"I'm very impressed with the level of research Dr. Friedman has done and how he's integrated this information to helping people, including me! With so much confusion and contradictions on what we should and shouldn't be eating, *Food Sanity* sets the record straight! His blueprints for eating will add more years to your life and life to those years."

—**Jack Canfield,** *New York Times* best-selling author of the *Chicken Soup for the Soul* book series and *The Success Principles*. Featured teacher in *The Secret*

"Food has the power to heal or make us sick. Dr. Friedman does a magnificent job of pulling back the curtain, exposing hidden chemicals, biased agendas, and the profits behind them. *Food Sanity* gives you a definitive guide to eating your way to a life of total restoration and longevity."

—**Suzanne Somers,** health advocate and best-selling author of 23 books

"Hippocrates said, 'Let food be your medicine,' and Dr. Friedman has the prescription! *Food Sanity* delivers an infinite, crystal-clear message on how to identify the good and eliminate the bad from your diet. This book is a must read for anyone that eats."

—**Dr. Josh Axe,** *New York Times* best-selling author of *Eat Dirt* and *The Real Food Diet Cookbook*. Founder of the second-most visited natural health website in the world: DrAxe.com

"In *Food Sanity,* Dr. Friedman gives you impartial, unbiased information that helps you make up your own mind. He doesn't take the 'It's my way or the highway' approach of so many other authors."

—**Harvey Diamond,** #1 *New York Times* best-selling author of *Fit for Life*

"Dr. David Friedman has published an eye-opening review of some of the most controversial nutrition topics, helping to answer the 'Should we or shouldn't we eat it?' debate as it relates to a number of different foods, including beef, chicken, and fish. He takes a deep dive, analyzing scores of scientific research to give readers a clear bottom line so they can make educated personal food choices."

—**Joy Bauer, MS, RDN,** health and nutrition expert for NBC's *TODAY* show, best-selling author of *From Junk Food to Joy Food* and founder of Nourish Snacks

"*Food Sanity* delivers a no-holds-barred, well researched look into the shameless tactics used by the food industry that rob us of good health. Dr. Friedman shows you how to make the healthiest food choices for you and your family."

—**Vani Hari,** *New York Times* best-selling author of *The Food Babe Way*. Founder of FoodBabe.com.

"*Food Sanity* is much more than a guide on what we should and shouldn't eat. Dr. Friedman shares why the right food choices are the first line of defense for preventing and reversing disease and quite literally saving our planet!"

—**Jordan Rubin,** author of 25 health books including *The Makers Diet*, which spent 47 weeks on the *New York Times* bestseller list

"Food and fitness go hand in hand and I believe Dr. Friedman' s book *Food Sanity* will help everyone eat properly to fuel their bodies and optimize their performance!"

—**Denise Austin,** world-renowned health and fitness expert and author of 12 best-selling books

"It's sad how the food industry puts product and profits first and the needs of the people last. Regardless of what type of diet you follow, *Food Sanity* will show you the good and the bad, and help guide you down a healthier path."

—**Kim Barnouin,** #1 *New York Times* best-selling author of *Skinny Bitch*

"Dr. Friedman does a brilliant job of shattering many of today's popular food myths. If you want to live a healthier life, this book is for you."

—**Lyssie Lakatos & Tammy Lakatos (The Nutrition Twins),** *New York Times* best-selling authors of *Veggie Cure*

"Dr. Friedman takes the term 'Food for Thought' to a new level! Before buying a house, you hire an inspector to go through every nook and cranny and document any damages hidden inside the walls. *Food Sanity* gives you the same detailed insight on what's hiding inside your food. Before you take another bite, I strongly recommend you read this book!"

—**Devin Alexander,** author of several *New York Times* best-selling books, including *The Biggest Loser Cookbook,* host of *Healthy Decadence* (Discovery Health and Fit TV) and chef of NBC's *The Biggest Loser*

"*Food Sanity* is one of the first books I've seen that takes into account how valuable sleep really is to the metabolic process. Restorative sleep is crucial to how well we digest our food and it ultimately affects our weight, hormonal system, and mood. I am excited to see this and I know it will help everyone who reads it."

—**Dr. Michael Breus, AKA "The Sleep Doctor,"** best-selling author and clinical advisory board member of *The Dr. Oz Show*

"Dr. David Friedman has done a wonderful job of explaining a healthy diet, and ideal way of life, which leads to longevity and optimal health. Everyone who is eating the Standard American Diet (SAD) needs to read *Food Sanity* and keep it in your ready reference library."

—**Dr. Earl Mindell,** best-selling author of over a dozen books, including the #1 bestseller *The Vitamin Bible, The Happiness Effect,* and *Healing with Hemp*

"If Dr. Friedman tells you what to eat for better health, you can take that advice to the bank."

—**George Noory,** host of the nationally syndicated show *Coast to Coast,* the most listened-to late-night program in America

"Dr. Friedman does a wonderful public service of exposing unhealthy and hidden ingredients in our food supply. *Food Sanity* is a much-needed culinary protest to a biased food industry that puts profits before people! Dr. Friedman has created a recipe for attaining optimal health using just a fork and spoon."

—**Dr. Jayson & Mira Calton,** best-selling authors of *Rich Food Poor Food*

"*Food Sanity* provides an in-depth, detailed review of the latest science to make sense of the diet and disease connection and how you can achieve your ideal health."

—**Erin Palinski-Wade,** best-selling author of *Belly Fat Diet For Dummies* and *2-Day Diabetes Diet*

"Food and sex are our two basic instincts and everyone knows how to have sex, but not everyone knows how to feed the body with nutrition and satisfy our insatiable appetites, until now! Dr. David Friedman's *Food Sanity* will educate and empower you to choose foods you should be eating for optimal health."

—**Dr. Ava Cadell,** author of 10 books on love & sex, global speaker, and celebrity clinical sexologist

"Dr. Friedman has written a valuable book for learning misleading and dangerous information about foods. *Food Sanity* is revealing, enlightening, and offers a fresh source and insight that is crucial for a healthy life."

—**Gary Epler, MD,** considered among "The Best Doctors in America," renowned Harvard Medical School professor, and author of *Food: You're the Boss*

"*Food Sanity* contains brilliant ground-breaking information that will change your life. Dr. Friedman reveals the myths, clears up the ever-present confusion with diet and nutrition, and provides solutions using the latest research to help you create optimal health."

—**Lori Shemek, PhD,** leading health and weight-loss expert, best-selling author of *How to Fight FATflammation* and *Fire-Up Your Fat Burn!*

"As a holistic plastic surgeon, I'm a firm believer that what we eat greatly affects how we age. Dr. Friedman's recommendations go more than just skin deep! *Food Sanity* is a great guide to help you look and feel young again!"

—**Dr. Anthony Youn—AKA *America's Holistic Plastic Surgeon*™,** best-selling author of *THE AGE FIX*, and voted best plastic surgeon by *US News & World Report & Harper's Bazaar*.

"Read this book and you will never eat the same again—and that's a good thing! In *Food Sanity*, Dr. Friedman melds science with common sense to expose the fallacies in diet fads, food myths, and food propaganda that have, in one way or another, caused each of us to eat differently and to harm ourselves unwittingly. In one fell swoop, *Food Sanity* rights the wrongs and brings good food back to the table."

—**Jonathan Emord Esq.,** America's leading Food and Drug lawyer who's defeated the FDA more times in federal court than any other attorney in American history

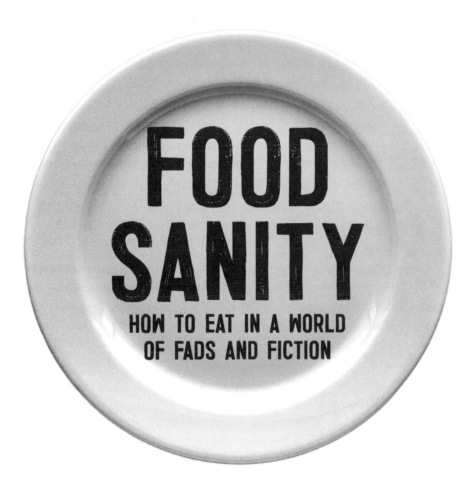

FOOD SANITY

HOW TO EAT IN A WORLD OF FADS AND FICTION

DR. DAVID FRIEDMAN

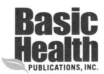

Basic Health
PUBLICATIONS, INC.

Turner Publishing Company
Nashville, Tennessee
New York, New York
www.turnerpublishing.com

The information contained in this book is based upon the research and personal and professional experiences of the author. It is not intended as a substitute for consulting with your physician or other healthcare provider. Any attempt to diagnose and treat an illness should be done under the direction of a healthcare professional.

The publisher does not advocate the use of any particular healthcare protocol but believes the information in this book should be available to the public. The publisher and author are not responsible for any adverse effects or consequences resulting from the use of the suggestions, preparations, or procedures discussed in this book. Should the reader have any questions concerning the appropriateness of any procedures or preparation mentioned, the author and the publisher strongly suggest consulting a professional healthcare advisor.

Cover design: Maddie Cothren
Book design: Tim Holtz

Library of Congress Cataloging-in-Publication Data
Names: Friedman, David Ross, 1965- author.
Title: Food sanity : how to eat in a world of fads and fiction / Dr. David
  Friedman.
Description: New York, New York : Basic Health Publications, an imprint of
  Turner Publishing Company, [2018] | Includes bibliographical references
  and index.
Identifiers: LCCN 2017054001 (print) | LCCN 2017055159 (ebook) | ISBN
  9781683367291 (e-book) | ISBN 9781683367277 (paperback : alk. paper)
Subjects: LCSH: Nutrition. | Diet.
Classification: LCC RA784 (ebook) | LCC RA784 .F75 2018 (print) | DDC
  613.2--dc23
LC record available at https://lccn.loc.gov/2017054001

Printed in the United States of America
18 19 20 10 9 8 7 6 5 4 3 2 1

CONTENTS

FOREWORD

I magine how everyone felt after Christopher Columbus proved the world was round and not flat. What many people believed at the time to be true, he exposed as false. Dr. David Friedman is a modern-day Christopher Columbus. In *Food Sanity* he looks at many of today's so-called common health and nutritional "truths" and exposes them for the fallacies they are. He then goes a step further, pulling back the curtain to educate the reader and expose some of the conflicts of interest and money trails that all too frequently are behind many of today's health recommendations.

Nearly three decades after my book, *Fit for Life*, was published, our industrialized food industry continues to sweep important, lifesaving information under the carpet. Even though it's our consumer money—and our tax subsidies—that keep them in business, Big Pharma, Big Agra, and Big Dairy certainly do not have our best interests at heart. Back in the 1980s, the food industry was promoting partially hydrogenated vegetable oil (better known as trans fats) as a healthy alternative to saturated fats. I was ridiculed when I warned everyone about the dangers of eating this artificial food additive. Research now shows ingesting just two grams a day of trans fats, the amount contained in just one donut, increases your risk of heart disease by 23 percent! Many people berated me when I spoke out against the dairy industry in *Fit for Life* and showed the detrimental health effects that drinking milk can cause, especially in children! Fast forward three decades, and the dangers of milk, particularly from the hormones and antibiotics it contains, are common knowledge. Even so, the dairy industry still runs massive advertising campaigns to fool us into believing that milk promotes strong bones—when unbiased scientific evidence now shows just the opposite. In *Food Sanity*, Dr. Friedman traces back the little-known but very profitable dairy industry/government partnership that began almost a century ago.

There's no denying it; dis-ease in the body comes from the bad food choices we make! The health advocates who shout the loudest are the ones who can make a difference in the lives of millions of innocent consumers. In *Food Sanity*, Dr. Friedman grabs his megaphone and shouts from a mountaintop. His message is loud and clear: Take action and reclaim your own health! What I enjoyed most about *Food Sanity* is the way Dr. Friedman gives you impartial, unbiased information that helps you make up your own mind. He doesn't take the "it's my way or the highway" approach of so many other authors. He points out how scientific studies are often anything but objective—many are sponsored by the very corporations that have vested interests in producing the most profitable outcome. It is a sad commentary, but opinions, scientific data, and legislation can all be purchased for the right price. Dr. Friedman shows you how to follow the money behind the science and decide for yourself where the truth really lies.

Fit for Life was originally rejected by numerous publishers; many told me the book had no information that would be of interest or of worth to the reader. I was told my "peculiar theories" on how to eat were outlandish. But belief in my message and unshakable perseverance were rewarded when Warner Books saw the potential of the book. Fourteen million book sales later, *Fit for Life* remains one of the best-selling health books of all time! It held the #1 position on the prestigious *New York Times* bestseller list for an unprecedented forty consecutive weeks. The book earned a coveted position on the *Publisher's Weekly* list of Top 25 Best-selling Books in Publishing History, along with *Gone with the Wind* and the Bible. Changing how you eat will (not might) heal and prevent disease. In addition to learning how to make the right food choices, *Food Sanity* does a wonderful job of exposing the dangerous chemicals commonly used to process, color, preserve, and tenderize our food. You won't find many of these ingredients listed on a food label or restaurant menu—but thanks to *Food Sanity*, you'll now be able recognize and protect yourself from them.

When the first edition of *Fit for Life* was published in 1985, obesity was not the epidemic it is today. At present, 70 percent of the population is now overweight and obesity has become the leading health affliction in history! Why is the United States the fattest developed country in the world? We have access to thousands of diet books, weight-loss programs, diet pills, and diet shakes; our grocery store shelves are filled with sugar-free, fat-free, and low-calorie foods. Dr. Friedman makes the point well—no matter what type of fad diet or program you go on, although you may initially lose weight, more often than not, six to twelve months later, chances are even greater that you will not only regain the weight you lost but you will likely end up heavier and even more unhealthy than before. The key to achieving permanent weight loss is to embrace a healthy lifestyle—not a fad diet or product. *Food Sanity* gives you the information you need to attain permanent weight loss, improve longevity, and reach optimal health.

I was one of the first health advocates encouraging people to at least cut back, if not eliminate entirely, red meat from their diet. The question is frequently asked, "If humans weren't designed to eat red meat, why then did our Stone Age ancestors eat so much of it?" Dr. Friedman does an admirable job revealing forensic proof that cavemen ate a widely varied diet that only rarely included red meat.

As we all journey our way through this thing called life, we are, on occasion, blessed by crossing paths with those whose integrity and desire to do good in the world is exceeded only by their genuine caring for the well-being of others. Just such a person is Dr. Friedman, who is the supreme personification of these high ideals. Before Dr. Friedman began writing this book, he asked me as a friend if I would share the secret to creating a national bestseller. I told him, "Just be yourself, share your passion, and most importantly, don't talk over the heads of your readers. If you share your knowledge on a level everyone can grasp, they will embrace your vision." I'm pleased to say, he took my advice! *Food Sanity* gives you a wealth of important information in a way that's easy to follow, with lots of great stories gleaned from his considerable experience with his many patients. I'm honored to write the foreword to a book that is destined to enhance the lives of millions. Some of what you read here may make you angry, some may make you laugh, but every chapter will inform and inspire you. You'll come away with the understanding that we cannot rely on our health care system or on prescription drugs; we must take charge, take back control, and reclaim our own health!

—**Harvey Diamond**, #1 *New York Times* best-selling author of *Fit for Life*

INTRODUCTION

ESCAPE FROM THE LAND OF CONFUSION

"You are what you eat," my mother said with a finger wave, as she watched me sink my teeth into the center of a warm, squishy Pop-Tart. I ran into the bathroom and looked in the mirror. I hadn't yet turned into a strawberry toaster pastry but decided to really put her statement to the test. Since I was vertically challenged (aka short for my age), I asked Mom to buy Jolly Green Giant vegetables, hoping they would make me taller. Unfortunately, I never did become a giant. But I did learn from an early age that our food choices really do determine what we eventually become. I would ultimately share this message with millions of people as a syndicated radio host and weekly health expert on Lifetime Television. For more than fifteen years, I've had the privilege of interviewing hundreds of world-renowned health advocates, scientists, doctors, and *New York Times* best-selling authors. My goal has always been to share cutting-edge topics and advice to help my audience reach their optimal health. Unfortunately, that's not what happened. Instead, every guest I interviewed would end up leaving my audience (and me) more and more confused. Each expert would share opinions, research, and health advice that was as different as night and day compared to the previous guest.

I interviewed Robb Wolf, *New York Times* best-selling author of *The Paleo Solution*. He told everyone that if you want to live a long and healthy life, you need to eat meat like our caveman ancestors did. "Not so fast," says best-selling author and vegan, Dr. Neal Barnard, who told my listeners, if you want to be healthy, "Don't eat anything with a face." He said if everyone ate a whole-food, plant-based diet, they would be healthy. Okay, that's easy to grasp. Then I interviewed cardiologist Dr. William Davis (*Wheat Belly*) who shared with my listeners that eating grain was not a good idea.

In fact, he said that avoiding wheat is the best thing you can do to prevent and reverse diseases like allergies, cataracts, diabetes, obesity, heart disease, arthritis, etc. For decades we've been told that whole grains are good for us. The compelling information presented in Dr. Davis's book shows that avoiding wheat is the most crucial thing we should do to combat disease and achieve optimal health. Well, not according to *New York Times* best-selling author JJ Virgin (*Sugar Impact Diet*). She believes that sugar is the root of all evil. In fact, she shared profound information on how sugar leads to inflammation, the catalyst leading to most disease. Okay, let's recap: Eat meat; don't eat meat; avoid sugar; and eat a plant-based diet including grain. On second thought, better stay away from grain. But wait! There's another item to add to the "Do Not Eat" list—salt!

We've all heard about the dangers of too much salt in the diet. In fact, if you have high blood pressure, the first thing your doctor will prescribe is a low-sodium diet. Salt is also linked to obesity and cardiovascular disease. According to Morton Satin, vice president of science and research for the Salt Institute, this is not true. He shocked my radio audience when he told them we need *more salt* in our diet to prevent heart disease! He backed this up with some credible science. According to research conducted at Albert Einstein College of Medicine, heart patients that were put on a low-salt diet had a *higher* incidence of heart disease. In another study, the *Journal of the American Medical Association* (JAMA) published findings that showed people with the lowest salt intake had the highest rate of death from heart disease. That's right: eating less salt *increases* the risk for cardiovascular disease! That's not all. Research also shows sodium reduction *increases* the risk of death. This totally goes against what doctors have been telling their patients for decades!

But, when it comes to food, the one thing that seems to confuse us the most is butter. In the late 1970s, consumers were told to stop using butter and switch to margarine because scientific studies showed it was a healthier alternative. A decade later, researchers found that margarine contained dangerous partially hydrogenated oils (trans fats) that were far more harmful than the saturated fat in butter. So we went back to eating butter. In 1990, butter was once again getting bad press as being the most dangerous type of fat, raising cholesterol levels more than vegetable oils. We went back to eating margarine, which was considered a healthier option than olive and canola oils. Fast forward to 2010, when a new study showed butter was healthful, and no evidence linked the saturated fat found in butter to heart disease. But wait! A year later, scientists discovered flaws in this study and warned us that a connection between butter and heart disease may exist after all. Then in 2014, new research revealed that butter is healthful for us. I had Dave Asprey on my show, author of the *New York Times* bestseller, *Bulletproof Diet*. He shared with my listeners how putting butter in coffee every day can help you achieve optimal health and lose weight![1]

All of this type of flip-flopping brings me back to chauffeuring my backseat-driving grandmother, "Go left at the light. Yes, I'm sure. Wait a minute. No, take a right. Yes, a right. This time I'm positive." If we listened to the advice of all these experts, we would have absolutely nothing left to eat!

In spite of all the differences of opinion, one thing every expert does seem to agree on is that the food we consume will either make us healthy or sick. Sadly, even for us health-minded people, the best food options aren't always easy to find. Hiding within our food supply are unnatural binders, fillers, preservatives, pesticides, hormones, artificial coloring, and chemicals. So, if we are what we eat, then we are fake! Even the soil in which our *organic* vegetables grow has been stripped of their vital minerals. It's no wonder the "land of opportunity" has turned into the land of the sick, overweight, and dying.

During my twelve years of college and ongoing continuing education courses, I learned from some of the very best teachers and paid their knowledge forward in my practice. Unfortunately, I would later discover, much of what I learned from these so-called experts was wrong. The way I see it, in addition to all the conflicting opinions, two other culprits are to blame for misinformation: books and biased research.

Books

It's awkward to write that books could be part of the problem, considering they are our primary source of attaining knowledge. However, it is important to note that on the day a college textbook is published, 20 percent of the material is already considered obsolete. Doesn't sound like much? Imagine that the last seventy-seven pages of *The Hunger Games* went missing.

In 2003 physics professor John Hubisz checked the accuracy of information presented in dozens of middle school science textbooks.[2] Hubisz and his team uncovered an alarming amount of information that was inconsistent or incorrect—even the answers in the teacher's editions were full of errors. His work received widespread media attention because it showed our children are being taught misinformation. Not much has changed since then. College textbooks are also filled with inaccuracies. State boards of education have no processes for receiving complaints of inaccuracies or conducting public open reviews of complaints, nor do they require textbook publishers to correct misinformation for the millions of textbooks in circulation. Textbook writers and academic reviewers are not contracted to review for accuracy and are not penalized for producing erroneous textbooks. Many textbook publishers are no longer American-owned, which makes the information they contain even tougher to mandate.

We have a tendency to put clinicians, scientists, authors, and teachers on an expert pedestal, yet most of them gained their education from books containing outdated information. *Gray's Anatomy*, the most respected textbook studied by doctors, is now in its forty-first edition. That means doctors who learned from the first forty editions were taught some information that is antiquated by today's standards. In our ever-changing world, a lot of what we consider the facts of today becomes tomorrow's fiction.

Biased Research

New discoveries come to us by way of scientists conducting research that often contradicts the standard and accepted information taught in textbooks, making it newsworthy. But is it reliable? Much scientific research turns out to be anything but objective. In fact, many scientists are supported, i.e., funded, by lobbyists, Big Pharma, and Big Agra. Not surprisingly, their work is often biased in favor of the companies who pay for it. So, if a scientific study funded by the American Dairy Association proved that milk was healthy, should you trust the findings? Probably not. But since these financial incentives are concealed from the general public, why wouldn't you think their conclusions are anything but solid? Sadly, some of today's leading university researchers, doctors, and other scientists have a little-known conflict of interest . . . money.

Scientists are paid big dollars by organizations to ensure favorable results. These vested interest groups have the power of, what I like to call, *moneypulation*! It's not a bad thing that universities require funds to conduct their research; after all, nobody works for free. But it's who is behind the money trail that can be troublesome. This funding often comes from sources such as the National Institutes of Health, Big Pharma, Big Agra, and various political parties. Too often scientists are hired by these organizations to create figures that either prove or disprove, depending on whether it's the funder's product or one from the competition.

PLOS Medicine journal did an interesting study on the correlation between the funding source and the researcher's conclusion. They analyzed 206 scientific studies regarding nutrition-related articles and looked at the relationship between the findings and the group conducting the research. The results of this study was staggering! When the group conducting the research had a vested interest in the outcome, the results were *four to eight times* more favorable than when the group conducting the research was an independent third party.[3] As the saying goes, "He who pays the piper calls the tune." One of my goals in writing this book is to help you decipher all of the information you are being bombarded with and help you make your own educated choices.

With all the confusion about what we should and shouldn't eat, at least we can turn to dietary supplements to fill the void. In college, I had to learn the recommended daily allowance (RDA) for all vitamins and minerals published by the Institute of Medicine. I lived by these recommendations. From 1973 to 1980 the RDA for calcium was 1,000 milligrams per day for people age four through adulthood, so that's exactly how much I consumed. Then, in the 1980s, the RDA for calcium was increased to 1,200 milligrams, so I added more calcium. In 1994, research showed that 1,200 milligrams was not enough to achieve optimal bone mass. The National Institutes of Health increased that recommendation to 1,500 milligrams per day.[4] Still I added more calcium to my daily regimen. Then, in 2008, the journal of *Cancer Epidemiology Biomarkers & Prevention* found that men with high levels of calcium in their blood are more likely to die of prostate cancer.[5] Wait a minute! I was taking high levels of calcium! Two years later, the *British Medical Journal* published a comprehensive study that showed calcium supplements increase the risk of heart attacks by

30 percent.[6] This sure wasn't what I learned in the textbooks I studied in college! The supplement I was taking to strengthen my bones was increasing my risk of having a heart attack and dying of prostate cancer. No, thanks. I no longer take calcium supplements.

But, I was doing something right. I was taking vitamin E. Medical research shows daily vitamin E supplementation, between 400 and 800 International Units (IU), reduces the risk of cardiovascular disease, which was awesome news considering I was taking 800 IU every day. (That's probably what saved me from having a heart attack from all the calcium I had been taking.) Now comes the flip-flop! In 2005, startling research by Johns Hopkins University, published by the *Annals of Internal Medicine*, showed evidence that vitamin E supplementation increases a person's risk of *dying* from all causes![7] Huh?! I was taught that vitamin E would keep my heart healthy and increase my lifespan, and now it was killing me?! The research showed that the dangers of vitamin E begin with 400 IU, the dosage of most vitamin supplements on the market.

Next up: vitamin D. Research has shown a lack of this vitamin can lead to rickets, cancer, heart disease, depression, weight gain, and many other maladies. The Vitamin D Council, a scientist-led group promoting awareness of vitamin D deficiency, suggests vitamin D is also helpful in treating or preventing autism, autoimmune disease, chronic pain, depression, diabetes, high blood pressure, flu, neuromuscular diseases, and osteoporosis.[8] The Institute of Medicine recommends that adults take 800 IU of vitamin D daily. So that's what I took. But of course there's one big D-lemma! Researchers began reporting that too much vitamin D *increases* the risk of cancer. In 2006, *Cancer Research* published findings of scientists at the National Cancer Institute in Rockville, Maryland, that indicated high blood concentrations of vitamin D are associated with a 300 percent increased risk of pancreatic cancer.[9] Let's see. On the one hand, vitamin D *protects* us from getting cancer, and, on the other hand, it *causes* cancer. During the same year, the *New England Journal of Medicine* published findings that postmenopausal women who take supplements containing vitamin D with calcium to improve bone health increase their risk of getting kidney stones.[10]

Then there's vitamin C, the number-one-selling nutritional supplement in the world. It's considered by nutritionists, medical doctors, and scientists to be vital for a healthy and strong immune system. I listened to these experts, read their research, and personally took 3,000 milligrams of vitamin C every day. Who doesn't want a strong immune system and a longer life?

The top proponent for vitamin C supplementation is Dr. Linus Pauling. He was the chemist, biochemist, peace activist, author, and educator who received numerous awards and honors during his career, and is the only person to win two unshared Nobel prizes, one for chemistry and one for peace. Pauling is considered one of the most influential chemists in history and ranks among the most important scientists of the twentieth century. He reportedly took 12,000 milligrams of vitamin C daily and published research and documented studies showing that mega-doses of vitamin C are effective in preventing and curing cancer. Dr. Pauling did live a long life but died in 1994 from . . . *cancer.*

Now comes the de-C-eptive flip-flop! Research from New York City's Mt. Sinai School of Medicine revealed that taking only 500 milligrams per day of vitamin C could cause genetic damage to your genes and offspring.[11] Great! So here I am, taking 3,000 milligrams a day of vitamin C for my immune system, and it's destroying my DNA—the genetic blueprint of every cell in my body. Doctors following the research of Pauling have preached for decades that the secret to outsmarting a cold is to double the dosage of vitamin C at the first sign of one. Perfect timing! Damage your cells when they're at their weakest and most vulnerable.

Are you confused? Frustrated? Welcome to my world.

Food Sanity will finally give you a *common sense* meets *common science* approach on how to eat right in a Paleo, Mediterranean, vegan, GMO, gluten, sugar-addicted, salt-fearing nation.

Facts, Fads and Fallacies

Shortly after cell phones came out in the mid-eighties, the Federal Aviation Administration (FAA) imposed strict rules that cell phones had to be turned completely off before takeoff and stay off until the plane had landed. It was believed that the cell phone's radio frequency could interfere with cockpit communications and wreak havoc on the plane's navigation equipment. Even laptops, Kindle e-readers, and iPads were prohibited until the plane had reached ten thousand feet. During my years of traveling, I have seen many confrontations between crew and passengers who didn't turn off their portable electronics. On one flight, a frustrated flight attendant told a little boy, "You need to turn off your game now, or we can't take off." The little boy responded, "Why can't the plane fly while I play Super Mario Brothers?" She told him, "Because it will cause the plane to crash, and we could all die!" A few years ago, I was sitting next to a person who was kicked off an airplane because he refused to shut off his cell phone after being told twice.

In October 2013, the rules were changed and the FAA announced that passengers would now be allowed to operate their smartphones and portable electronic devices, read e-books, play games, and watch videos during all phases of flight, with the phone in airplane mode. Many international airlines now let passengers make calls, text, and browse the web.[12] Wait a minute! For three decades we were told cell phone use would cause the plane to crash and now it's perfectly safe?! The rules changed after Delta Airlines conducted analysis on hundreds of thousands of electronic interactions and concluded there were no detrimental effects from the frequency emitted by handheld devices.

In the food, diet, and nutrition arena, I have seen decades of similar myths and fallacies. Things people wholeheartedly believe today as the truth are, in reality, complete fabrications or unproven theories. I will not only break through this misinformation but will also teach you the process of doing the same.

Fewer subjects raise more controversy and heated opinions than food politics. The omnivore-herbivore-carnivore diet debate is as diverse as Republicans, Democrats, and Libertarians. While vegetarians believe a diet void of meat is the secret to reaching optimal health and longevity, proponents of the very popular Paleo diet say we need to eat meat like our caveman ancestors did.

In chapter 1, you will see how this belief is based on a serious distortion of human history. Cavemen were not the predator *hunters* they have been portrayed to be. In fact, we'll explore evidence showing that they were the *hunted*. The superhero, big, strong, beef-eating carnivorous caveman image was the brilliant marketing creation of the beef and cattle industry, designed to sell more red meat. This book will answer the three-million-year-old question, "What did our ancestors really eat?"

One of the biggest food fallacies, spanning more than fifty years, is the perceived need for cow's milk to keep our bones strong and supply us with the calcium our bodies need. Despite decades of government and industry propaganda about the health benefits of milk and dairy products, the truth is, milk does a body bad!

Contrary to all those milk-mustache ads, milk doesn't build strong bones. In fact, unbiased research shows milk causes brittle bones (osteoporosis).[13][14][15] We are brainwashed as children into believing that if we want to grow up big and strong we need to drink milk. The fact is, children who drink milk get more chronic ear infections, have more allergies, are more likely to be overweight, and are at greater risk of diabetes. Humans don't have the enzymes to break down the high amount of casein, a protein found in milk. While casein makes up approximately 20 percent of the protein found in human breast milk, cow's milk contains 80 percent, which is far more than humans are designed to break down.[16]

Why then does the federal government mandate milk in the school lunch program? In chapter 2, I share new evidence why a product full of pus (yes, pus!), antibiotics, and hormones is not good for us, and I offer some healthy alternatives.

I find it rather interesting how beef and milk from a cow have become part of the government's dietary guidelines, while fish seem to be the redheaded stepchild of food. (We'll explore the reason for this favoritism.) We've been told that eating fish—especially tuna, mackerel, marlin, orange roughy, shark, and swordfish—can cause dangerous mercury toxicity to the body. There's definitely something fishy going on here! We hear all the time how polluted our waters are and how eating fish has turned into a game of Russian roulette when it comes to our health. First of all, the earth is 70 percent water, and our oceans go seven miles deep (326 million trillion gallons)! When we consider basic chemistry and the law of dilution, there simply is not enough pollution taking place on the earth's 30 percent surface to ruin our oceans. Also, the oceans contain self-sufficient microorganisms that work like Pac-Man, eating toxic debris and pollutants, which is why it's now safe to eat fish and shrimp that are caught in the area of the 2010 BP Gulf of Mexico oil spill.[17][18]

If polluted water is your reason for not eating fish, why do you eat food from polluted land? Pollution takes place *on land*, where humans live.

Emissions from industries and crop-dusting, fumigating homes, household cleaning products, painting supplies, insect/pest killers, factories, trucks, trains, cars, and other environmental pollutants all put harmful chemicals into the air and ground. We breathe this land pollution. It ends up in the soil; on plants, fruits, and vegetables; and ingested by the cows, pigs, and chickens we eat. Why does the topic of fish always come up when discussing polluted food?

As for the mercury concern when it comes to fish, the oceans are not the mercury-laden cesspools we've been led to believe. In chapter 5, I debunk this popular mercury fish myth by exploring cultures around the world that eat fish daily, sometimes three times a day. Their blood tests show no mercury toxicity, and they are the epitome of good health. Pregnant females have been told to avoid certain types of fish because they supposedly contain mercury that can "harm the unborn fetus." There is simply no credible research to support this. In fact, evidence shows quite the opposite. Cultures where pregnant females eat a diet primarily of fish (mostly tuna) have healthier children with higher IQ scores than mothers avoiding fish.[19] [20] Eating fish gives us vital omega-3 fatty acids, which fight inflammation, the underlying cause of chronic illnesses such as arthritis and heart disease. The only type of fish you need to stay clear of is the farm-raised variety. In this book, you will learn how to purchase healthy, wild-caught, sustainably harvested fish.

With all the confusion and conflicting opinions regarding what we should and shouldn't eat, most health experts do agree that everyone should eat fruits and vegetables as part of a healthy diet. However, they still have differences of opinions on whether we should eat them GMO free, organic, refrigerated, room temperature, raw, cooked, steamed, or juiced. In chapter 7, I share answers to these matters and more. And finally, no book on food would be complete without exploring the skinny on diets. Hundreds of options are available, from the cabbage soup diet to eating bacon on the Atkins diet, to adding up points on the Weight Watchers diet. The word *diet* is derived from the Greek word *diatia*, which means "way of living." Sadly, most people think the definition of diet means counting calories, drinking meal-replacement shakes, and taking a handful of the latest weight-loss pills they saw advertised on TV. These things only bring temporary results because they have not addressed the real meaning of the word *diet*.

Two-thirds of the American population is overweight. Today, we have more access to information and diet programs than ever, yet we continue to get fatter and fatter. I will expose some of the health risks of many of today's fad diets and share my three easy-to-use, safe, and effective ways to lose weight and keep it off!

DIG for the Truth

Between all the conflicting opinions, outdated books, and biased research, I just knew I couldn't be alone in my land of confusion. I wanted to find a way to decide on my own terms what was valuable and what could be harmful, what was misinformation and what was an outright lie; so I developed a three-tier system to uncover the truth. I call it DIG: **D**iscovery, **I**nstinct, and **G**od.

You don't need to have any prior knowledge of the world of health to make the DIG system work for you. Think of it as somewhat like the Socratic method. By asking yourself questions based on three simple categories—science (discovery), common sense (instinct), and blueprints of our creation (God)—you will learn to assess warning labels, ingredient lists, newsworthy "findings," packaging practices, and so on. You will be able to make personal choices about what you eat and drink and how to supplement your diet without relying on the ideas of anyone else—expert or no expert.

Let's take the first category of the acronym DIG. The **D** stands for "discovery." Discovery is synonymous to the science behind what you are reading or hearing from the experts. Their conclusions or opinions change frequently (sometimes weekly), but if the science is based on unbiased research, it does give us a foundation and the most current objective viewpoints. In this book, I share published research from respected, peer-reviewed journals. However, I don't ever rely solely on the accuracy of research to make my points, unless the findings also make common sense.

That brings us to the **I** in DIG, which stands for "instinct." Instinct helps you get in touch with, and give credence to, what your gut is telling you so it can be your guide. For example, if you read a study that says people in Florida purchase more ice scrapers than anywhere else in the country, would your instinct allow you to believe it?

Finally, the **G** in DIG represents "God," which is a way of saying we need to make sure the facts as we interpret them follow the blueprints of our creation. God could represent anything you choose to believe in—a higher power, Mother Nature, angels, an infinite spirit, universal life force, and on and on. In this book, I will use the word *God* when talking about how our bodies and minds are comprised, and the nature, or entity, that formed them. Whatever anyone's beliefs, I base my healing philosophy on our innate and brilliantly designed bodies, which are designed to thrive and be healthy. The human body is a spectacular living machine with a powerful innate ability to adapt, reproduce, grow, and heal. Every cell of your entire body relies on absorbing the nutrition of the foods you feed it, so it can operate on all cylinders.

Ultimately, DIG is a formula that cannot be compartmentalized. All three must work together in order for a conclusion to be made: Take your **D**iscoveries, then add your **I**nstincts, and see if they correlate with the unique and complex design of the body created by **G**od. There's no two out of three here. It's all or nothing.

The DIG method in this book will be applied in each chapter (indicated with the following symbol: [I]), and by the book's end, you will have a blueprint for determining   the validity of what you learn and it will help you understand the facts when it comes to diet, disease, and the deceptions that have kept you from achieving optimal health, wellness, and longevity.

A healthy person is an informed person. And you are about to become both. Can you DIG it? Then, let's get started.

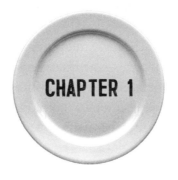

THE CAVEMAN DIET
IS OUR HEALTH BEING STONEWALLED?

A severe stomachache woke me from a sound sleep and kept me doubled over until I could get to the hospital. I was only twenty-two, in the middle of my third year of college. Tests confirmed I had an acute appendicitis. After explaining to me that this diagnosis meant my appendix was inflamed, the doctor asked me, "David, do you eat a lot of red meat?" *Why would he ask me that?* He didn't ask me if I ate a lot of vegetables, chicken, or eggs, nor was he remotely curious about how much pizza I consumed. He specifically asked me if I ate red meat. I told him that I was indeed a beef lover—making it my meal of choice at least three times a week. When I asked the surgeon, who would later be removing my appendix, how he knew I ate a lot of red meat, he replied, "Red meat doesn't contain fiber, and eating too much of it can lead to digestive difficulties and inflammation inside the gut."

Weeks later, I was feeling back to my old self and planned on resuming my regular diet. But I couldn't help but wonder: If the human body has such a hard time digesting red meat, why do we eat it? This question, which I asked myself three decades ago, has led me on a lifelong professional and personal obsession with understanding what exactly our bodies are meant to ingest, digest, and process in order to achieve optimal health and longevity. My research began with me, simply by doing nothing other than eliminating red meat from my diet. As a result, by the end of my third year in college, I had lost a needed ten pounds, had more energy, and even improved my skin complexion. Most important, I never made a trip to the ER again.

The results I witnessed by simply removing a specific food group from my diet inspired me to investigate: Are there any other common foods we aren't designed to eat? I changed my major from journalism to pre-med so I could better understand the complexities of the human body, its ability to heal itself, and how certain foods play a role in this healing.

I became a chiropractic physician and doctor of naturopathy with a post doctorate degree in neurology. The nature of my practice focuses on facilitating the body's innate ability to restore and maintain optimal health. By helping create a healing internal and external environment, my role as a holistic physician is to identify—really dig into the whole lifestyle of the patient—and remove barriers that inhibit good health. My first act in doing this was removing the barrier of red meat from my own diet and experiencing positive side effects. It was those results that fueled my interest in exploring the body's ability to self-heal—the nature of disease and the profound role food plays on our health, attitude, weight, and longevity.

I opened my office in North Carolina and treated many frustrated, confused, and ailing patients with conditions that were not relieved through conventional drugs, ranging from migraine headaches to bursitis to sciatica. One day a patient named Eric came in complaining of chronic lower back pain, a condition for which I had a tremendous success rate. But in this particular case, I was failing. I tried spinal traction, physical therapy, and exercise, but no matter what I did for Eric, his back pain continued to intensify. His pain was so bad that he couldn't put on his own socks. He was growing impatient and on the verge of considering surgery. One day his growling stomach sparked some small talk that revealed after his treatment he'd be heading to his favorite steak restaurant for lunch.

"How often do you eat red meat?" I asked Eric, duly noting the irony of my question. "Pretty much every day," he answered.

Whether it was a hamburger, steak, or a beef taco, red meat was a huge part of Eric's diet. Could the red-meat consumption, which was the cause of my painful and inflamed appendix back in college, also be causing inflammation of Eric's muscles and spinal joints? I turned this idea into a hypothesis and put the theory to the test.

"You've been coming here for several weeks and not seeing any reduction in your symptoms," I told Eric. "Rather than throw in the towel, let me make you a two-week challenge. If you commit to the terms and don't feel better afterward, I'll personally call and get you an appointment to see the best orthopedic surgeon in town."

He was in unbearable pain and would have agreed to try anything to get better. I asked him to completely remove red meat from his diet for two weeks. He agreed. To our mutual astonishment, after two weeks of taking treatments in my office and abstaining from all beef, Eric's back pain completely resolved. He changed nothing except his diet during those two weeks. It wasn't long before I recognized the direct correlation to my patients' diets and their ability or inability to heal.

Then there was Stephen, a patient who came in one day looking amazing. He had lost twenty-eight needed pounds in less than a month! Stephen was excited to show me that he was wearing his belt two notches tighter thanks to the Atkins Diet, which reduces carbohydrate consumption while emphasizing protein and fat. Stephen was eating *steak and bacon every day*, which are both high in saturated fats (the bad kind). While it would appear that Stephen's new diet of limiting carbs while eating red meat was improving his health, *looks can be deceiving.*

A few months later Stephen came in for his follow-up treatment, but this time he wasn't feeling or looking so good. While he still maintained his new weight, he told me he felt weak, and all he wanted to do was sleep. What Stephen didn't realize was that the diuretic effect of a low-carb, high-protein diet can result in someone losing a gallon of water (8.5 pounds) per week.[21] Yes, Stephen was losing mostly water weight. Additionally, when the body is unable to metabolize glucose (blood sugar) into energy, it burns fat instead, and this produces a chemical called ketones. Stephen's beef-friendly, low-carb diet had also put his body into a state of ketosis, in which it must resort to burning fat for energy rather than the quick and easy energy of carbs. Because the liver is responsible for metabolizing this fat for energy, this diet was making Stephen's liver work on overdrive!

I referred Stephen to an internist who did a full blood and urine panel, and CAT scan. His tests revealed he was suffering from inflammation, which was affecting his liver. His C-reactive protein (CRP) level was 5.5

(above 3.0 is considered high). The CRP level rises when there is inflammation throughout the body. Stephen's aspartate transaminase (AST) was 90 U/L (normal is 8 to 48 U/L), and his alanine transaminase (ALT) was 82 U/L (normal is 7 to 55 U/L). Elevated liver enzymes usually indicate inflammation of or damage to cells in the liver. Stephen's liver was failing, despite the fact that he didn't consume alcohol.

Stephen shared with me the first question his doctor asked him after reviewing his test results: "Are you eating a lot of red meat?" There was that question again. The internist shared with Stephen how red meat can be a major contributing factor to inflammation by explaining that the liver is the processing center of the body. It designates nutrients such as proteins and fats for use and sends the toxins that result from protein breakdown to the kidneys. However, excess red meat can cause the liver to slow down. According to the *Journal of the National Cancer Institute*, red meat is associated with a higher risk of chronic liver disease.[22] Because Stephen ate a daily diet consisting of red meat, his liver function never had time to recoup.[23] He stopped eating red meat, and within three months, his blood levels returned to normal.

As a teacher of neuroanatomy (the study of the nervous system), I've shared with thousands of students the intricate blueprints of the human design. Our brain and nerves control everything in our body, from our organs, muscles, and glands to our reproductive system. I remember a student asking me, "Dr. Friedman, if the brain and nerves control everything in the body, what controls our brain and nerves?" This was an interesting question, and one I had never been asked, but it was an easy one to answer. The thing that strengthens or weakens our nerves is *food*. What we eat, and whether we are designed to eat it, creates either proper function or a dysfunction inside the brain, spinal cord, and nervous system.

The Food Feud

While many fad diets have come and gone over the decades, today's most popular craze, the Paleo diet (aka the "caveman diet") doesn't seem to be losing any steam. Proponents of the Paleo diet say we should eat like our ancestors did, when food was pure, void of chemicals and unnatural additives. I'm on board with that. They also tell us that low-carb diets are close to the ancestral diet of the humans who lived before the dawn of agriculture, thereby making modern humans genetically adapted to diets low in carbo-hydrates and high in meat protein, which includes red meat, pork, and poultry. The popular Atkins diet, while not claiming to be a "caveman diet," has a lot of similarities to the Paleo diet in that both promote low carbs and a diet high in animal protein. The Ketogenic diet is starting to gain a lot of popularity. It's actually a repackaged version of the Atkins diet. The premise behind this diet is that fat consumption almost entirely replaces carb consumption. It induces the body into a state of starvation which triggers ketosis. First, it's important to note that, for the time being, I am going to focus on the health detriments of eating a diet that is high in red meat since, in both the Atkins and Paleo diets, red meat is ubiquitous when it comes to the high protein intake that is recommended. Even the most popular Paleo diet cookbook has a picture of a big juicy hamburger on the cover. Second, carbs include both good and bad carbs, and while high-protein diets tend to allow consumption of some low-glycemic "good" carbs, they tend to oversell the necessity of eating either a lot of red meat or processed meats.

Good carbohydrates include whole grains, vegetables, fruits, and beans, so wouldn't it make sense to theorize that our ancestors chose to eat these things when they were plentiful in their environment? Instead, it is a common belief that close relatives of modern *Homo sapiens*, such as Neanderthals, had a diet that was almost exclusively carnivorous.[24] It is believed that, when given a choice, "the caveman" chose to eat lion over legumes and venison instead of vegetables.

Based on my own experience with inflammation and red meat, as well as the indisputable results of so many of my patients like Stephen and Eric, before choosing to eat like a caveman, maybe we should first explore what they really ate. The remainder of this chapter focuses on compelling scientific evidence that reverses everything we imagined about our mammoth-hunting, flesh-ripping ancestors; implementing that knowledge today can give us guidelines for our modern-day diet and create a pathway to achieving optimal health.

Meats vs. Beets

If you really want to follow the diet of our *original* ancestors, you should eat only fruits. From about 24 to 5 million years ago, hominids were fru-givores (fruits eaters). In fact, science shows that the *Australopithecines*, predecessors of *Homo erectus*, had a diet that consisted almost exclusively of prehistoric fruits.[25] After the divergence of the human and ape lines (which occurred between 7.5 and 4.5 million years ago), our ancestral feeding pattern included vegetation and a very small amount of animals.[26] Studies of carbon isotope signatures of teeth show that these humans' diet was primarily ground fruits, vegetables, shrubs, trees, and other plants. Between 2.5 and 1.9 million years ago, as the rains became less abundant, so did the fruits, vegetables, and other plants. Not having access to the plant-based foods they were used to eating, it's during this time that scientists have hypothesized the dietary shift to eating animals.

Interestingly, while our proto-humans chose to eat animals when vegetation was sparse, the ancestors of chimps and gorillas never did.[27] Our closest living relatives are the chimpanzees. In fact, there is only about a 1.6 percent difference between chimpanzee DNA and ours.[28] Chimpanzees are actually considered frugivores (fruit eaters). Their diet is 95 percent plant-based, with the remaining 5 percent filled with insects, eggs, and baby animals.[29] They will eat meat but only if they are left with no other choice.

The hands and feet of chimpanzees include five digits and fingernails rather than claws. They have fingerprints and an opposable thumb, and their eyes are located a few inches apart on the same plane of the face, which allows depth perception and the ability to see in three dimensions just as humans do. Their reproductive systems are similar (the gestation period is approximately nine months) and stomach pH and gut size is also similar to humans. Chimpanzees have thirty-two teeth just like humans. They are also the only species except for humans that is able to use tools.[30] There have been many important fossil discoveries in Africa, which may connect chimpanzees to the prehistoric days of the caveman.[31] The genus of chimpanzees is called *Pan*, and this is considered to be part of the subfamily *Homininae* to which humans also belong. Biologists at Wayne State University School of Medicine in Detroit, Michigan, provided new genetic evidence that lineages of chimps (currently *Pan troglodytes*) and humans (*Homo sapiens*) are so similar that chimps should be reclassified as *Homo troglodytes*. That would make chimps full members of our genus *Homo*, along with Neanderthals.[32] This begs the question, if scientists have proven beyond a shadow of a doubt that humans are so closely related to chimps, why aren't these scientists telling us to eat like them?

It is the Neanderthals who existed 200,000 to 300,000 years ago that are closely related to modern humans, and whom we are expected to eat like, differing in DNA by only 0.12 percent.[33] So this will be the species we'll explore when answering the question, what did our ancestors eat? Neanderthals (often referred to as "cavemen") attached stone tips to wooden shafts to create deadly hunting spears. But were our Paleolithic ancestors biologically designed to eat animals or was their diet based merely on circumstances and survival? If given a choice, would they have preferred animal or plant foods? If modern humans do follow a genetic carnivorous trait, exactly which animals are we supposed to eat?

Can You DIG This?

If we truly believe the concept that cavemen were primarily carnivorous hunters, and we should follow their diet, why eat beef? Cows are grazing, docile animals. Have you ever heard of anyone "hunting cows in the wild"? If cavemen hunted wild game for survival, their kills would have included fox, lions, tiger, and deer—not cows. I've not yet seen a Paleo diet cookbook that shares recipes for wild animals. I can't find even one result when I Google "How to sauté a lion."

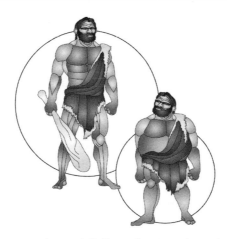

Figure 1: How cavemen are depicted (left) vs. their actual size (right).

Cavemen—The Hunters?

Cavemen are portrayed as big, strong, savage hunters able to stab and kill mammoth-size animals and carry their dead carcasses over their shoulders.

That may be how the cartoons and movies portray them, but it is far from the truth. Cavemen were actually short and stocky. In fact, they were not much taller than 5 feet.[34] In 2010, analysis of twenty-six specimen showed the average weight for male cavemen was 171 pounds.[35] The size of their bodies was an evolutionary adaptation for cold weather, since this extra fat consolidated heat. According to the National Institutes of Health, a male between 5 feet and 5 feet, 5 inches tall, weighing 171 pounds, is classified as clinically obese.[36] A person measuring 6 feet tall, weighing 171 pounds would be considered at an ideal body weight.[37] It definitely raises the question of whether a short, stocky man had the speed and endurance needed to run fast enough to hunt and kill a mammoth, lion, or bear.

After scientists found fossils of stone-tipped wooden spears they were led to the conclusion that our Neanderthal ancestors hunted animals for their meat. This hypothesis was really *put into stone* when archeologists found fossils of wild animals that had signs of being stabbed by sharp weapons. Cavemen did make the weapons by which these animals were killed, and therefore it stands to reason that they must have eaten them. Case closed. Or is it? This entire theory is based on circumstantial evidence. I've watched enough Hollywood courtroom scenes to know that in order to prove someone guilty, putting him at the scene of the crime is not enough. You still have to show a motive.

There is no denying that cavemen made weapons. However, was it their intent to *kill animals*? Or were these weapons made primarily for self-defense against larger animals and other cavemen? A short, stocky man was probably no match for a vicious sharp-toothed animal five times his size. The same can be said about a seven-foot-tall man with arms of steel. Would he really antagonize a wild beast? Anthropologists at Washington University in St. Louis analyzed the cortex of adult Neanderthal fossils and found their skulls and arm bones commonly exhibited evidence of fractures and trauma.[38] It was hypothesized that these injuries took place while hunting animals like mammoth, wild boars, and tigers. But, what if the fractures of the arm and broken frontal bones of the skull are consistent with someone holding their arms up in a defensive position while being attacked by a larger combative animal or person? If someone were to attack you in an alley, it is human nature to hold your arms up in front of your head to protect your face.

Is the caveman's nature to hunt and have a diet primarily of animal meat based on anything besides speculation? Yes. Forensic analysis of cavemen's bones has shown high protein levels, which researchers believe came from eating meat. Proceedings of the National Academy of Sciences suggested that the Neanderthal's diet consisted of land animals and deemed insignificant any protein in their diet coming from plants.[39] The caveman's perceived reliance on red meat is also what some experts feel was the reason they became extinct, with one hypothesis being the Ice Age killing off large animals, leaving cavemen with nothing to eat.

We don't have access to food diaries of our ancestors to really know exactly what they ate; however science does show us enough to make a few educated decisions.

Anatomy 101: Vegetarians or Carnivores?

Before we delve more into the science exploring whether or not cavemen primarily ate a carnivorous diet, let's first look at real carnivores—lions, tigers, and bears. There is no doubt that these animals are designed to eat meat. So when deciding whether or not humans are also designed to be carnivores, we need to examine their anatomy and compare it to ours.

Comparing the Mouth and Jaw

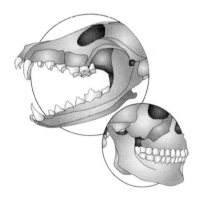

Carnivorous animals such as the lion, tiger, and bear have wider mouths relative to the size of their heads, which allows them to kill and dismember their prey.[40] The jaw of a carnivore is similar to a hinge joint and doesn't move forward or from side to side like a human's jaw does. Humans can freely move their jaws, conducive to chewing and grinding of vegetables and fruits. When the jaw of a carnivore closes, the sharp blade-shaped molars slide past each other creating a scissor-type connection that is perfect for tearing meat from bone. The carnivore's facial muscles are also quite different when compared to those of humans. In order for a meat-eating animal to prey on another intact animal, its facial muscles must be limited so not to get in the way of opening its mouth. Humans, on the other hand, have

9

intricate and complex facial muscles prohibiting the mouth from opening widely, which is why we prefer to eat our food in bite-sized pieces as
opposed to whole carcasses.

Comparing Teeth and Saliva

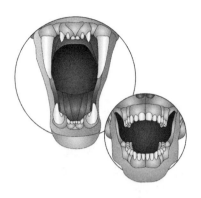

Human teeth closely resemble those of
chimpanzees and apes, both which live
largely on fruit and plants.[41] Carnivores,
on the other hand, have short, pointed
incisors that are necessary for grasp-
ing and shredding meat. Their canines
are elongated and razor sharp, ideal for
puncturing flesh, tearing apart, and kill-
ing their prey. Their back molars are triangular with jagged edges that function like serrated-edged blades. Compare that to the front teeth of humans,
which are flat and more conducive to crushing and grinding berries, fruits,
and seeds. The human incisors are flat, ideal for peeling, snipping, and bit-
ing soft materials like vegetables, beans, and legumes. Next to the incisors,
humans have cuspids, sometimes referred to as "canine" teeth. Some people argue that having canine teeth is proof we were designed to eat meat.
First of all, human canines look nothing like the canines of a carnivorous
animal. And horses have similar canine teeth as humans, and they don't eat
meat. Our canine teeth are triangular, dull (not sharp), and primarily used
to separate the back teeth from excessive amounts of force when chewing.
Finally there's the human molars, which are flat, perfect for crushing and
grinding foods like rice, oats, wheat, and barley. Carnivorous animals have
no need to floss because their teeth are discretely spaced so as not to trap
any animal debris. When humans eat red meat, strands of the animal tissue
gets stuck between their teeth. This is not the case with fish and chicken.

In humans, food is broken down in the mouth before it travels through
the thin esophagus. Carnivores have a larger esophagus to allow big pieces
of animal to freely travel from the mouth directly to their stomach. Because
the human mouth cannot process red meat unless it is thoroughly chewed,
meat can lodge and get stuck in the esophagus. The number one reason
people require the Heimlich maneuver for choking is because a piece of
undigested *red meat* has gotten stuck on the way down.[42]

Carnivores do not chew food, nor does their saliva contain digestion enzymes, as does the saliva of humans. Instead, a carnivorous animal eats its prey quickly and then gorges itself. Carnivores don't digest their food beginning in the mouth like humans do because protein-digesting enzymes in their saliva would cause digestion of their own oral cavity. This is the reason they bite off huge chunks of meat and swallow them whole. Human saliva contains carbohydrate-digesting enzymes which easily break down food molecules while food is still in the mouth.

Comparing Stomach and Colon

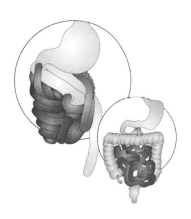

The stomach volume of a carnivore represents 65 percent of the total capacity of the digestive system.[43] The stomach volume for humans represents only 23 percent of the total volume. Since, on average, carnivores kill and eat prey only once a week, their stomachs require more room to allow the animals to quickly gorge themselves when eating, taking in as much meat as possible, and digest their food later. Humans have a smaller stomach so food can exit quickly, allowing room for another meal in just a few hours.

Carnivores have short intestinal tracts and colons that allow meat to pass through the animal relatively quickly, before it has time to putrefy and cause illness. Humans' intestinal tracts are much longer than those of carnivores of comparable size. Longer intestines allow the body more time to break down fiber and absorb the nutrients from plant-based foods. The bacteria in red meat has extra time to multiply during the long trip through the human digestive system, increasing the risk of food poisoning. In a typical Western diet, up to 12 grams of protein from meat can pass through the colon of humans undigested. These undigested particles cause putrefaction in the lower part of the colon, which can turn into ammonia and become toxic.[44] [45] This could be why we see more colorectal cancer lower down. In addition to length, human bowels have pockets and curves. Red meat can get caught in these twists and turns and cause inflammation and constipation, thereby increasing the risk of colon cancer.[46] The reason meat doesn't flow through human intestines efficiently like plants, fruits, and vegetables is because, unlike plant-based foods, meat contains absolutely zero fiber. Fiber is important because it acts like a broom in the intestines, sweeping out the remains of food. Because of their smooth bowels, carnivorous animals don't require fiber like humans.

Comparing Hands and Claws

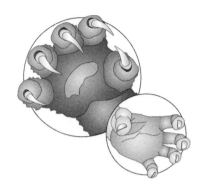

Carnivores have large paws and razor-sharp claws, which enable them to hunt, chase, and trap their prey. It's not uncommon for a tiger to puncture another animal's jugular vein with just one quick swipe of his claws. Humans, on the other hand (pun intended), have five fingers and soft nails. Animal flesh and hide cannot be torn by a human hand because the hand was made for picking plants, vegetables, and fruits.

Comparing Livers

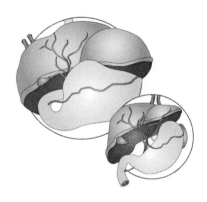

Carnivores have large livers compared to humans because the liver works to break down fats, something of which red meat contains a lot. If carnivores had a human liver, they would not be able to break down all the fats necessary, which would lead to them becoming overweight, to the detriment of their speed and ability to hunt. In order to break down the fat in meat, a carnivore's liver produces massive amounts of enzymes, powerful enough to break down all the fat. Additionally, in order to break down animal meat, uric acid is needed. A carnivore's liver has the capacity to emit ten times more uric acid than a liver of a human or any other plant-eating species. If humans were designed to eat as much beef as a carnivore, their livers would be larger and able to produce the enzymes and uric acid required to metabolize it. This might explain why my patient Stephen's liver malfunctioned after eating beef every day.

Alkaline vs. Acidic

Now let's look at pH. In chemistry, pH is a measurement of the acidity or basicity of an aqueous solution. Solutions with a pH less than 7 are said to be acidic, and solutions with a pH greater than 7 are basic or alkaline. When we compare the gastric pH, humans are at a 5 (acidic), which happens to be ideal for the digestion of plant-based foods. The gastric pH of carnivorous animals stays around 1 (very acidic). This acidic pH is necessary to facilitate protein breakdown and to kill the dangerous bacteria often found in decaying flesh foods. Pathogens like salmonella, E. coli, campylobacter, and other parasites can't thrive in the stomach of a tiger, thanks to high acidity. However, if humans were to eat uncooked meat, these pathogens could indeed survive, causing sickness and even death. The Centers for Disease Control and Prevention says that, on average, more than one million Americans are poisoned every week by something they eat, and food poisoning kills about five thousand people each year.[47] According to the United States Department of Agriculture (USDA), meat contaminated with dangerous bacteria is the cause of 70 percent of food-borne illnesses in the United States, costing $2.9 to $6.7 billion in annual healthcare costs in America.[48]

The Argument of Geography

This is not to say our Paleo ancestors were vegetarians. Some civilizations ate animals. When we look at those who lived closer to the equator, they would have probably consumed more plants and not as many animals. Those groups living at higher latitudes with less access to plants may have consumed more animals. Scientists who analyzed fossils concluded that our Stone Age ancestors received 80 percent of their protein from meat, and their diets included only a small amount of vegetative foods. It was also claimed these hunting societies typically ate all of the animal for protein, including the organs, fat, and bone marrow.[49] These theories were debunked, however, by a study published in November 2012 by the *American Journal of Physical Anthropology*, which revealed that the animal protein intake of our ancestors was not as high as we've been led to believe. The study's author, Tamsin O'Connell, a University of Cambridge researcher, explains that had modern humans consumed as much meat as their early ancestors were previously thought to have consumed, they would have been poisoned by such a protein-heavy diet.[50] Since protein is the only macronutrient that contains nitrogen, in order to determine what cavemen ate, archaeologists measure the ratio of heavy-to-light nitrogen isotopes in fossilized bones. Because the body naturally stores a greater number of heavier isotopes of nitrogen, scientists also had to calculate an offset to adjust for that tendency when determining what a person actually consumed. When using this offset, current research shows that our Stone Age ancestors had a diet that was only 45 percent protein.[51] The question remains, was this protein derived from meat?

In the book *The Rise and Fall of the Third Chimpanzee*, Jared Diamond describes how he was invited on a hunt by a tribe in New Guinea who had retained Stone Age technology and habits. Their total catch for the day was two baby birds, a few tiny frogs, and a lot of mushrooms. Although the men of the tribe frequently bragged of the large animals they had killed, when pressed for details, they admitted that killing large animals was rare and that a hunter was lucky to achieve only a few big kills in his lifetime. This tribe's hunting tools were far more advanced than the stone tools found on prehistoric sites.[52] This makes it very unlikely that prehistoric hunters could have seen a higher success rate than present-day hunter-gatherer tribes. This also makes for a good case that Neanderthals had a diet that consisted mostly of vegetation, with some small prey like birds and fish.

In 1991, "Ötzi the Iceman" was found in a glacier in the Alps, near Hauslabjoch on the border between Austria and Italy. He was mummified and well preserved. At 5,300 years old Ötzi is not considered a Neanderthal; however, DNA analysis shows he has a 5.5 percent Neanderthal genome, meaning he shares a larger genetic link to Neanderthals than do modern-day humans. Ötzi was found with a bow and arrow and wore clothes made of animal skin, which made many assume that he died while hunting around 3300 B.C. Remarkably, there were still a few body hairs intact on this prehistoric man. Hair analysis is an objective way to analyze a nutritional composition and learn what type of diet a person follows. The chemical composition of Ötzi's hair shows that he was primarily vegetarian, eating little if any meat.[53] Another archaeologist named Stanley Ambrose of the University of Illinois at Urbana-Champaign says that the results of the hair analysis shows that Ötzi's diet consisted of approximately 10 percent meat, supporting Macko's claim that he was primarily a vegetarian. That small percentage of meat found in Ötzi's system was goat.[54] Ötzi's teeth showed considerable internal deterioration from cavities, which would have been brought about by his grain-heavy, high-carbohydrate diet.[55] A far cry from what the high-protein diets advocate.

In his book *The Man in the Ice*, Konrad Spindler revealed that Ötzi experienced a traumatic episode a few days before his death. They found an arrowhead embedded in his shoulder blade. This led experts to the conclusion that Ötzi was perhaps the victim of a raid on his village.[56] Scientists have always assumed the weapons that our ancient ancestors carried were used to hunt large animals. It appears that our ancestors may have carried weapons to protect themselves from *dangerous people*.

Psychologically Speaking

Okay, let's finish up our comparison of carnivores and humans by exploring their psychological differences. Carnivores are predators and have an innate need to hunt and kill other animals. When a tiger sees a furry animal, instincts signal his brain to tell the body to attack. Instead of attacking, killing, and eating it, when a human sees an animal, he's more likely to get the video camera out and film it. The sight of a wounded animal and scent of its blood arouses carnivores. On the contrary, most humans are grossed out by blood and the sight of raw flesh. When hearing horrid screams from an animal being ripped to pieces, most humans will cringe, yet these sounds motivate and fuel an attacking carnivorous animal. Yes, people eat red meat, but if a grocery store or butcher shop didn't sell it with the blood removed and cut, trimmed, neatly processed, and nicely packaged, the sight and smell would be repulsive to most humans. On the other hand, if a hyena found a dead animal on the ground, it would seize the opportunity to devour it. If *you* saw a dead animal on the side of the road, would you say to yourself, "Yummy! I think I'll pull the car over and stop for some carcass"?

Another psychological factor to consider is, when a carnivorous animal is hungry, he is at his best. This hunger mechanism activates strength, speed, and focused precision. Quite the opposite holds true for man. When a human is hungry, it would be difficult for him to hunt for an animal. A starving man would be weaker and have a lack of speed and focus. Hunger spurs a carnivore to go hunting while it inhibits a human's physical ability to do so.

When humans put on their camouflage gear and hunt bear, deer, or elk, what do they do after they kill it? They don't devour the animal like a carnivore would. Instead the hunter carries that dead carcass to his truck, brings it home, cleans it, removes the fur, skin, all the blood, and then cooks it. If a hunter ate that meat in the forest *raw*, like a carnivorous animal, it would make him sick and could potentially kill him. Quite the opposite holds true for carnivorous animals. If they eat *cooked* meat, they could get sick and die. Even domesticated circus lions have to eat raw meat to keep them from starving to death.

One of the largest studies on raw versus cooked foods with animals was conducted by Dr. Francis M. Pottenger, using nine hundred cats. The ten-year study revealed dramatic findings on the advantages of raw foods for the carnivorous feline. In this experiment, cats that were fed raw meat produced healthy kittens year after year with no ill health or premature deaths. The cats that were fed the same meat, but this time cooked, developed heart disease, cancer, pneumonia, kidney and thyroid disease, tooth loss, arthritis, birthing difficulties, diarrhea, liver problems, and osteoporosis. Here's the irony. Uncooked red meat is dangerous for humans, and cooked meat is dangerous for carnivorous animals.[57] If a deer is burned in a forest fire, a carnivore will *not* eat its flesh. Carnivorous animals won't eat cooked meat.

Dr. William C. Roberts, editor of the *American Journal of Cardiology*, sums it up nicely: "Thousands of years ago when we were hunter-gatherers, we may have needed a bit of meat in our diets in times of scarcity, but we don't need it now. Although we think we are, and we act as if we are, human beings are not natural carnivores. When we kill animals to eat them, they end up killing us, because their flesh, which contains cholesterol and saturated fat, was never intended for human beings, who are natural herbivores."[58]

Can You DIG This?

Archaeological and scientific evidence now shows us that Prehistoric man was mostly vegetarian. Perhaps they only resorted to eating meat when plants, fruits, vegetables, and legumes were not available.

The *Real* Caveman Diet

Thanks to advancements in modern technology, the diet of our ancestors is now better understood. Information presented on November 12, 2010, in the *Proceedings of the National Academy of Sciences* revealed that fossilized grains of plants and vegetable material had been found in the teeth of cavemen, and some of it was cooked. Microscopic particles trapped in the teeth did not contain meat but rather residues of plants, barley, beans, roots, and tubers, as well as palm dates.[59] This is an interesting finding considering that proponents of the Paleo ("caveman") diet tell us that we should boycott foods that our caveman ancestors didn't eat, which they say include grains and beans. Considering these fossils prove cavemen did eat beans, which offer a significant amount of protein, the assumption that their dietary protein came solely from red meat is no longer accurate.[60] Science does show that our Neanderthal ancestors did occasionally eat red meat, fish, fowl, and even eggs, but their diet was primarily plant based.

Dr. Dolores Piperno, of the Smithsonian National Museum of Natural History in Washington, D.C., said, "Neanderthals made use of the diverse *plant foods* available in their local environment and transformed them into more easily digestible foodstuffs, in part through cooking them, suggesting an overall sophistication in Neanderthal dietary regimes."[61]

So, if short and stocky Fred Flintstone lived today, he would probably drive past the local steak house and go for the all-you-can-eat salad bar.

What started off as a college quest has led me to the understanding that we are not designed to eat the same diets that carnivorous animals do. What's more important is that our caveman ancestors didn't think so either. Thanks to grocery stores, packaging, refrigeration, technology, and innovations in farming, modern-day humans have gravitated toward a diet that is high in beef, pork, chicken, dairy, and eggs. Are there any nutritional benefits to eating these other food groups? What else can we unlock about food, nutrition, and how our choices relate to disease prevention? Each chapter in the rest of this book is dedicated to digging in and finding out.

 Discoveries: According to forensic science analyzing teeth, bone, and mummified hair particles, humans' ancestors ate a diet that was primarily plant based with a small amount of animal foods.

Instincts: The sight of a wounded animal and scent of its blood arouses carnivores. The horrid screams from an animal being ripped to pieces are sounds that bring joy to an attacking carnivorous animal. If humans were supposed to primarily eat a carnivorous diet, why do these things repulse most of us?

God: When analyzing the human anatomy, we find that we are not designed to indulge in a high-meat diet. Human teeth, saliva, stomach pH, colon, and the size of the liver are not conducive for eating and digesting large quantities of meat. Humans have the same teeth, hands, and digestive system as a chimpanzee, our closest living relative. Do chimps eat bears, lions, deer, or cows? No, they do not.

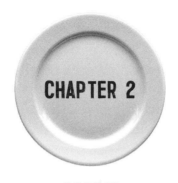

MILK
IT DOES A BODY GOOD?

"Milk is nature's perfect food—but only if you are a calf."
—Dr. Mark Hyman

A patient came to my office experiencing back pain after stepping off a curb. Her X-ray showed advanced osteoporosis and a severe compression fracture in her lower back. When I showed her the X-ray, she told me there was no way she could have brittle bones because she drank two glasses of milk every day. Like this patient, millions of people have been told, "If you want to have strong bones you need to drink your milk!" After all, milk is a great source of calcium, strengthens teeth, keeps the heart healthy, and protects against weak and brittle bones (osteoporosis). Actually, that's not true. Here's what they *don't* tell you in those milk-mustache ads—information that will be the focus of this chapter:

1. Pasteurized cow's milk is not a good source of calcium. One of the worst side effects of pasteurization is that it renders most of the calcium contained in raw milk insoluble.[62]
2. The benefit of the vitamin D, which is touted as one of milk's essential ingredients, is insignificant. Replace with: We will learn later that human blood levels of vitamin D are only minimally affected by dietary sources such as milk.[63]

3. Milk is the most common allergy, affecting eight out of ten adults with symptoms they don't even associate with their dairy consumption. Intolerance and allergy to cow's milk is also a factor in sudden infant death syndrome.[64]

4. Babies who consume cow's milk are fourteen times more likely to die from diarrhea-related complications and four times more likely to die of pneumonia than breastfed babies.[65]

5. Milk ages the body and weakens bones.

In Defense of Milk

Am I against milk? Absolutely not. I think every mammal on Earth should drink milk—during infancy, and from its own species.

Milk in infancy. We are the only species on Earth that drinks the milk of another animal in adulthood. Have you ever seen an adult chimp nurse from an elephant or a fully-grown cat nurse from a horse? No! Because it's just not natural. All other mammals nurse their own species for a short period of time immediately following birth. Once the offspring are weaned, they never drink milk again. In nature, there is no species in the world that drinks milk in adulthood. So why does the average adult in America drink 21 gallons (181 pounds) of milk per year?[66]

Species-specific milk. The nutritional requirements for young mammals are met by the unique qualities of the milk produced by that particular species. A cow supplies her calf with hormones, protein, enzymes, and antibodies to prevent disease and support metabolism and growth *specific to the species*, just as a human mother supplies her child with these same species-specific constituents.

For example, casein is the primary protein found in cow's milk. This protein is what makes a 100-pound baby calf grow into a 2,000-pound cow. The average human baby weighs less than 8 pounds and grows into a 170-pound adult. Here's a common-sense question for you: Would you use rocket fuel in the gas tank of your moped? Why would you put gargantuan-size cow fuel inside a human body?

Science has proven that infants need *human* breast milk. A baby that is not breastfed has ten times the risk of being hospitalized in her first year, sixty times the risk of contracting pneumonia, and may have signifi-cantly lower IQ as well as behavior and speech difficulties. The baby will also have a higher risk of asthma, allergies, digestive problems, infections, type 1 diabetes, eczema, and developing lymphoma and leukemia later in life. A child that is not breastfed also has a greater risk of obesity.[67]

Here's the irony: Many of the health conditions that are *prevented* by human breast milk are *caused* by drinking cow's milk. In the mid-1800s, human breast milk was replaced with cow's milk for emergency situations (such as when a mother died in childbirth). As a result, most of the infants died. The high-protein content of the cow's milk forced fluid out of the infant's kidneys, causing dehydration. In 1994, over a century later, *The Lancet* reported that cow's milk was still killing babies! Researchers stated, "Babies that consumed cow's milk were fourteen times more likely to die from diarrhea-related complications and four times more likely to die of pneumonia than were breastfed babies. Intolerance and allergy to cow's milk products is a factor in sudden infant death syndrome."[68]

Because of the side effects, including *death*, infant formulas were developed with added water to dilute the milk and sugar and so reduce the massive protein concentration. When given unpasteurized milk, like cows naturally drink, an infant could die of infection because unpasteur-ized milk contains dangerously high levels of bacteria that only a calf can tolerate. When a calf is given pasteurized milk, like humans drink, he will die within sixty days, because most of the nutrients needed for survival are altered during the heating process.[69]

Here's something to ponder. If you were in the hospital and needed a blood transfusion and you had the option of choosing cow's blood, how would you feel about that? Probably not something you would consider, right? Why not? Could it be because your instincts would immediately put up a red flag that the content of cow's blood probably serves a differ-ent purpose and doesn't contain the red and white blood cells, enzymes, and antibodies that human blood contains? Then why do you drink cow's milk? Why don't your instincts step in? It's the same concept, but instead of fluid from cows' veins entering your body, it's the hormonal fluid secre-tions from their nipples.

Several years ago, a patient of mine was appalled to discover that the day care staff fed her baby someone else's breast milk. "Oh, my God,

Dr. Friedman! Disgusting!" she said. "Can I sue them? What if my little baby catches something from her and gets sick? How do I know the mother doesn't have germs or diseases? What if she's on medications? Or worse, has an illegal drug habit or is an alcoholic!" This mother was so distraught that she wrote a letter to the editor of the local paper and reported the day care center to the Better Business Bureau. Was she right to be so upset? Her baby did drink a total stranger's breast milk.

Here's the odd part. This same mother doesn't think twice about drinking a nice tall glass of cow's milk or pouring it over her older child's cereal. Why is that acceptable and not considered "disgusting"? Drinking milk from an animal that stands in its own feces is gross. I bet the mother of the breast milk her child drank doesn't stand in her own excrement. I also would bet anything that she didn't have bleeding ulcerated sores on her nipples, as many cows have on their udders. I bet this lady took a shower that day—which is something a cow never does.

Why is society so brainwashed into believing that drinking the milk from an animal and giving it to our children is perfectly okay? Why do we think milk is a pure product that doesn't contain any medications, illegal drugs, or germs, when, as you will learn, it does?

Milk Mustaches and the Media

It's time to ask the billion-dollar question. If cow's milk is so unhealthy for humans, why does the media tout it as a fantastic healthy drink? Ever hear of supply and demand?

The dairy industry consists of some very large organizations. The Dairy Farmers of America (DFA) has sixteen thousand farmers who produce about 62 billion pounds of milk a year and net $8 billion in sales. Then there's the National Dairy Council (NDC), whose mission statement says it works in collaboration with those committed to taking a leadership role in promoting child health and wellness through milk campaigns.[70] Then there's the American Dairy Association and Dairy Council, Inc. (ADADC), which has an interesting goal. When I looked at the corporate website, it didn't take long for the motives to become quite apparent. (Italics and bold letters have been added for emphasis.)

Mission: "The ADADC, Inc., is funded and directed by dairy farmers *for the purpose of increasing sales of and demand for dairy products*. ADADC,

Inc., works closely with Dairy Management Inc.™ and is *responsible for increasing demand for U.S.-produced dairy products ...*"

Purpose: On behalf of U.S. dairy farmers, *drive increased sales of, and demand for,* U.S. dairy products and ingredients.

Role: Work proactively, and in partnership with leaders and innovators, to increase and apply knowledge that *leverages opportunities to expand dairy markets.*

Vision: To initiate forward thinking, aggressively seek new opportunities, and implement cutting-edge programs *that build a stronger market for dairy products.*[71]

So, the mission, purpose, role, and vision of the ADADC are focused on just one thing: making money! The verbiage expresses motivations that are all about increasing sales, building stronger markets (not bones), and leveraging opportunities to expand those markets. Why doesn't the mission statement say anything about helping humanity? Feeding the poor? Building stronger bones and muscles or helping people lose weight? That type of dairy hype is left to advertising agencies. Cows aren't the only ones being milked here.

Dairy—No Bones About It

One of the leading causes of death in the elderly is hip fractures, which are more common than the combined risk of breast, uterine, and cervical cancer.[72] Worldwide, an osteoporotic fracture is estimated to occur every three seconds! One in two women over the age of fifty, and one in eight men, will experience an osteoporosis-related fracture. Seventy-five percent of those over the age of sixty-five who fracture a hip or leg bone die within ninety days.[73][74] Many believe drinking milk offers calcium that helps build strong bones. Actually, if you drank it directly from the cow, you would get some *usable* calcium; however, before milk gets to your glass, it goes through a heating process called pasteurization, which is required to destroy harmful bacteria. Most milk you purchase at the grocery store is ultra-pasteurized, which means it's heated to 280°. While exposing milk to excessive heat does help to kill off harmful bacteria, it also damages the calcium content, making the mineral *unusable* by the body.[75] Grocery stores in America are prohibited from selling unpasteurized (raw) milk. But what if raw milk was available? Would unheated cow's milk offer you a good source of calcium to support the health of your bones? To find that answer, ask yourself, where do cows get the calcium for *their* big strong bones? From the plants and grain they eat. Plant-based calcium also has a large amount of magnesium, a mineral that cows also need for their bodies to absorb and use calcium. Without the proper amount of magnesium, calcium is useless to a cow, just as it is for humans. So, even if you did drink unpasteurized milk, you would still need to make sure you have enough magnesium in order for your body to absorb the calcium it contains.

Many nutritionists recommend people take a ratio of two parts calcium to one part magnesium in dietary supplements for bone strength, which is why most contain 66 percent calcium and 33 percent magnesium. In the plant kingdom, the ratio is closer to the needed 1 to 1 ratio. The calcium in cow's milk has only a 9 to 1 ratio (90 percent calcium/10 percent magnesium), meaning it contains an insufficient amount of magnesium for the calcium to be absorbed and used by the bones.

What about human breast milk? It actually contains slightly *less* magnesium than cow's milk: 91 percent calcium/9 percent magnesium. That means our own mother's milk doesn't contain enough of the magnesium required for an infant to adequately utilize the bone-building calcium it contains. That's because milk is not where humans were intended to get their calcium—nor is it where cows get theirs. We need to get our calcium from the same place that cows do—from plants!

Through plants, we can attain the perfect balanced ratio of calcium and its synergistic partner, magnesium. Sources like almonds, summer squash, sesame seeds, and spinach offer almost a perfect 1 to 1 ratio of calcium to magnesium. These ratios allow the two bone-building partners to do their job. Cow's milk, pasteurized or not, is a lousy source of magnesium and therefore does not help build strong bones.

You may be thinking, since mother's milk is supposed to provide infants with all the nutrients they need, why wouldn't it contain a perfect balance of magnesium/calcium required for an infant's bones? Great question. To answer that, I'll need to share a little human biology 101. Newborn babies *don't have fully ossified bones*. Their bones start off as soft cartilage in the womb, and most of the skeleton is still cartilage at the time of birth. If you have ever touched the crown of a baby's head, then you have felt the "soft spot." This is a growth plate. Babies have many growth plates on bones throughout their entire body. As cartilage develops, tiny cells called osteoblasts begin to form along the lining of the cartilage. Babies' arms and legs, and even their spinal vertebrae, are separated by cartilaginous pieces that eventually calcify over the years. Even a baby's kneecaps don't start turning into bone until after his second year, when he begins to walk. Since breastfeeding is generally recommended for newborn infants during their *first six months of life*, this is a time when bone growth is not a primary function of the body. Calcium/magnesium for bone growth is not on the infant's list of top nutrient requirements. Top on the list are nutrients for brain function, in particular, the development of the senses and language.

Breast milk does contain the proper balance of every nutrient essential for the development of a newborn infant, but by design, that happens to not include the calcium/magnesium bone-building duo.

An Elixir for Aging and Brittle Bones

As we grow into adulthood, we get the needed calcium/magnesium duo required by our bones from our diet. If you're drinking cow's milk as a source of calcium, this can lead to degenerative disease and accelerated aging. You read that right: milk makes you age more quickly. The powerhouse cell of the body is called the mitochondria. It's what helps control the body's growth. Every time these cells produce energy, they use something called a calcium pump, which is located inside the cell's membrane. This pump needs a sufficient amount of magnesium to function properly. If there's too much calcium and not enough magnesium, only a minimal amount of energy is produced, and the pump stiffens up and becomes much less effective. This causes the mitochondria to calcify, which ages the cells of the body.

Simply put, think of a boat that has barnacles forming along the bottom of the hull. They eventually spread to the propeller and then around the outboard motor. How much power would this boat have if you tried to start it? Would it even start? This same type of calcification process can take place in the body when you drink cow's milk, traveling to your muscles, ligaments, and ultimately stimulating degeneration of the body and accelerate aging. You do not get a proper balance of calcium and magnesium from milk and this resulting lack of energy production leaves your cellular powerhouse stuck in first gear.

Surely with so much hype about dairy products helping to strengthen bones, there has to be *some* research backing up these claims? Actually, there is, if you consider biased research credible.

In September 2000, two researchers compiled a review of the fifty-seven studies on dairy products and bone health, which had been published in the scientific literature since 1985. This review was published in the *American Journal of Clinical Nutrition*. The majority of this research was funded by the dairy industry. Surprised? The researchers reported that 53 percent of the studies showed no benefit from dairy. Then they excluded studies with weak evidence or poor techniques, which eliminated more than half of the studies. Of the remaining twenty-one studies, 57 percent again showed no benefit from dairy, and another 14 percent found that dairy products actually weaken bones. That means 71 percent of the research touted as "supporting evidence" for the health benefits of cow's milk is bogus. In fact, these very studies showed evidence that cow's milk can actually harm the body.[76]

No concrete evidence proves milk helps build strong bones, but there is a plethora of evidence showing quite the opposite—milk *causes* osteoporosis. The *British Medical Journal* reported that calcium intake is completely irrelevant to bone loss.[77] [78] It's not a lack of calcium that causes bone loss, but rather too much animal protein in the diet. Guess what milk is? Animal protein. To me, this is like brushing your teeth with fluoride toothpaste that also has cavity-causing sweeteners added to it.

How exactly does cow's milk *cause* bone loss? Milk has sulfur-containing amino acids, which are metabolized to sulfuric acid. Milk provides predominantly acidic precursors, which stimulates premature osteoclastic activity and inhibits osteoblastic formation. This causes a rapid and premature aging of the bone.

All right, enough geek talk. Here's how bones form in simpler terms. Remember the video game Pac-Man? Imagine an evil Pac-Man inside your bones, eating holes in the cortex. This is what an osteoclast cell does. These cells break down calcium to be used elsewhere in your body, sort of like how a termite eats wood. Now imagine Super Mario (osteoblast) coming along and filling up those holes with a protective compound, similar to spackling holes in sheetrock. Up until the human body reaches the age of thirty, Super Mario (osteoblast) outnumbers the Pac-Man (osteoclast), and you build more bones. After you reach thirty, your Pac-Man gets the upper hand, and you gradually lose bone mass through the normal aging process. Milk creates a higher number of Pac-Men, which leads to premature bone destruction.

Can You DIG This?

If you look at global research, countries with the highest consumption of dairy products, such as the United States, Sweden, Israel, Finland, and the United Kingdom, have the highest levels of osteoporosis-related hip fractures.[79] [80]

Places in the world with low intake of dairy, such as Hong Kong, Singapore, and some countries in Africa, have the lowest incidence of osteoporosis.[81] Women in many countries in Africa average only 350 milligrams of calcium per day, 70 percent less than the recommended U.S. daily calcium allowance, yet osteoporosis is almost nonexistent among them. Regardless of how much calcium they get each day, they have a diet that is extremely low in animal protein, so (as the hypothesis goes) their bones remain stronger. On the other hand, the Inuit people in the Arctic have the highest calcium intake in the world, far surpassing the recommended daily allowance, but due to their high animal protein diet, they have one of the highest rates of osteoporosis.

In an attempt to see if the claims are true that milk helps protect against bone fractures, researchers from the long-running Nurse's Health Study looked at milk consumption among 78,000 women nurses. Because more women than men suffer from osteoporosis, most of the studies conducted on the disease are female based. The results were surprising: The women who drank more than one glass of milk a day had a 45 percent *greater* chance of hip fractures.[82] Those who took in the same amount of calcium from nondairy sources saw no increase or decrease in the risk of fractures. Researchers decided to do a similar study on men, this time focusing on the long-running Health Professionals Study run by the Harvard School of Public Health. They found that men who drank three or more glasses of milk per day, compared to one glass or less per week, had slightly fewer hip fractures; however, these were balanced by slightly more arm fractures.[83]

Elderly woman are more prone to hip fractures. Females sixty-five to sixty-nine who break a hip are five times more likely to die within a year than women of the same age who don't break a hip.[84] The *American Journal of Epidemiology* published a study on elderly women and found that those with the highest dairy product consumption actually had double the risk of hip fractures compared to those with the lowest consumption.[85]

You are probably wondering, if so much unbiased research shows milk does not benefit bones as the milk-mustache ads claim, why isn't this documented research shared with us by the National Osteoporosis Foundation? I'll share with you a little-known secret, and then perhaps you can answer that for yourself. A big financial supporter of the National Osteoporosis Foundation is a company called Bozell Worldwide, which happens to be the marketing firm that created the successful milk-mustache campaign for the dairy industry. Do you think the National Osteoporosis Foundation would risk losing a big chunk of their money by making this information public and going against the message pushed by one of their largest financial supporters? What do your instincts tell you?

If milk doesn't give us strong bones, what does? Eating a diet rich in natural foods such as vegetables, beans, seeds, and nuts offers the body sufficient bone-building calcium along with the needed magnesium. Research has proven that eating more of these plant-based foods will actually strengthen your bones.[86] The protein in cow's milk causes calcium to be excreted in the urine, which is not the case with plant-based calcium sources. (We'll discuss this further and explore calcium supplements in chapter 9.)

Vitamin D-ceit

Vitamin D has many beneficial functions; one is ensuring adequate serum calcium levels to aid in building strong bones. Two common bone diseases are caused by a lack of vitamin D: rickets (in children) and osteomalacia (in adults).[87] Both lead to diffuse body pains, muscle weakness, and fragile bones. Technically, vitamin D isn't a vitamin—it's a steroid hormone produced by the body when it's exposed to sunshine. Our bones need vitamin D, because without it, calcium can't do its job. (In chapter 9, I will share why people are so "D-ficient" and offer solutions.) One thing is for sure: drinking milk is not the answer to low vitamin-D levels. I find it appalling that the milk industry is brainwashing everyone into thinking liquid from a cow is the perfect source of vitamin D. I saw a milk commercial once that dubbed milk "liquid sunshine." Great! Now the milk industry is telling us that the white fluid from a cow's nipples is better for us than sunshine.

The dairy industry would love for you to believe that vitamin D is naturally present in milk, but it's actually added at the processing factory. Historically, this dates back to the 1930s, when rickets among poor children caused by an inadequate diet and lack of sunshine was a real public health problem. The dairy industry got this great idea to add vitamin D to milk to help solve the problem and increase sales.

More than 90 percent of the vitamin D in the human body is produced by sunlight. Research shows that human blood levels of vitamin D are only minimally affected by dietary sources such as milk.[88] [89] Even if milk were a good source of vitamin D, you would have to drink more than a gallon of it every day to get the vitamin D you'd get from ten minutes of sunshine exposure.

Milk Maladies

Now that we've debunked the strong bones myth, let's explore if there are *any* health benefits to drinking cow's milk. For that answer, let's DIG a little deeper into the research, top it off with good old common sense, and put an instinct cherry on top.

The Casein Against Milk

Casein is the predominant protein found in cow's milk. When humans drink this casein, our bodies see this protein as being harmful and produces antibodies to attack it.[90] Casein from cow's milk is also used to make glue to hold together wood (think of the cow logo on Elmer's Glue) and a polymer used to make plastics. If you were to swallow glue, your body would consider this an invasion and attack it. When you ingest casein, or glue made from milk, your body attacks it by producing histamines, which cause mucus production that can lead to bronchitis, allergies, asthma, influenza, sinus infection, ear infection, irritable bowel syndrome, and diarrhea, just to name a few. Numerous studies, including data from the World Health Organization (WHO), have also linked consumption of casein with increased risk of heart disease, high cholesterol, type 1 diabetes, sudden infant death syndrome, and neurological/behavior disorders.[91]

One of the world's foremost nutrition researchers is Dr. T. Colin Campbell. His national best-selling book, *The China Study*, is considered the most comprehensive study of health and nutrition ever conducted. Campbell lists casein from milk as *the most relevant cancer promoter ever discovered*. Campbell states, "Casein, which makes up 87 percent of cow's-milk protein, promotes all stages of the cancer process."[92] He concluded that cancer growth could be controlled based on the amount of casein in the diet.

Casein has also been linked to schizophrenia and autism. In a 1996 paper, Dr. Kalle Reichelt, of the Institute of Pediatric Research at the University of Oslo, Norway, cited more than two hundred international scholarly sources that advanced the theory that schizophrenia and related affective disorders are caused by "food constituents (casein) that may have disease-promoting effects and cause behavioral changes."[93] The theory originated in the 1960s when people with schizophrenia were put on casein-free diets under double-blind conditions. The results were astounding! Many of the patients returned to normal and were able to return home from locked mental hospital wards.[94] Reichelt found dramatic learning and behavior improvements in autistic children who were put on a casein-free diet.

Milk—Not Such a Hearty Drink

In 1991, the headlines read, "Milk lowers the risk of heart attacks." Peter Elwood conducted a lifestyle study on five thousand men, ages forty-five to fifty-nine, and found those who drank the most full-fat milk and ate the most butter had a lower risk of having a heart attack.[95] This was big news at the time, but researchers later questioned the findings. They rightly pointed out that the difference could have been due to an overall healthier lifestyle on the part of the milk and butter consumers.

In the same year, Stephen Seely, M.D., a cardiologist and researcher, wrote an article, "Is Calcium Excess in Western Diet a Major Cause of Arterial Disease?" published in the *International Journal of Cardiology*.[96] This study showed quite the opposite of Elwood's reported findings. Seely showed that in countries where the daily calcium intake is 200 to 400 milligrams, coronary artery disease is almost nonexistent. In countries where the daily calcium intake is 800 milligrams, coronary artery disease is the leading cause of mortality.

The correlation between milk consumption and mortality from coronary artery disease is strong. Through the years, more research continued to debunk Elwood's findings. The *Journal of Nutritional and Environmental Medicine* published several studies on the connection between milk consumption in different countries and the death rates from coronary heart disease (CHD). This investigation showed that countries with reduced milk consumption also had lower rates of CHD death, while countries such as Portugal, with higher milk consumption, had an increased rate of CHD death.[97] *Hypertension* published evidence on the correlation of milk consumption and high blood pressure.[98] Lower dairy consumption is correlated with lower high blood pressure, which is a precursor to CHD.

In his book *Don't Drink Your Milk!* Dr. Frank Oski, of the Johns Hopkins Children's Center, states, "The fact is: the drinking of cow's milk has been linked to iron-deficiency anemia in infants and children; it has been named as the cause of cramps and diarrhea in much of the world's population, and the cause of multiple forms of allergies as well; and the possibility has been raised that it may play a central role in the origins of atherosclerosis and heart attacks."[99]

Okay, so milk does a heart bad, but why? Cow's milk actually causes lesions in the arteries, which the body tries to heal by laying down a protective layer of cholesterol. The end result is scar tissue, calcified plaque, and cholesterol deposits. This is known as atherosclerosis (artery clogging) and arteriosclerosis (artery hardening).[100] A leading cause of millions of heart attacks could be the consumption of milk and dairy products.

Got Pus?

Yes, I'm talking about that nasty stuff you used to pop out of your zits when you were a teenager. How many pus cells would you be okay drinking? A dozen? A hundred? None you say? Well, you better put down that glass of milk! According to *Hoard's Dairyman*, the magazine of the National Dairy Farm, milk contains millions of pus cells![101] One liter (approximately a quart) of milk from California contained 298 million pus cells. In Alabama, milk contained 444 million pus cells, slightly more than Nevada, which came in at 443 million. But at the top of the list was Florida's milk, with a whopping 548 million pus cells per liter! Sound like a lot? These states still fall below the USDA's allowable 750 million pus cells per liter. Yes, you read that right—*allowable* pus. One cubic centimeter (about half a teaspoon) of commercial cow's milk is allowed to have up to three quarters of a million somatic cells and twenty thousand live bacteria.[102] All right, milk has pus, but why?

When factory farms force cows to be on hormones and produce much more milk than they normally would, the cows become more susceptible to a type of udder infection called mastitis. Milk from a cow with mastitis will have extra somatic cells, along with bacteria, cellular debris, serum, and other gunk—better known as pus. Farmers aren't required to test the milk from each cow for bacteria and somatic cells. All they have to do is test the combined batch of milk from all their cows. So, as long as the pus-filled milk from a cow with mastitis is combined with the milk from a lot of other healthier cows, the total somatic cell and bacteria count for the batch is still within the USDA limits.

Milk Contains Growth Hormones

A cow normally produces eight to ten gallons of milk per day. To increase milk production and make more money, farmers inject cows with bovine growth hormones (BGH). To be certified organic, milk can't come from cows that have been treated with BGH. Research at Cornell University has shown that daily injections of BGH increases milk yield by as much as 41 percent.[103] That means an annual average yield of 2,920 gallons per cow turns into 4,117 gallons per year with the use of BGH, which translates into much more production and more money!

BGH is available for farmers to inject into their cattle, despite the fact that the hormone has been shown to cause many consumer health risks. Humans ingesting BGH has been linked to hormonal imbalances and other health issues, ranging from early puberty to thyroid disease to cancer. Many countries have banned the use of BGH, including Canada, Japan, Australia, New Zealand, and all twenty-seven countries of the European Union. However, it is still widely used in the United States. Later in this book, we will look at the strongest organization in the world, Monsanto. I compare this company to a corporate mafia kingpin who controls a large part of the food industry. Monsanto has tremendous political power and is represented by numerous lobbying associations, hired-gun lobbyists and scientists that act as their mouthpiece to keep BGH legal. Monsanto often displays publicly staged partnerships with environmental organizations to deflect from their unsavory activities.

Within every human body is *human* growth hormone, which is vital for our *human cells* to grow properly. Consuming milk that includes hormones designed to increase the growth of a *cow's cells* causes human cells to grow at a dangerously accelerated, unregulated pace, and can lead to disease. Remember: cows' growth hormone helps them grow to a whopping two thousand pounds! Cows have larger stomachs, lungs, livers, hearts, etc. Do you want the hormones that enlarge their organs to be inside your body, potentially enlarging yours?

Milk Contraband?

I once saw a bumper sticker that said, "Get antibiotics from your doctor, not your milk." Udder infections caused from over-milking cows are treated with antibiotics; residue from these drugs shows up in the milk you buy at the grocery store. In fact, milk contains traces of up to eighty different antibiotics![104] According to a Food and Drug Administration (FDA) report, dated April 19, 2011, 87 percent of antibiotics used in animals are either never, or very rarely, used in human medicine.[105] [106] Shouldn't we be concerned about the safety of these drugs for human consumption?

The push to eliminate antibiotics in milk was highly publicized in December 1989 after *The Wall Street Journal* shared results of a study showing 20 percent of milk tested had *illegal* antibiotics present.[107] Then in May 1992, a *Consumers Reports* feature showed 38 percent of milk was adulterated with illegal antibiotics.[108] Since then, the FDA has set up protocols that require all raw milk be checked for drug residues before it is received by the dairy plant. However, farmers are more motivated by economic incentives and don't have much motivation to prevent antibiotics from reaching the consumer. Today drugs continue to be used because they know it won't be tested. It's a vicious cycle. Growth hormones are used so the cow can produce an abundance of milk, which leads to the cow being milked ten times more than normal. This causes infections of their udders, which then require antibiotics. This is *udderly* ridiculous!

Milk Makes You Fat!

Ever wonder why cows have four stomachs? It's so they can eat and eat and eat all day. They don't get full because by the time stomach number four gets full, stomach number one is empty. No wonder cows are so big! When humans drink the fluid designed for an animal that has four times more room in its stomach, that fluid now entering only one small human stomach also make us want to eat and eat!

The dairy industry spent hundreds of millions of dollars between 2003 and 2007 promoting the statement that milk causes people to *lose weight*. Who was the mastermind behind this media blitz? An organization called Dairy Management Inc. (DMI), a group dedicated to promoting the sale of milk and cheese. They work with state and regional dairy promotion organizations to ensure the future success of dairy by integrating marketing, public relations, and education with nutrition, product, and technology research programs.

In a series of confidential agreements approved by agriculture secretaries in both the George W. Bush and Barack Obama administrations, DMI has worked with restaurants to expand their menus with cheese-laden products to increase profits. DMI, whose annual budget is $140 million, is largely financed by the government. Documented records show major conflicts of interest in the USDA's historical roles as both marketer and rule maker of agriculture products.[109] The USDA runs a "dairy check-off program," which levies a small assessment on milk (15 cents for every hundredweight of milk sold or used in dairy products) and raises hundreds of millions of dollars annually. DMI uses some of this money to promote products such as milk and cheese. In fact, the DMI used these "check-off" funds to help pay for the "Got Milk" campaign. DMI also includes members of the National Dairy Promotion and Research Board and the United Dairy Industry Association. Heading up DMI is CEO Thomas P. Gallagher, who reportedly made a hefty $633,475 annual compensation in addition to receiving first-class travel privileges, according to federal tax filings.[110]

In 2003, the government classified obesity as a disease. At the same exact time, they also funded the "Drink Milk and Lose Weight" campaign. Coincidence? I don't think so. Obesity was now *the* topic in the media.

DMI's weight-loss campaign appeared in magazines, newspapers, and TV news features. While these dairy advertisements were sweeping the nation and convincing overweight people to drink more milk, researchers were finding absolutely no proof to substantiate these claims. Every time the deceptive claims were questioned, the DMI lawyers would reply with, "The USDA has reviewed, approved, and is continually overseeing the program." A physician's advocacy group finally had enough of the lies and relentlessly pursued a claim against the dairy industry for deceptive advertising. They proved in a court of law that there was no supporting evidence showing a weight-loss benefit from drinking milk.[111] In fact, an abundance of double-blind research shows quite the opposite: people who drink the most milk gain the most weight.

Researchers from the Harvard School of Public Health and other institutions studied the weight and milk consumption of 12,829 kids ages nine to fourteen from across the country. They concluded that the more milk children drank, the more weight they *gained*. Those consuming more than three servings each day were about 35 percent more likely to become overweight.[112] After the truth was finally made public, the U.S. dairy producers had no choice but to stop making these bogus claims. But did people really need this research made public before realizing that milk causes a weight gain? Get in touch with your instincts. They are usually right. A calf drinks cow's milk so he can grow up to weigh 1,500 pounds!

The Skinny on Nonfat Milk

For people watching their weight, the terms "fat-free" or "skim" milk may seem like a better choice than whole milk. Not so, says Dr. T. Colin Campbell, world-renowned biochemist from Cornell University, who specializes in the effects of diet on long-term health. During a radio interview I conducted with Dr. Campbell, he shared his thoughts on milk with me: "Skim milk is a serious problem. In skim milk or low-fat milk, the fat is skimmed away, but we end up with a higher concentration of protein. Skimmed-down cow's milk can actually be worse for you than whole milk."[113]

Animal protein in milk, particularly casein, may lead to serious health issues, not necessarily just its fat content. Is there any evidence that skim milk helps with weight loss? No. In fact, evidence shows quite the opposite. When farmers feed skim milk to pigs, they gain more weight. When pigs are fed whole milk, they actually stay leaner.[114] This paradox holds true for humans as well. One study of more than twelve thousand adolescents over the course of three years found that drinking reduced-fat and skim milk was associated with weight gain.[115 116]

Cow's Milk and Kids

For many decades this nation has been bombarded with media propaganda that states that milk helps our children grow up to be big and strong. The evidence shows that our children are growing up weak, sick, and over-weight—thanks in part to milk—and that these conditions continue into adulthood. In addition to being tied to allergies, cow's milk also has been linked to a variety of health problems, including hemoglobin loss, heart disease, atherosclerosis, arthritis, kidney stones, mood swings, depression, and irritability.[117]

Milk causes allergies in young children that continue through adult-hood.[118] The journal of *Pediatric Allergy and Immunology* states: "Most for-mula-fed infants developed symptoms of allergic rejection to cow milk proteins before turning one month old. About 50 to 70 percent experi-enced rashes or other skin symptoms, 50 to 60 percent had gastrointesti-nal symptoms, and 20 to 30 percent showed respiratory symptoms. The recommended therapy is to avoid cow's milk."[119]

Another report published in *Natural Health* stated: "At least 50 percent of all children in the United States are allergic to milk, and many go undiag-nosed. Dairy products are the leading cause of food allergies, often revealed by constipation, diarrhea, and fatigue. Many cases of asthma and sinus infec-tions are reported to be relieved and even eliminated by cutting out dairy."[120]

More than twenty well-documented studies have shown a link between milk and type 1 diabetes, which is also called juvenile diabetes because most people get it in childhood or early adolescence.[121] The *New England Journal of Medicine* states that cow's milk can contribute to juvenile diabetes and autoimmune diseases by impairing the ability of the pancreas to produce insulin.[122]

Some say it's just genetics, but this is not so. The common hypothesis that DNA plays a role in type 1 diabetes has been debunked by analyzing people who move from one country to another and change their diets. Native-born Polynesians who moved to Australia were found to have a two-time increase in the risk of type 1 diabetes, after shifting their diet from fish protein to cow protein.[123] Children given cow's milk formula in the first three months were 52 percent more likely to develop type 1 diabetes than those that weren't fed milk. Compare that to breastfed infants, who have a 34 percent *lower incidence* of type 1 diabetes than formula-fed infants.[124]

Even if proactive parents keep cow's milk out of their kitchens, most schools today are required to have it available as part of the USDA's National School Lunch Program. Why? Four billion dollars—that's why! This is not the first time the USDA has "partnered" with multibillion-dollar industries (more on them later). McDonald's even added milk to the Happy Meal as a "healthier alternative" to soda. The healthier alternative to soda and milk is called water.

After the age of five, most kids gradually lose their ability to produce the enzyme lactase, which is needed to digest lactose, the form of sugar found in milk. That's perfectly normal; once kids stop drinking breast milk, they no longer need the enzyme. When you don't make lactase, you have trouble digesting milk and dairy products such as ice cream—you get gas, cramps, bloating, and diarrhea from these foods. This is called being lactose-intolerant, but that's a misleading way to look at it. A more accurate view of this is to consider the minority of people in the world, who are lactose-tolerant, as genetic mutants. Around the world, only most people of northern European ancestry and people from some areas of Africa continue to produce lactase and can still digest milk past childhood. School kids who aren't of northern European heritage—meaning most of them—are being made sick several times a day when they're given milk or ice cream at breakfast, lunch, and snack time. The government continues to mandate milk in the school lunch program, however, and supports that mandate with low prices.

On top of that, the dairy industry actively promotes milk to kids, including flavored milks and yogurt with a lot of added sugar. If your kid isn't doing well in school, seems to have frequent digestive upsets, or is cranky a lot, milk could be the culprit. After all, it's hard to concentrate in class or feel like having fun when you've got cramps, bloating, and gas from the milk you just drank. And if you can't figure out why your kid is gaining too much weight, check to see if the school is serving flavored milks. A small carton of chocolate milk is loaded with sugar and contains 226 calories!

Ear Infections

If you are a parent, you probably have experienced a child suffering from a middle ear infection (otitis media). A common medical procedure for chronic ear infections is to insert drainage tubes into the child's ears. Every year, about 500,000 children have holes surgically drilled into their eardrums and plastic hollow tubes implanted. Doctors are quick to do this for children who have repeated ear infections or who have fluid behind the eardrum after antibiotic therapy.

When a doctor surgically inserts tubes into a child's ear, the hole drilled into the eardrum causes scar tissue that can lead to partial deafness. Parents, if a doctor tells you otherwise, he or she is not being truthful. If you cut your skin and it heals, a scar forms. When you pierce through an eardrum, it too heals with a scar. Because scar tissue doesn't reverberate, that part of the eardrum won't transmit sounds, leading to a partial deafness. When a doctor puts surgical tubes through an eardrum, it drains the fluid behind it. Mission accomplished? Actually, that's like draining excessive water from a boat without stopping the cause of the leak. The tubes eventually fall out of the eardrum but, if the underlying cause is not addressed, the infection comes back and the procedure is repeated with another set of tubes, causing even more scar tissue to form. Drilling holes in a child's eardrum is not a solution to the problem. Could the solution to chronic ear infections be as simple as eliminating dairy from a child's diet?

In *Healing Childhood Ear Infections: Prevention, Home Care, and Alternative Treatments*, Dr. Michael A. Schmidt presents more than sixteen scientific studies suggesting that many cases of chronic ear infections are due to food allergies.[125] He lists dairy as the number-one contributor to childhood ear problems. A child can't digest the milk that is created by nature for a big baby cow to drink. This can create fluid/mucus buildup behind the eardrum. The American Academy of Allergy, Asthma, and Immunology lists cow's milk as the leading cause of food allergies in children.[126]

Healthy Milk Alternatives

For those of you who love milk, I have good news for you. You can still enjoy it! Just not cow's milk. Here are three healthy alternatives:

Almond milk. Created from ground almonds, this delicious alternative to cow's milk contains antioxidants, protein, calcium, magnesium, manganese, selenium, and vitamin E. Almond milk can be used as a substitute for cow's milk in most recipes. Commercial almond milk products come in plain, vanilla, or chocolate flavors. The two brands I recommend are Silk Pure Almond (www.silkpurealmond.com) and Almond Dream (www.tastethedream.com). All-natural, almond-based nondairy frozen desserts are a good alternative to ice cream.

Hemp milk. Made from the seeds of the edible part of the *Cannabis sativa* plant, also known as marijuana, hemp milk does not contain THC, the component of the herb that can get you high. The seeds are used to make milk that has a delicious nutty flavor and is a terrific alternative to cow's milk with your morning cereal. It provides many health-enhancing nutrients, including omega-6 and omega-3 essential fatty acids, magnesium, beta carotene, calcium, fiber, iron, potassium, phosphorus, riboflavin, niacin, and thiamin. Hemp milk is creamier than soy and rice milk and works great in coffee and dessert recipes. The one I recommend is called Tempt from Living Harvest (www.livingharvest.com).

Rice milk. This tasty beverage is made from brown rice. It is naturally sweet, light, and refreshing and is loaded with vitamins, minerals, and protein. Drink it by the glass, pour it on your morning cereal, or use it in your favorite recipes. The two brands I recommend are Rice Dream (www.tastethedream.com) and Growing Naturals (www.growingnaturals.com). Rice milk is organic, vegan, gluten-free, lactose-free, and a delicious alternative to cow's milk.

Cashew Milk. This has become a very popular alternative to cow's milk because of its versatile, creamy texture. Cashews are also great to use in recipes for vegan cheeses and other mock-dairy recipes. Cashews are a good source of healthy fats and plant-based protein, and are high in the minerals magnesium and potassium, which are needed for good cardiovascular health. A great option is Silk (www.silk.com).

Coconut Milk. This dairy alternative contains healthy medium-chain fatty acids, which are used by the body as energy rather than storing it as fat. Coconut milk also provides the body with needed protein, vitamins, and minerals. Coconut milk also helps reduce the appetite. If you enjoy the thick and rich, creamy texture of dairy, you'll love using coconut as a milk alternative. A great company I recommend is Califia Farms (www.califiafarms.com).

Discovery: Unbiased research from major universities, scientists, doctors, and authors have found a link between drinking milk and certain diseases, including cardiovascular disease, osteoporosis, ear infections, allergies, diabetes, and cancer. Cow's milk contains blood, bacteria, growth hormones, and antibiotics. Biased research, corrupt legislation, and conflicts of interest line the pockets of corporations, Big Pharma, Big Agra, politicians, and corporate scientists. These are the people telling us to drink milk.

Instinct: Try to ignore what your elementary school teacher taught you when you were an impressionable child learning the government's biased food pyramid. Try to leave behind the major conflict of interest funding of the milk-mustache advertisements with your favorite sports figure, model, singer, actor, or politician. Okay, now look at the simple fact that a cow is a four-legged animal, and the milk it produces is *species specific* for a calf, not humans, to drink. You would cringe at the idea of a baby calf sucking the nipples and drinking the milk from a lactating woman. Why aren't you cringing at the thought of a human child drinking the milk from a cow? Trust what your stomach is telling you (that gut feeling) about drinking from an animal that has four stomachs.

God: Every baby mammal that exists on this planet drinks milk from its own mother because it contains the *perfect balance* of hormones, enzymes, and nutrients to promote growth. The milk from a cow is, by design, created to help a calf grow to a half-ton, four-legged animal. All species except humans drink milk only in their infancy, never as adults. All of God's creatures (including human babies) are weaned off their mother's milk before the age of one. Children, teenagers, and adults no longer need milk from their mothers; why should they continue drinking milk from an animal's mother?

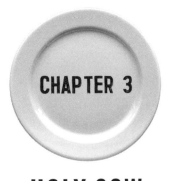

CHAPTER 3

HOLY COW
WHAT'S THE BEEF?

"I am living without fats, without meat, and feeling quite well this way ... man was not born to be a carnivore."
—Albert Einstein

Whether you're an athlete, a pregnant woman, or simply a person trying to lose weight, eating a high amount of protein has been touted as the best way to gain muscle, speed metabolism, lose weight, increase energy, and improve health. For many people, when they think protein, they think red meat, which includes beef, venison, and lamb. Though meat consumption in the United States has dropped slightly in recent years, at 270.7 pounds per person a year, we still eat more meat per person here than in any other country on the planet.[127]

Seventy percent of this meat consumption is beef. That means, in a lifetime, the average American will eat over ten thousand pounds of beef (five tons of cow carcass per person)! Since the most commonly eaten red meat in America is beef, this will be the focus of this chapter. One thing that puzzles me is how much red meat body builders eat to help them build muscle. Why do humans feel the need to eat cow muscles to help their human muscles grow? This just doesn't make sense.

Plants: A Plethora of Protein

Americans have been extremely misled about the need for protein derived from red meat. Research confirmed by hundreds of studies around the world shows that vegetarian diets can provide sufficient human protein requirements.[128] On the contrary, excessive protein from red meat has been linked to osteoporosis, arthritis, and cancer.[129] [130] [131] Protein from plant sources has never been found to be unsafe, and it is better assimilated into the bloodstream than protein derived from animals.

How much protein do we really need? According to the *American Journal of Clinical Nutrition*, we only need 2.5 percent of our daily calories from protein.[132] [133] That means if you eat the recommended 2,000 calories per day, only 50 calories should come from protein sources. It's quite easy to get that much protein from fruits, vegetables, beans, nuts, and grains.

See Table 3.1 for the protein content of several foods.

Table 3.1: Protein content of foods as a percentage of total calories

Food	Protein Value	Food	Protein Value
Spinach	50%	Pumpkin seeds	21%
Watercress	46%	Whole wheat	17%
Broccoli	45%	Lemons	16%
Kale	45%	Oats	15%
Bean sprouts	43%	Walnuts	13%
Cauliflower	40%	Honeydew melon	10%
Bamboo shoots	39%	Brown rice	8%
Mushrooms	38%	Strawberries	8%
Lettuce	34%	Oranges	8%
Chinese cabbage	34 %	Cherries	8%
Wheat germ	31%	Apricots	8%
Zucchini	28%	Watermelon	8%
Navy beans	26%	Grapes	8%
Cabbage	22%	Pecans	5%

As you can see, a variety of plant foods can offer sufficient amounts of protein. 100 calories of ground beef has 10 grams of protein; 100 grams of baby spinach has 12 grams of protein. Additionally, spinach contains 30 percent protein and zero fat, while ground beef contains 40 percent protein, but 60 percent fat. One cup of navy beans contains nearly 16 grams of protein. Add in 3 ounces of pecans for another 10 grams or so, and you can see how a vegetarian diet provides plenty of protein. And we're not talking about just for the average person. This also goes for athletes and bodybuilders who are intent on building lean muscle. If it sounds counterintuitive that bodybuilders could grow muscle to the extent that they can compete professionally simply by eating a diet strictly of plant-based protein, I ask, how does an elephant grow to 10,000 pounds by eating nothing but plant food? They couldn't grow so big if plants weren't loaded with enough protein. Some of you may be thinking, "Well, of course elephants get enough protein from plants, because they eat much more than humans do!" Actually, that's not so. Once you adjust for body weight, elephants actually eat *less* than we do. A typical American eats about 3 pounds of food per day per 100 pounds of body weight. Even though elephants are much larger than humans (weighing up to 20,000 pounds,) they eat only 1.9 pounds of food per 100 pounds of body weight.[134]

In addition to lifting weights to increase body mass, bodybuilders follow a very strict diet to achieve muscle growth and fat loss. You might not expect to find a vegetarian among the world championship bodybuilders, but Andreas Cahling, a Swedish bodybuilder, who won the 1980 Mr. International title, is a long-time vegetarian. When he first came on the scene, it was reported that "Cahling's showings at the Mr. Universe competitions and at the professional bodybuilding world championships, give insiders the feeling he may be the next Arnold Schwarzenegger."[135] Andreas Cahling went on to win many more bodybuilding titles. His famous physique has been featured on hundreds of magazine covers around the world. He's still a vegetarian.

Even after his career in movies and in politics, Arnold Schwarzenegger remains an icon in the world of bodybuilding and as a leading expert on the topic. Earning the title of "Mr. Olympia" seven times, Arnold certainly knows the type of diet that is required to help build strong muscles. In his book, *Arnold's Bodybuilding for Men*, he writes, "Kids nowadays tend to go overboard when they discover bodybuilding and eat diets consisting of 50 to 70 percent protein, something I believe to be totally excessive and unnecessary."[136] Arnold goes on to recommend 1 gram of protein for every 2 pounds of body weight. That means if you are a bodybuilder with a goal of building stronger muscles, eating spinach, broccoli, and almonds can give you Arnold's suggested daily protein requirement. Of course, most bodybuilders also supplement their diet with branched-chain amino acids, L-glutamine, creatine, etc.

Can You DIG This?

The following athletes are world champions and vegetarians:
- Hank Aaron, baseball's home-run champion
- Bill Pearl, four-time Mr. Universe
- Carl Lewis, ten-time Olympic champion; named Sportsman of the Century by the International Olympic Committee
- Tony Gonzalez, tight end for the Atlanta Falcons
- Keith Holmes, middleweight boxing champion
- Billie Jean King, tennis champion
- Martina Navratilova, tennis champion
- Ed Templeton, professional skateboarding champion
- Kenneth Williams, America's first vegan bodybuilding champion
- Ricky Williams, running back for the Miami Dolphins
- Desmond Howard, Heisman Trophy winner, former wide receiver for the Green Bay Packers
- Robert Parish, former Celtics star
- James Southwood, kickboxing champion

Unlike plant-based protein, excessive animal protein in the diet can lead to dehydration, which inhibits performance and can cause serious health problems. In studies of athletes eating high-protein diets and drinking equal amount of fluids, hydration levels go down as protein intake goes up. Because as little as a 2 percent decrease in body water has been found to negatively affect athletic performance and cardiovascular function, the results of the study suggest that red meat is not necessary for athletic performance and could even be inhibitive.[137]

IRONing out the Wrinkles

In addition to being told red meat is needed for protein, another popular but false belief is that we have to eat red meat to get the iron our body needs. Iron is important because it's what enables red blood cells to carry oxygen from the lungs to the entire body. Contrary to what we have been taught, a well-balanced vegetarian diet does provide enough iron for good health. Iron deficiency is no more common in vegetarians than non-vegetarians.[138] But what about children, who need iron for their growing bodies? Children who are strict vegetarians also show no greater incidence of iron deficiency.[139]

Plant foods that are rich in iron include beans and legumes such as kidney beans, chickpeas, and lentils; nuts and seeds, such as cashews, hemp seed, and sunflower seeds; whole grains such as whole-wheat bread and oatmeal; and other foods, such as raisins, tomato juice, and molasses.

When you eat plant foods, you're also eating a lot of vitamin C, because it's found in abundance in vegetables and fruits. Vitamin C, which is needed to enhance iron absorption in the body, enables more absorption of iron from plant foods than from red meat.[140] The reason for this is because vitamin C isn't found in beef. Also, people who wash their beef down with a nice tall glass of milk create a real source of IRONy. Casein, the protein in dairy products, binds with iron molecules and carries them out in the stool. That means dairy products combined with red meat can create an iron deficiency (such as when you put cheese on your hamburger).

Where's the B12?

The major reason we are told we need to consume red meat is for its vitamin B12. This vitamin is crucial for normal metabolism in every cell of our body. It's also needed for DNA synthesis and cell division, and for the formation of normal blood cells. The body can't make vitamin B12, so it needs to come from food or supplements. Although animal foods, such as beef, contain vitamin B12, it's not made directly by the animal. Instead, bacteria in the animal's gut creates the vitamin.[141] Inside the animal's body, vitamin B12 attaches to a protein molecule. When you eat beef and other animal foods, like eggs, you consume vitamin B12.

Plants can't make vitamin B12, which means that very strict vegans who eat no animal products at all can become deficient. Does that mean vegans are doomed to becoming deficient in vitamin B12 if they don't eat red meat? Not really. Very small doses of vitamin B12 are required for good health—the recommended daily amount for adults is only 2.4 micrograms. If you used to eat red meat, you've probably got a reserve of the vitamin that could last for up to thirty years.[142] In fact, a healthy vegetarian's risk of developing a disease from B12 deficiency is extremely rare—less than one chance in a million.[143]

To increase B12 reserves, eating red meat is not necessary. You can easily get the daily requirement (and then some) from eggs, certain breakfast cereals, sea vegetables, and yeast-extract products. Nutritional yeast products are sold in powder or flake form. They have a nutty and cheesy flavor and creamy texture, which makes for a great dairy-free cheese substitute. If none of these appeals to you, you can take B12 supplements.

Heart Attack, Stroke, and Death . . . Oh, My!

The three major factors contributing to strokes and heart attacks are inflammation, cholesterol, and plaque buildup, which just so happen to be the three things red meat has been said to cause in the human body. You're better off indulging in some A1 steak sauce without the steak. Here's why.

Heart disease is the leading cause of death for men and women in the United States. Cardiovascular disease and strokes account for about a third of all U.S. deaths.[144] Red meat consumption is a major culprit associated with an increased risk of heart disease and mortality.[145] [146] [147] [148] Red meat is high in calories, protein, and saturated fat, which in excess have been linked to inflammation, weight gain, and increased cholesterol levels and the ultimate killer—the formation of plaque in the arteries that feed the heart and the brain. When plaque in the heart ruptures, it blocks the flow of blood through the artery and causes a heart attack. Similarly, when plaque in the arteries to the brain ruptures, it causes a stroke.

In August 2011, the *American Journal of Clinical Nutrition* published the largest study to date on the relationship between stroke and red-meat consumption, which showed the higher the intake of red meat, the higher the risk of heart disease and stroke.[149] In the same year, a study published in *Stroke: A Journal of Cerebral Circulation* showed that women who consume at least 102 grams (3.5 ounces) of red meat per day have a 42 percent higher risk for strokes than those who eat 25 grams (less than 1 ounce) of red meat daily.[150]

Red meat also increases your risk of death. A ten-year study analyzed people who ate the most red meat (about 62.5 grams per 1,000 calories per day, equivalent to a quarter-pound burger or small steak per day). The group eating the high amounts of red meat had a 30 percent greater risk of dying compared to those who consumed the least amount of red meat. The researchers estimate that 11 percent of deaths in men and 16 percent of deaths in women could be prevented by reducing consumption of red meat.[151]

Eating more than eight servings of red meat per month is associated with a 52 percent increased risk of cardiac arrest and sudden death.[152] Results of a case-controlled study published in the *European Journal of Clinical Nutrition* found that frequent red-meat consumption significantly increases the risk of unstable angina, plaque rupture, blood clot formation, and heart attack.

Red Meat Causes Colon Cancer

Everyone knows by now that smoking is a major cause of lung cancer. No *ifs*, *ands*, or *butts* about it. Even with the warnings on cigarette labels, people still have the right to smoke and choose to take the risk. Before it was mandated for Big Tobacco to inform people of the harms of smoking cigarettes, smokers weren't able to make educated decisions prior to lighting up. Where is the law when it comes to mandating the cattle industry to label the risks of eating red meat and its link to colon cancer? Among all victims of cancers, colon cancer is the second-leading cause of death among women and men. Every nine minutes, someone dies from colon cancer, meaning more deaths in one year are caused by colon cancer than by car accidents, breast cancer, and murder combined.

In 2005, Europe and the United States conducted two extensive studies.[153] The research from Europe tracked 478,000 men and women who were found to be free of cancer at the start of the study. During nearly five years of follow-ups, those who ate the most red meat (about 5 ounces a day or more) were a third more likely to develop colon cancer than those who ate the least amount of red meat (less than an ounce a day, on average). In the United States, researchers looked at 148,610 adults between the ages of fifty and seventy-four and found those with high levels of meat consumption were at a 50 percent greater risk for colon cancer than those who consumed less meat, even when weight, activity level, fiber intake, and vitamin supplements were taken into consideration.[154]

I have seen far too many patients who have either died from colon cancer or have had friends or family members die from the disease. When a patient tells me someone they know was just diagnosed with colon cancer, I ask if that person eats a lot of red meat. Without fail, I *always* get the same response, "Yes, he loves his steak and hamburgers. Why? Is that bad for you?"

In May of 2011, the most authoritative report on colon cancer risk to date was published by the World Cancer Research Fund International (WCRF International), confirming that red meat increases the risk of colon cancer. The research concluded that 43 percent of colon cancer could be prevented if people ate less red meat.[155]

The beef industry was livid when this WCRF International study was released. In a collaborative attack, the National Beef Association (NBA), the National Sheep Association (NSA), and the National Farmers' Union (NFU) accused the WCRF International of misleading the public with factually inaccurate and potentially defamatory comments. However, all the evidence was based on published research conducted by world-top scientific journals, following careful scientific peer reviews, with no conflict of interest.[156]

Is there any research out there showing that red meat *doesn't* cause cancer? Actually, Exponent, a consulting firm made up of multidisciplinary scientists, conducted an independent, large-scale examination of the epidemiological literature pertaining to meat consumption. This included total meat, red meat, processed meat, and factors related to eating meat and its relationship to cancers of the colon, breast, prostate, pancreas, kidney, and stomach. After evaluating more than fourteen thousand published scientific studies that have linked eating beef to causing cancer, they found, "No conclusive evidence of a causal relationship between red meat and any form of cancer. Available data from the relevant epidemiologic studies was not sufficient to conclusively support a causal association for red meat and processed meat being linked to colon or stomach cancer because of inconsistencies."[157]

Case closed! Fourteen thousand studies were wrong! Well, before you make that assumption, let's follow the money. This scientific panel debunking all of the research linking red meat to causing cancer was funded by none other than the National Cattlemen's Beef Association. I refer to that as *buyased* research. Does this remind you of the way the tobacco industry presented "their" evidence before Congress, saying that tobacco was not addictive and did not cause lung cancer?[158]

Why Does Red Meat Cause Colon Cancer?

The evidence is unequivocal, but exactly why does red meat cause an increased risk of colon cancer? And why doesn't the same thing happen when eating chicken or fish? We can look at several research studies to understand this. In one study, healthy volunteers agreed to stay in a metabolic research unit, where their diet could be carefully controlled while all of their fecal waste was collected and analyzed. (Your day job isn't looking so bad now, is it?) The volunteers ate one of three test diets for a period of fifteen to twenty-one days. The first diet contained 14 ounces of red meat per day. The second diet was strictly vegetarian, and the third contained a combination of both red meat and dietary fiber. Stool specimens from the twenty-one volunteers who consumed the high-meat diet contained high levels of N-nitroso compounds (NOCs), which are potentially cancer-causing chemicals.[159] [160]

The twelve volunteers who ate vegetarian food excreted low levels of NOCs, and the thirteen who ate the meat and high-fiber diets produced intermediate amounts. The researchers analyzed cells from the lining of the colon that are normally shed into the stool with every bowel movement. The stool samples from the group that ate the most red meat contained a large number of cells that had NOC-induced DNA changes. The vegetarians' stools had the lowest number of genetically damaged cells, and people who ate the high-meat, high-fiber combination diet produced intermediate numbers of damaged cells.[161] Red and processed meats are associated with increased risk of colon cancer because they create high levels of NOCs in the body. Chicken and fish, because they don't produce these high levels of NOCs, have actually been associated with a decreased risk.[162] [163]

In the first chapter, we looked at the anatomy of our ancestors and the biology of carnivorous animals compared to that of humans. This provides us with a common-sense and common-science viewpoint that humans weren't designed to consume large quantities of red meat. Another thing to consider: humans are the only animals that have a higher risk of cancer when it comes to eating red meat. Other carnivores eat red meat naturally with no ill side effects. A unique sugar called Neu5Gc, which is found in most mammals but not in humans, triggers an immune response that in turn causes inflammation. Most other carnivores' bodies are built to process this sugar, but human bodies are not.[164] When humans eat red meat, this sugar molecule triggers the immune system to constantly produce antibodies to fight it off. This can lead to chronic inflammation, which has been shown to promote tumor growth that may lead to cancer.

Also, because humans have longer intestinal tracts compared to carnivores, the remnants of red meat remain in the colon longer, leading to putrefaction in the lower part of the colon, which can turn into ammonia and become toxic.[165] [166] Also, when red meat putrefies, it produces a waste product called uric acid. This acid can destroy the intestinal flora in the small intestines, making you more prone to colon cancer. If this uric acid remains stagnant in the colon for too long, it will get absorbed into the bloodstream, which can contribute to arthritis, hypertension, and increased risk for type 2 diabetes.[167] [168]

Compared to other animal foods, red meat is the most difficult to digest. Fish takes 30 minutes to digest, chicken takes 1½ to 2 hours, and red meat (beef, lamb, and pork) takes 3 to 5 hours.[169] Red meat is protein-dense animal muscle, and, in comparison to fish and poultry, it requires better chewing for optimal digestion, more acid secretion by the stomach's parietal cells, and more active enzyme secretion by the pancreas. Remnants of red meat can cling to the walls of the intestines for fourteen to twenty-one days. However, if a person has constipation, the rotting meat can stay in the intestines for months. A person should have two to three healthy bowel movements per day—one after each meal, just as babies do. If your frequency is less than that, you are constipated. Think about the pipes in your house getting a buildup of slime or debris that clogs them up. When animal protein and fat build up, your colon accumulates a thick, sticky mucus surrounding the poorly digested food debris. Just as a narrow passageway of the pipes in your house would slow down the flow, a buildup in your colon does the same thing.

The three major causes of constipation are eating red meat, not eating enough dietary fiber, and not drinking enough water. Dr. H. Aviles, a cancer biochemist, found after seeing 7,715 cancer patients over fifteen years that 99 percent suffered chronic constipation and the degree of malignancy was parallel to the intensity of their constipation.[170]

Red Meat Can Cause Gallstones

More bad news for red meat lovers, found by researchers at the University of Kentucky Medical Center after conducting a sixteen-year study, revealed that excess heme iron (the kind of iron in red meat) is correlated with gallstones.[171] Gallstones are common in Western countries and increasingly are a major cause of abdominal morbidity. Surgery to remove the gallbladder is one of the most common procedures in the United States today—more than 500,000 people have this organ removed every year.[172]

Beef Increases the Risk for Diabetes

A Harvard study published in the *American Journal of Clinical Nutrition* in 2011 suggests that eating as little as one serving of red meat a day is associated with a 50 percent increased risk of type 2 diabetes, compared with people who eat it less than once a month.[173] Several reasons were cited:

- The high iron content of red meat can increase inflammatory chemicals, which may destroy insulin-producing beta cells in the pancreas.
- The nitrates in processed meats may also be toxic to beta cells, which could explain why processed meats contributed even more to the risk of type 2 diabetes.
- The people who eat the most red meat also tend to gain more weight, which is a risk factor for diabetes.

Obviously, the results from this study were met with some criticism from those in the beef industry. Shalene McNeill, executive director of human nutrition research at the National Cattlemen's Beef Association, rebutted the study, saying, "A significant body of research showed red meat could actually lower the risk of type 2 diabetes. There is simply nothing in this recent Harvard study that should change how people enjoy nutrient-rich beef as part of a healthy, balanced diet."[174]

McNeill never did produce evidence that eating beef reduces the risk of getting type 2 diabetes. Should we just believe her biased opinion?

This was not the first time a Harvard study showed a correlation between eating red meat and the onset of type 2 diabetes. Another example is a study from the ongoing Women's Health Study, which looked at rates of type 2 diabetes among 37,309 participants. At the start, the women were all more than forty-five years old and free of cardiovascular disease, cancer, and type 2 diabetes. The researchers completely leveled the playing field by adjusting for age, body mass index (BMI), total energy intake, activity level, alcohol intake, cigarette smoking, and family history of diabetes. After nearly nine years of following these women, Harvard's findings showed a positive correlation between intake of red meat and the onset of type 2 diabetes.[175]

A similar study on males included 42,504 male participants between the ages of forty and seventy-five. The criteria for this study included only men who did not have diabetes, cardiovascular disease, or cancer, since these diseases might have affected their dietary habits. They also made sure their caloric intake was greater than 800 calories and no more than 4,200 calories per day. During a twelve-year follow-up, the results showed that the more red meat and processed meat in the diet, the more risk of type 2 diabetes.[176]

Genetically Altered Meat: What's Really at Steak?

Imagine being able to alter the DNA of cows, control the exact time of conception, the date the calves are born, and even their size. It's actually happening every day. To ensure profitability, a rancher has only about fourteen months to get a calf to grow from 100 pounds to more than 1,500 pounds, so beef cattle are treated with growth hormones, which help them grow up to 20 percent faster than untreated animals.[177] Growth hormones also pack on more weight, which means the animal makes it to the slaughterhouse in record time. Of course, the most profitable solution for the cattle farmer isn't the healthiest for consumers.

Synthetic hormone use in cattle dates back to 1956. In the 1970s, the FDA approved six hormone growth promotants (HGPs). These included three naturally occurring hormones—estradiol, progesterone, and testosterone—and three synthetically prepared hormones—zeranol, trenbolone, and melengestrol. When humans eat steaks and hamburger made from cows that have been treated with growth hormones, they also consume the hormones the animals were given. While circulating around the human body, these hormones still perform as intended—they promote growth. Research shows they increase the growth of tumors.[178]

At Ohio State University, cancer researchers mixed human breast cancer cells with trace amounts of zeranol. This resulted in a significant spurt in tumor growth, even at hormone levels thirty times lower than what the FDA maintains as safe.[179] The reason for an increased growth in tumors is because growth-promoting hormones circulate through the body, searching for any immature cells. When they find dormant, immature cancer cells, they attach to them and make them grow. If you have dormant skin cancer cells and you consume growth hormone, those sleeping cells could awaken, and your skin cancer could spread.

Some of the growth hormones used in cattle are made of synthetic estrogen, similar to the hormone that women produce naturally. Sixty years ago, estrogen in its natural form was usually produced by females after the age of fifteen, at the onset of puberty. Today it's not uncommon for a girl to start her menstrual cycle at the age of ten, and in some cases, earlier.[180] When girls are raised on a vegan diet from birth, which has no animal products, they usually begin their menstrual cycle after the age of fifteen.[181] In fact, in rural China today, where very few animal products are consumed, the average age of puberty is seventeen to nineteen. In areas of the world where westernized fast-food restaurants are becoming the norm, puberty in girls proportionately starts earlier. For boys, an increase in estrogen can cause enlarged breasts, known as gynecomastia. Other conditions include loss of muscle tone, shrinking testes, depression, fatigue, lower energy levels, and poor memory.

The FDA says the current hormones being used in the beef and poultry industry are safe. The FDA is the same organization that told us in the 1950s and 1960s that the hormone diethylstilbestrol (DES) was safe. DES was used as a growth hormone in the beef and poultry industries. After laboratory tests definitively showed DES was a serious carcinogen, it was banned from use as an animal growth promoter in 1979 by the FDA.[182] This left the drug companies with a massive inventory of DES. So, rather than destroy it, the manufacturers shipped it to farmers in less-developed parts of the world, promoting the fact that DES would help their livestock and poultry grow faster. One of these places was Puerto Rico.

Many Puerto Rican farmers supplemented their cattle and poultry with DES, and they were excited about the results. Just as they were told, the DES produced bigger cows and chickens. It wasn't long, however, before the Puerto Rican health authorities discovered a horrid after-effect. Thousands of babies and children were showing full sexual maturity. Five-year-old girls were found with fully developed sexual glands, pubic hair, and even menstruation![183]

This "gift" from the U.S. drug manufacturers would eventually leave an aftermath in Puerto Rico of cancer and death. Again, DES was once deemed a "safe" growth hormone for cattle by the FDA. This should make you wonder if you should trust them now with their adamant position that growth hormones used today are safe, when so much evidence continues to show quite the opposite.

Can You DIG This?

Ninety percent of all calves are given hormones,[184] despite the fact that the National Institutes of Health considers too much estrogen and progesterone probable carcinogens.[185] Ingesting estrogen has been linked to breast cancer in women, and progesterone has been found to increase the growth of ovarian, breast, and uterine tumors. Exposure to growth hormones from beef also puts people at risk for infertility. Women who routinely eat beef are far more likely to give birth to boys who grow up to have lower-than-normal sperm counts. In fact, sperm concentration has been found to be 24.3 percent higher in sons of mothers that had low to no beef consumption.[186]

Scientists are also concerned about the environmental impacts of hormone residues in cow manure. Growth-promoting hormones not only remain in the meat we consume, but also pass through the cattle and get excreted in their feces. When manure enters the surrounding environment, these hormones can contaminate land and groundwater and can have a negative impact on residents living near these feedlots.[187] Aquatic ecosystems are particularly vulnerable to hormone residues. When these hormones contaminate the water, they can also have a major effect on the gender and reproductive capacity of fish, interrupting their natural cycle.[188] [189] In spite of the worldwide research presented to the FDA showing the potential dangers of hormones in our beef, the position remains that the levels of hormones used is not high enough to be unsafe to humans.[190]

Beef Contains Antibiotics

We've all been there, sitting at the doctor's office with a sore throat. He takes out his little flashlight and tells you to say "Ahhh," then informs you that you have strep throat and prescribes an antibiotic. There are enough pills in the bottle to last you ten to fourteen days. Ever wonder why people don't take antibiotics for several weeks? Let's look at the word *antibiotic* for that answer. The word *anti* means "against" and *biotic* means "life." So, by definition the word *antibiotic* means "against life" (i.e., death). And death is exactly what these drugs cause. They circulate and destroy the bacteria in your body, and within ten to fourteen days, more of the bad bacteria are destroyed than the good bacteria.

But what if you were to take antibiotics every single day for your entire life? Imagine the effect a constant bombardment of antibiotics would have on your body. Folks, welcome to the life of a cow. They are fed these "against life" drugs every day. Why daily? Obviously, one of the reasons is because of their constant exposure to bacterial infections on their udders caused by the milking machines, as we covered in chapter 2. But ranchers and farmers have another reason for this daily dose of medication. Small doses of antibiotics administered daily have been shown to increase the weight of the animal by as much as 3 percent. Remember, the heavier the cow, the more profits to be made. The daily antibiotics make cows gain weight by changing the natural flora that would normally be found in the animals' intestines. This allows the cow to utilize its food more effectively.

While the annual use of antibiotics is not information you'll read in the daily headlines, 15 to 17 million pounds of antibiotics are used in the cattle industry each year.[191] Whether you swallow antibiotic pills prescribed by your doctor or swallow beef that has been tainted with trace elements of the drugs, it still gets into your system. But here's the scary part: a licensed doctor, trained in medicine, is the only person allowed by law to prescribe antibiotics for humans, yet 93 percent of the drugs approved for animals can be administrated by the owners of livestock, without veterinary supervision.[192] Cat and dog owners are *prohibited* from giving antibiotics to their pets without first seeing a veterinarian, yet the law says ranchers and farmers, untrained in administering prescription drugs, are free to do so for cattle.

When farmers give cattle sub-therapeutic dosages of antibiotics that are also used to treat human illnesses, it can pose health risks to the people who eat the meat. The bacteria inside the cattle can eventually become resistant to antibiotics. When humans ingest these resistant bacteria and become ill from them, they may not respond to antibiotic treatment. In a study published in the *New England Journal of Medicine* in 2002, researchers found that people who were sick with bacteria resistant to the antibiotic Cipro had acquired the bacteria by eating meat that was contaminated with salmonella bacteria.[193] Twenty percent of ground meat sold in supermarkets contains salmonella. Eighty-four percent of that contaminated meat is resistant to at least one form of antibiotic.[194]

The World Health Organization recommends a drastic reduction in the amount of antibiotics used in livestock. Many other countries have followed their lead and banned the use of non-therapeutic antibiotics, including Sweden, Finland, Belgium, Denmark, and Canada. However, in the United States, such use is still legal.[195]

Cow's Meat Contains Pesticides

Insecticides are chemicals used to control, repel, or kill insects and other pests; herbicides are used to kill unwanted plants (weed killer). Both are types of pesticides. Eighty percent of all herbicides and insecticides in the United States are sprayed on corn and soybeans, which are then used as feed for cattle and other livestock. The saying "you are what you eat" turns into "you are what you eat eats." When these chemicals are consumed by animals, the substances accumulate in their bodies, and, in turn, end up being consumed by humans. Chemicals in both insecticides and herbicides can cause an array of symptoms, ranging from a simple skin rash to death. The pesticide industry has made false or misleading claims about the safety of their products. In 1996, Monsanto Company, the industry's largest manufacturer, agreed to change its advertising after pressure from New York Attorney General Dennis Vacco. Monsanto claimed that herbicides, including the company's brand, Roundup, were safer than table salt and "practically nontoxic" to mammals, birds, and fish; Vacco deemed them misleading.[196]

Roundup is the most popularly used herbicide and contains toxic ingredients which, when ingested, even in small concentrations, have been found to kill human embryonic, placental, and umbilical cells in vitro.[197] Another popular herbicide called Tordon 101 is manufactured by Dow Chemical Company. They claim that Tordon 101 has no effects on animals and insects, despite evidence of strong carcinogenic activity of the active ingredient.[198][199] Paraquat, another popular herbicide, has been linked to Parkinson's disease.[200]

In 2005, The National Research Council of the National Academy of Sciences (NAS) found that beef contains the highest concentration of herbicides of any food sold in America. The NAS also found that beef ranks second only to tomatoes as the food posing the greatest cancer risk due to pesticide contamination and ranks third of all foods in insecticide contamination.[201] Meat contains fourteen times more pesticide residue than plant foods, and five times more than dairy products.[202]

Cow's Meat Contains Bacteria

Cattle are bombarded with so many antibiotics throughout their lives that they build up tolerances to many of these organisms, which means harmful bacteria remain in their bodies. Eating certain bacteria from cow's meat can lead to permanent health afflictions, including renal failure, brain/spinal cord damage, and miscarriage.

The good news is, most bacteria in raw meat get killed during the cooking process. However, the bacteria on large pieces of meat can survive, if not heated throughout. Cooking a thick steak on a grill, for instance, kills only the bacteria on the outside surfaces, if the steak is served rare or medium rare.[203] Any pink part remaining can still harbor bacteria. Cooking a burger or steak at less than 160 degrees Fahrenheit won't kill off all the bacteria living within the meat. But even if you do cook your burger at the right temperature, and until it's no longer pink inside, there is still the issue of cross-contamination.

You can't judge a burger by its color. According to the USDA, one in four burgers turns brown before it reaches 160 degrees. To really make sure your burger is fully cooked at 160 degrees, you need to insert a meat thermometer. Keep in mind that, once you stick the thermometer into the meat to see if it's cooked to the right temperature, the thermometer is infected with bacteria—if the meat isn't cooked through—and should not be used again (without proper washing) as the meat continues to cook. Another form of cross-contamination occurs when using a spatula or tongs to place or remove your burger or steak on the grill; these instruments make contact with that raw meat. If you then pick up your fully cooked, bacteria-free burgers with these instruments, you can contaminate the meat with the bacteria they used to have. The same is true of cutting boards and serving platters. If you put your cooked burger or steak on the same tray you used to bring the raw ones out to the grill, you have contaminated the meat with bacteria.

Overcooking your steak or hamburger helps to "burn off" dangerous pathogens, making it safer to eat; however, this comes at a price. Men have a higher risk of developing aggressive prostate cancer if they frequently consume meat that is grilled well-done. In fact, those who prefer their burgers and steaks well-done have double the cancer risk. When meat is cooked and charred at high temperatures over an open flame, a reaction occurs that causes the formation of two chemicals: polycyclic aromatic hydrocarbons (PAHs) and heterocyclic amines (HCAs).

These chemicals are linked to breast cancer in women and prostate cancer in men.[204] Researchers at the University of Minnesota School of Public Health and Masonic Cancer Center state that regular consumption of well-done, charred meats can also boost the risk of pancreatic cancer by a frightening 60 percent.[205]

Foodborne Organisms Live in Red Meat

Each year, an estimated 48 million people in the United States experience a foodborne illness, which leads to three thousand deaths annually.[206] Foodborne illnesses come in the form of infections of the gastrointestinal tract and are caused by food that contain harmful bacteria, parasites, or viruses. Common symptoms of foodborne illnesses include vomiting, diarrhea, abdominal pain, fever, chills, and death. Below are the most common foodborne organisms in red meat.

Escherichia coli bacteria

Also known as E. coli, this bacterium is the most commonly talked about foodborne organism. E. coli bacteria are found in the lower intestinal tract of most warm-blooded animals, humans included. These organisms are already inside of the body and help digest the food you eat and aid in the production of beneficial vitamin K. This bacterium also helps protect us from various diseases of the intestines. How did E. coli get such a "crappy" reputation? This bacterium exits from warm-blooded animals through fecal matter. E. coli can be passed from person to person, but serious E. coli infections are more commonly linked to food contaminated with the bacteria (cow poop in your food!). How does that happen? Manure is often used for fertilizer, and sometimes contaminated water is used to irrigate crops. Cows literally stand all day in their own manure in feedlots. Their entire bodies are sometimes covered in it. It is very difficult to completely clean a cow before it is slaughtered and the meat can get contaminated during the slaughtering process.

These microscopic organisms can cause very serious food poisoning in humans. Every year, hundreds of thousands of pounds of beef products are recalled because of E. coli contamination. One of the largest recalls to date took place in October 2007 when Topps Meat Company recalled 21.7 million pounds of hamburger meat because of potential E. coli contamination, which put the company out of business. E. coli is responsible for an estimated 74,000 illnesses per year.[207] Ground beef is the food most commonly contaminated with E. coli. Care for a little ketchup with your doo-doo burger? Of course, there have been some reports of E. coli and other pathogens contaminating spinach, berries, and other produce. Researchers aren't 100 percent sure how these fruits and veggies became infected with the pathogens.

Shigella bacteria

This little bugger is actually considered a subgenus of E. coli and is usually found in meat contaminated with fecal matter. This time it's usually human fecal matter being eaten. Most infections occur from contaminated fingers coming into contact with the mouth. The bacteria can also come from food contaminated due to poor hygienic practices in farming and harvesting produce. Flies are also known vectors of Shigella from feces to food. Shigella bacteria produce toxins that can attack the lining of the large intestine, causing swelling, ulcers on the intestinal wall, and bloody diarrhea. Shigella can lead to kidney failure and is implicated as one of the causes of reactive arthritis worldwide.[208]

Bovine spongiform encephalopathy (BSE)

More commonly known as mad cow disease, BSE is the most fatal neuro-degenerative disease in cattle. The disease is most often seen in the United Kingdom, but a handful of cases have been reported in the United States. This disease is not caused by eating bacteria. Instead, it's transmitted to humans from cattle that have eaten the meat, brain, spinal cord, or digestive tract of infected carcasses. Research shows that BSE developed after cows were fed other cattle in the form of meat and bone meal. Cows are herbivores (plant eaters), and are not supposed to eat the organs and meat from another animal because it makes them sick.[209]

> "The beef industry has contributed to more American deaths than all the wars of this century, all natural disasters, and all automobile accidents combined. If beef is your idea of 'real food for real people' you'd better live real close to a real good hospital."
> —Neal D. Barnard, M.D., President, Physicians Committee for Responsible Medicine

Red-Meat Alternatives

We live in a beef-eating society. When I was a child, my mom would take us to McDonald's and Burger King on a weekly basis for hamburgers and French fries, and on the weekends my father would cook steaks on the grill. However, when we look at common science and good ole common sense, it's apparent that humans should choose an alternative when it comes to eating beef. The good news is there are a lot of healthy options.

Veggie burgers

All right, get that grimace off your face! Trust me—veggie burgers have greatly improved in taste over the years. In fact, I'll share a little experiment I conducted one day with a friend of mine who happens to be a big steak lover. I told him I was cooking salmon on the grill and invited him over. He grimaced and reminded me that he didn't eat fish. I told him I would make him a hamburger instead, so he happily accepted the dinner invitation. What he didn't know was, I actually cooked a veggie burger on the grill and created it the way he liked it, with all the fixin's. He *loved it!* After he ate the entire thing, I decided to break the news to him that his burger contained no cow's meat but was a veggie burger. Don't knock 'em til you try 'em. They are a delicious alternative to cow's meat. My personal favorite is Organic Sunshine Burgers (sunshineburger.com). They are produced without the use of toxic, synthetic pesticides or fertilizers and were the first veggie burger to be Non-GMO Project Verified. Throw a few mushrooms and onions on the grill with one of these, and you have a healthy burger (not) to die for!

Another tasty red meat alternative is Amy's Organic Texas Burgers (amyskitchen.com). Amy's brand of organic vegetarian products makes several types of veggie burgers, even in barbeque flavor.

Turkey burgers

You can do what I do and make your own turkey burgers from scratch. Just replace hamburger meat with organic, free-range ground turkey and then follow your usual recipe. If you want to go the premade route, one of the most popular brands is all-natural turkey burgers from Jennie-O (jennieo.com). You can grill or fry these juicy quarter-pounders.

Portobello mushrooms

These are often referred to as "the vegetarian's filet mignon" because they have the same consistency as a juicy and tender steak. You can add your favorite steak marinade and spices to these giant mushrooms and throw them on the grill. Serve them with a baked potato, and you will never miss your putrefied, bacteria-laden, hormone-laced, cancer-causing steaks again.

Healthiest Red-Meat Choices

If you still feel the need to add red meat to your diet, bison is a healthier option. While eating beef increases both triglyceride levels and markers of inflammation, eating bison involves a smaller increase in triglyceride levels and no increase in the markers of inflammation. Federal laws prohibit the use of growth hormones in bison, so consider this as a healthier alternative to beef.

If you still want to indulge in the occasional hamburger or steak, the healthiest choice is USDA certified organic. Cattle farmers with this certification are required to comply with strict guidelines to ensure you are not ingesting chemicals, pesticides, and hormones. The USDA grades are Prime, Choice, and Select, from best to worst, respectively. Many people believe that the higher the grade, the healthier the beef. This is not the case. Beef is graded by taste, texture, and amount of marbling, also called intramuscular fat. Marbling adds flavor and is one of the main criteria for judging the quality cuts of meat. In general, the more marbling it contains, the better grade of meat.

Certified Organic Beef

The word *organic* is not the same as *natural* or *grass-fed*. The USDA's Food Safety and Inspection Service (FSIS) allows the word *natural* to be used on a label for beef if it doesn't contain any artificial flavoring, coloring, or chemical preservatives. This definition only applies to how the beef was processed *after* the cows were harvested and doesn't apply to how they were raised. Grass-fed beef (sometimes referred to as "naturally raised") pertains to how the cattle were managed prior to harvest and the type of diet the cattle consumed. While most cattle start off eating grass and are moved to feedlots for grain-finishing, grass-fed cattle stay on a pasture and forage their entire lives. However, unless they are eating grass free of fertilizers, the grass-fed cows won't be certified organic. Only "certified organic" beef is required to pass strict regulations both on the farm and during processing. This class of beef is guaranteed to be fed organic grains and grasses and must have unrestricted outdoor access. The cattle can't be given antibiotics or hormones. When shopping for beef, always look for "USDA Certified Organic" on the label.

Table 3.2: Comparisons for Choosing Beef

Process Includes:	USDA Certified Organic	USDA Grades	Natural	Grass Fed
Humane Treatment	Yes	Not Regulated	Not Regulated	Not Regulated
Organic Fed	Yes	No	No	No
Antibiotics or Synthetic Hormones	No	Yes	Not Regulated	Not Regulated
Access to the Outdoors (Pasture)	Yes	No	Not Regulated	Yes

Process Includes:	USDA Certified Organic	USDA Grades	Natural	Grass Fed
Animal By-Products	No	Yes	Not Regulated	Yes
Fed GMOs	No	Yes	Not Regulated	Not Regulated
Synthetic Pesticides/ Herbicides Used	No	Yes	Yes	Not Regulated
Artificial Fertilizers to Grow Feed	No	Yes	Yes	Not Regulated

 Discovery: Science has proven humans don't need to eat cow's meat for protein. In fact, the protein derived from beef has been linked to diabetes, cancer, high cholesterol, hypertension, heart disease, and stroke. Red meat can also contain harmful bacteria, growth hormones, and antibiotics. The American Dietetic Association, the American Heart Association, the National Academy of Sciences, and the American Academy of Pediatrics all recommend people reduce their consumption of red meat. There is no health organization in the world that recommends reducing or eliminating the consumption of vegetables.

Instincts: People are eating cow muscle to support the health of human muscles. What does your gut say about that? Since childhood, you've heard that red meat gives you protein to help build strong muscles. If that were true, how can it be explained why many record-holding champion athletes are vegetarians? Don't they have strong muscles?

God: Red meat naturally contains things humans were not designed to digest which causes inflammation, hurts our immune response and composition of good bacteria, and raises cholesterol, which has been linked to various diseases. Commercialized red meat may also contain antibiotics and hormones, which are detrimental to the health of humans.

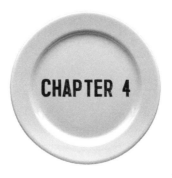

FOWL PLAY
ARE WE PLAYING CHICKEN WITH OUR HEALTH?

"Why did the chicken cross the road?
To get away from Colonel Sanders!"
—Unknown

If it looks like a chicken and clucks like a chicken, does it mean that the meat we're eating is really chicken? Unfortunately, the healthy farm-fresh chicken of the past has flown the coop. Today, chickens often contain dangerously high levels of contaminants like pesticides, appetite stimulants, insecticides, and bacteria. Add to the mix coloring agents and chemical preservatives, and it begs the question: What's really on our plate? But before I put the chicken before the egg, let's discuss some of the great health benefits of eating chicken, the way nature intended.

In the last chapter, I shared information about a sugar in cow's meat called Neu5Gc, which can cause inflammation and a lowered immune system. Poultry does not contain this inflammation-causing sugar. Also, chicken is low in fat and cholesterol, containing three times more polyunsaturated "good fat" than red meat. A chicken breast has half the fat of a trimmed choice grade T-bone steak, but watch out for the skin. Consuming the skin doubles your intake of saturated fat. If you are a chicken eater, I recommend removing the skin *prior* to cooking. Some people leave the skin on while cooking and remove it before they eat it, but by then, the fat from the skin has already soaked into the meat during the cooking process.

Poultry meat has several advantages over other meats. For instance, it's void of trans fats that contribute to coronary heart disease. Chicken and turkey are also low in calories, are virtually devoid of sodium, offer a great source of niacin, zinc, and selenium—all of which aid in lowering cholesterol, increasing circulation, and reducing the risk of heart disease and stroke.

Ever notice how everyone's usually in a good mood, stress free, and relaxed after eating turkey on Thanksgiving? That's because turkey meat contains high amounts of tryptophan, a precursor for serotonin, a neurotransmitter, which regulates the body's sleep patterns and mood. Its ability to raise serotonin levels has led to tryptophan being used therapeutically in the treatment of a variety of conditions including insomnia, depression, and anxiety.[210]

Chicken for Disease Prevention

We've explored how red meat is linked to colon cancer, but when we look at poultry, research shows quite the opposite. Eating chicken can actually *prevent* colon cancer. A study of more than 1,500 patients underwent baseline colonoscopies to remove existing polyps. At intervals of one year and four years, the group underwent follow-up colonoscopies to determine if any polyps had returned. Those who consumed diets higher in processed meat and red meats showed a marked increase in developing recurrent pre-cancerous growths (colorectal adenomas). Individuals consuming diets high in chicken were less prone to this risk. People with the highest risk of advanced adenomas, who also ate the most chicken, had 39 percent lower risk of these cancer-causing growths.[211]

In a fourteen-year study of sixteen thousand Swedish men and women, the foods found to have the highest risk of causing colon cancer were beef and lamb—not chicken.[212] And finally, one of the largest worldwide studies on the causes of colon cancer and the associated risks from eating meat was collectively funded by the Medical Research Council, Cancer Research UK, and the International Agency for Research on Cancer. The study revealed the risk of developing colon cancer greatly increases in people who eat red and processed meat. However, poultry did not influence the risk of colon cancer. Scientists theorize that selenium present in chicken could be the reason.[213] [214]

Selenium is a great antioxidant that helps stimulate the body's immune system. In fact, low selenium levels in the body have been linked to skin, prostate, and lung cancers.[215–222] The reason selenium may prevent or slow tumor growth is because components of the nutrient enhance immune cell activity and suppress the development of blood vessels to the tumor.[223] Selenium also has been found to reduce the risk of thyroid problems.[224] This is because selenium assists in the production of the thyroid hormone, triiodothyronine (T3), which regulates metabolism. Four ounces of chicken supplies 99 percent of the daily value for selenium.[225]

Chicken Combats Alzheimer's Disease and Age-Related Cognitive Decline

Let's face it. We all know someone getting up there in years who suffers from C.R.S. (Can't Remember Squat). Just like our muscles, hair, and skin wither as we age, so does our brainpower. But, there's good news for chicken eaters. Research published in the *Journal of Neurology, Neurosurgery, and Psychiatry* indicates regular consumption of niacin-rich foods, like chicken and turkey, can provide protection against age-related memory decline and even Alzheimer's disease. Scientists analyzed the diets of 3,718 people sixty-five years of age and older while testing their cognitive abilities over a six-year period. Individuals who received the most niacin from foods were 70 percent less likely to have developed Alzheimer's disease.[226] [227]

Chicken for Heart Health

Beef and pork have been associated with heart disease, but quite the opposite holds true when it comes to eating poultry. A nutrient called taurine, found abundantly in dark-meat poultry, has been found to significanlty lower the risk of coronary heart disease in women with high cholesterol.[228] Researchers also claim that taurine might also help protect against diabetes and high blood pressure. While many doctors recommend eating white or light meat instead of dark meat to avoid high levels of saturated fat, this study demonstrates how dark meat ultimately packs a healthier punch when combating heart disease. Being a good source of essential B vitamins, chicken is a great food choice for supporting the cardiovascular system by helping to maintain low levels of homocysteine, a molecule that damages blood vessel walls.[229] [230] [231] The higher our homocysteine levels, the more of a risk factor for hardening of the arteries and cardiovascular disease.[232]

Chicken Business—We're All Getting Clucked!

I wish I could just end this chapter on the obvious high note: *For cardiovascular, brain, thyroid, digestion, mood, and immense nutritional benefits, eat chicken!* But chicken is a business—a big one—and when you follow the money trail, you'll find that there's a general rule: the bigger the chicken, and the faster it can be grown, the bigger the profits. Put another way, the grocery stores don't charge you per chicken; you pay for chicken by its weight! It's in the interest of the chicken farms such as Tyson, Purdue, Foster Farms, and others, to do whatever it takes to fatten up their chickens—and fast! The easiest and most traditional way of accomplishing this feat would be to inject chickens with growth hormones; however, unlike cattle, chickens are protected from hormone use.

In the early 1950s, synthetic estrogens, in particular, diethylstilbestrol (DES), were also used to produce plump chickens. In 1970, DES was shown to be a cause of cancer. When the news hit, it made national headlines but didn't compel the FDA to act on this information. Once public pressure, including Congressional hearings, gained ground, the FDA was forced to issue a warning about DES in November 1971. Even then, the drug was not banned for human use; only a "contraindicated if you're pregnant" warning was issued a year later. In September 2000, almost three decades later, the FDA finally withdrew its approval of DES. However, it wasn't until February 22, 2011, that the FDA would release a three-page document acknowledging the devastating health consequences of DES, which, of course, includes death.[233]

Beware of Package Gimmicks

Since the ban of DES in poultry, the USDA prohibits manufacturers from advertising the phrase "no hormones added" on poultry product labels *unless* followed by the statement, "Federal regulations prohibit the use of hormones." Many semantics gimmicks are used on food packaging, so don't be fooled into paying more for chicken because you see "no hormones added" on the package when regulation has already stepped in to mandate such.

Why hasn't hormone use in cattle also been banned? Because the beef and dairy industries in the United States pack a very powerful political punch, both in the legislative and the regulatory arenas. They spend a ton of money on key lawmakers and regulators who have a direct impact on their business interests. Most of the companies involved in the beef and dairy businesses are represented by powerful cattle trade and lobbying organizations that have both a strong influence in Washington and the ability to sweep under the rug topics like the dangers of growth hormone use in cattle.

However, the ban on growth hormones didn't stop chicken farmers from figuring out another way to quickly grow and plump up a chicken using something else in Big Pharma's arsenal—antibiotics. Even without growth hormones, today's chickens are 2 to 3 pounds heavier than and reach maturity thirty-eight days sooner than chickens of the 1950s. What's the secret recipe? Take chickens, confine them to cages, deprive them of exercise, and pump them full of antibiotics. It actually makes sense. If you were confined to a small closet for your entire life, fed food, and deprived of exercise, wouldn't you gain weight? They don't call it "cooped up" for nothing. Cramming chickens together in cages doesn't just make them fat, it makes them crazy. With no turf to call their own, emotional stress in chickens rises, and, in an attempt to protect whatever territory they can claim, they viciously peck at each other to the point of inflicting bloody puncture wounds prone to infection, creating the need for antibiotics. Farmers quickly discovered that administering antibiotics to chickens destroys the "good bacteria" in their gut and disrupts digestion, causing them to grow faster and heavier!

Infected Chicken

"Two-thirds of Chickens Tested Harbor Dangerous Bacteria" read the headlines of a January 2010 edition of *Consumer Reports*. These findings showed that most chicken companies' safeguards are inadequate. *Consumer Reports* also found that most disease-causing bacteria sampled from contaminated chickens were resistant to at least one antibiotic, potentially making any resulting illness more difficult to treat.[234] The three common bacteria specific to birds are salmonella, campylobacter, and listeria. *Consumer Reports* had a third party test 382 chickens purchased from more than one hundred randomly chosen supermarkets in twenty-two states. The following was discovered:

- Campylobacter was found in 62 percent of the chickens, and salmonella was discovered in 14 percent. Only 24 percent of the birds were clear of both pathogens.
- Tyson and Foster Farms chickens were found to be the most contaminated with more than 80 percent containing both pathogens.
- Only 43 percent of store-brand organic chickens were free of campylobacter.
- Among all brands, 68 percent of the salmonella and 60 percent of the campylobacter organisms analyzed showed resistance to one or more antibiotics.

In this article, Jean Halloran, director of Food Policy Initiatives at Consumers Union, stated the following: "USDA has been pondering new standards to cut the prevalence of bacteria in chicken for more than five years but has yet to act. Consumers shouldn't have to play roulette with poultry; the USDA must make chicken less risky to eat."[235] Fast forward to four years later, and things got much worse. In 2014 *Consumer Reports* found 97 percent of the chicken breasts tested harbored dangerous bacteria. They analyzed more than three hundred raw chicken breasts purchased at stores across the United States and found potentially harmful bacteria lurking in almost all of the chicken, including organic brands.[236]

It is worth emphasizing that these findings were published by an independent, nonprofit organization whose mission is to work for a fair, just, and safe marketplace. They have no agenda other than the interests of consumers. Remember what the "D" stands for when you DIG for the truth: a discovery needs to be *unbiased*.

Big Pharma Has Bad Karma

As we explored in the last chapter, when an animal ingests antibiotics, this can cause them to build up a tolerance to many bacteria. In the United States, 80 percent of all antibiotics sold are administered to livestock animals, and most of these antibiotics are identical or closely related to drugs used for treating illnesses in humans. Consequently, many of these drugs are losing their effectiveness on humans. Antibiotic-resistant infections sicken millions of Americans each year and kill an estimated 23,000.[237] [238]

Chicken farming commonly uses four antibiotics: tetracycline, amoxicillin, ampicillin, and ciprofloxacin—all of which are also popular antibiotics administered to humans. Ciprofloxacin is one of the most powerful antibiotics on the market, yet two-thirds of the pathogens found in chickens are resistant to this powerful drug. Research shows that poultry, especially chicken, is the bridge that allows resistant bacteria to move to humans, taking up residence in the body and causing infections.[239]

Another class of antibiotic, antimicrobial drugs—nitrofurans—used to be commonly administered to chicken and turkey. In 1991, however, they were found to be carcinogenic, and the FDA withdrew approval for use of nitrofurans (furazolidone and nitrofurazones) in poultry. Well . . . not exactly.

The FDA allowed the use of these drugs in topical form, stating that there was no evidence that such application would reach edible tissues in animals.[240] Fast forward eleven years to February 7, 2002, when the FDA banned the topical use of nitrofuran drugs from use in food-producing animals because "the presence of carcinogenic residues was not shown to be safe."[241] Imagine that! It took more than a decade for the FDA to figure out that putting chemicals on the skin of animals could penetrate their tissue, which humans would later eat!

I find it rather odd that the FDA didn't have the knowledge that veterinarians have had for decades—topical flea and tick products and antibiotic creams and ointments applied to the skin are absorbed, enter the bloodstream, and are distributed throughout the body.[242] And even *if* I suspended my disbelief for a moment, what about all of the FDA-approved topical creams for humans? Like the ones to increase testosterone levels in the blood? Or how about the transdermal patches as a means of absorbing birth control, hormone replacement, and for the prevention of motion sickness? But, it's incomprehensible that nitrofuran drugs absorb transdermally in animals and could end up in their organs and muscles?

Isn't there some need for antibiotics in poultry? After all, birds do get sick. Actually, if poultry were raised in clean environments, with outdoor exposure, proper food, and no chemicals in their feed, the risk of them getting sick would be extremely low.

In an October 2000 USDA press release, the Food Safety and Inspection Service (FSIS) finally addressed the prevalence and levels of bacteria in chicken and stated the following: "Governments, local authorities, and international agencies need to take a greatly increased stance in combating the role of factory farming, commerce in live poultry, and wildlife markets which provide ideal conditions for a bacteria or virus to spread and mutate into a more dangerous form."[243] The FSIS's message seemed to fall on deaf ears because the lousy conditions at factory farms have continued and so has antibiotic use.

Then in May 2011, the Natural Resources Defense Council, the Center for Science in the Public Interest, the Food Animal Concerns Trust, and the Union of Concerned Scientists had enough and sued the FDA. This lawsuit was spurred by growing evidence that the worldwide spread of bacteria immune to antibiotics showed clear links to the overuse of antibiotics in the food industry. This coalition suit was filed to compel the FDA to take action on the agency's own safety findings, withdrawing approval for most nontherapeutic uses of antibiotics in animal feed. They also submitted evidence showing that antibiotic use in farming costs the U.S. health-care system $34 billion each year.[244]

On March 23, 2012, a court ruling stated that the FDA must act to address the growing human health threats resulting from the overuse of antibiotics in animal feed.[245] Since the ruling, the FDA has tightened its approval standards where new antibiotics for animal agriculture are concerned. And the FDA released new guidelines in an effort to phase out the use of antibiotics to promote animal growth—though the move was criticized largely because those policies remain "voluntary." That pretty much equates to something along the lines of, "We, the FDA, recommend you stop using antibiotics, but it's up to you to decide if you want to cease making hundreds of millions of dollars every year." That's one tough *voluntary* decision to leave in the hands of the agricultural industry. Since the FDA published its voluntary industry guidelines in 2012, antimicrobial use in livestock has actually increased. On September 12, 2016, the FDA announced that they are soliciting public comments on the issue until March 13, 2017.[246] Really? Public comments? Such stalling tactics would never be allowed if you or I were issued a court order.

Bacteria Commonly Found in Chicken

Salmonella leads to a potentially fatal disease called Salmonellosis, which affects 1.4 million people annually in the United States.[247]

Campylobacter bacteria is responsible for most pathogen-related cases of diarrheal illness in the United States (approximately 845,000 per year).[248] Long-term effects can include paralysis, appendicitis, and reactive arthritis.[249] [250]

Listeria is caused by contamination of food-processing plants. Listeria on infected chicken can grow and multiply even in the refrigerator. In the United States, thousands of people become seriously ill from exposure.[251]

Protect Yourself

- Most bacteria are killed off during the cooking process, so never eat undercooked poultry.
- Thoroughly wash your hands and anything poultry has come in contact with such as utensils, cutting boards, and countertops. Even touching a trash can lid after handling chicken can cause cross contamination.
- Keep uncooked chicken away from raw vegetables to avoid cross contamination.
- Store poultry at the proper temperature. Foodborne microorganisms grow much faster at temperatures between 70 degrees Fahrenheit and 135 degrees Fahrenheit. Freeze and heat above this temperature zone.

Arsenic in Your Chicken?

Most people are familiar with arsenic, a highly carcinogenic toxin—a.k.a. *poison*—used to kill rats, insects, and bacteria. We're not talking about the safe kind of arsenic that is naturally found in trace amounts in soil, sediment, and groundwater. For instance, environmental traces of arsenic are found in bananas and apples, and these are safe. We're talking about large amounts of arsenic that haven been intentionally put into poultry by Big Agra, which they get from Big Pharma, which is then ingested by humans. In 1944 an organic form of arsenic called roxarsone was added to chicken feed, and what's more disturbing, for more than seventy years, the government said it's okay. The FDA approved this poison to be used to kill intestinal parasites, artificially promote growth, and stain chicken's flesh a pink color rather than permit it to be gray, a color preference that apparently doesn't show well on the grocery store shelves. Roxarsone is manufactured by Alpharma LLC, a subsidiary of Pfizer. That's right; the same drug company that brought Viagra to market has also been making the chickens *bigger* by supplying them with poison. The drug has been used in more than 70 percent of all chickens raised for their meat.[252] Pfizer has always claimed roxarsone is safe because it contains *organic* arsenic, which is less toxic than the *inorganic* form, a known carcinogen. However, studies done by the Department of Chemical and Environmental Engineering and Duquesne University show that roxarsone arsenic becomes *inorganic* in fewer than ten days.[253] Unfortunately these findings didn't make any waves.

For seven decades, 1.7 to 2.2 million pounds of roxarsone has been given to chickens. Arsenic contamination spread through much of the 26 to 55 billion pounds of chicken feces or waste generated each year by the U.S. chicken industry and the communities where that waste is generated or dispersed. In the chicken-producing town of Prairie Grove, Arkansas, for example, dust in 4 percent of homes was found to contain at least two kinds of arsenic also found in chicken litter.[254]

The Institute for Agriculture and Trade Policy, an organization that works globally on policy and practices to ensure fair and sustainable food, farm, and trade systems, did what the U.S. government failed to do. They conducted the most thorough research to date, measuring arsenic content in the wings, thighs, legs, breasts, and livers of chickens. In 2006, the findings were published, along with an analysis of chicken from all the major brand names and fast-food chains, including some of the nation's largest chicken-producing companies and "premium" chicken products that were certified organic and kosher.

Most uncooked chicken products purchased at supermarkets (55 percent) contained detectable arsenic. Out of 155 samples, 65 percent showed signs of arsenic. Nearly 75 percent of the raw chicken breasts, thighs, and livers from conventional producers that were tested had detectable levels of arsenic. Even certified organic or other "premium" chicken parts, or whole chickens, had one-third detectable arsenic despite the fact that the use of arsenic in chicken feed is prohibited under organic standards.[255]

The Environmental Protection Agency investigated arsenic in chicken and shared findings with the FDA showing the long-term effects of arsenic exposure, which included bladder, lung, skin, kidney, and colon cancer, as well as the negative effects it has on the immunological, neurological, and endocrine systems.[256] This information didn't seem to influence the FDA's and poultry industry's stance that roxarsone "does not leave detectable amounts of arsenic in the parts of chickens consumed by people"; however, the FDA could no longer muffle the outcry from health advocacy groups and consumers and conducted its own tests on one hundred chickens that consumed feed containing roxarsone and compared the chickens to unexposed chickens. The results showed chickens that ingested the drug had high levels of inorganic arsenic. After the FDA shared this information with Pfizer, the drug company voluntarily suspended sales of roxarsone in the United States, even though its spokespeople did not concede that the arsenic in chicken was a health concern.[257]

After decades of the FDA's firm stance that roxarsone was safe, Michael Taylor, the FDA's deputy commissioner for foods, said this new study only raised "some concerns of a *very low* but completely avoidable exposure to a carcinogen."[258] Taylor was the person who worked for the law firm seeking FDA approval of Monsanto's commercial form of bovine growth hormone Posilac. Taylor was promoted, given a raise, and went on to take charge of the FDA's labeling guidelines. Can you say, "conflict of interest"?

Even though roxarsone is no longer approved for use in chicken, the arsenic you've been eating all these decades can still be in your system.[259] This is because arsenic is stored in the brain, bones, and muscles. Some people have no immediate symptoms, but even many years after exposure, cancer, diabetes, or long-term liver damage can occur.[260]

Pfizer pulled the toxic feed chemical off the shelves in the United States in 2011; however, reminiscent of the ban of DES, the drug company did not agree to remove it from feed products in other countries. Now roxarsone, which could lead to disease and death, is being fed to thousands of people overseas. Pfizer continues to claim that the arsenic in roxarsone is at such low levels that it's safe to eat.

Okay, mission accomplished! After this ruling, no more arsenic in U.S. chicken. High five? Not so fast. Consumers Union then asked the FDA to investigate nitarsone, another drug containing arsenic that is fed to chicken and turkey stock. Guess who manufactures *this* version of poison—Pfizer! Nitarsone is essentially the same as roxarsone and used for the same purposes in conventional agriculture, which means that most chicken meat continues to be intentionally contaminated with arsenic. The FDA's position on nitarsone is, once again, that it's safe for human consumption. Then on December 31, 2015, the FDA announced that nitarsone will no longer be used in food-animal production, even though they still consider it to be safe for human consumption.[261] [Until the next arsenic drug is released. To be continued . . .]

Additives, Flavorings, and Other Tricks of the Trade

Smelling your food is just as important as tasting it. If our noses tell us that somehow that sweet cinnamon rice pudding is one day away from becoming a science experiment, we won't eat it. This is biology at its finest; it's nature's way of helping us save our own lives by not eating food that could make us sick or kill us.

But now our sense of smell is being masked by science, and this is occurring most rampantly in modern-day poultry processing. During the manufacturing process, the flavor can be lost, which is why additional flavorings with pleasant smells are often added to enhance the chicken. Take McDonald's, which adds "chicken flavor" to Chicken McNuggets.[262] This artificial chicken flavor is made from a synthetic chemical that goes by the name methyl furanthiol. Yum! This is just one of the more than three thousand food additives that are currently approved by the FDA for use in the United States.[263] Once approved, a food additive is considered safe. But just how safe is "safe"? Many people are allergic to food colorings and flavor additives, and some have been linked to asthma, birth defects, and cancer![264]

The ingredients that make up food flavorings are a multibillion-dollar business.[265] The FDA requires that all ingredients be listed on a food's label, but additives are often hidden in products listed as "spices" or "flavorings," making it impossible for consumers to determine exactly what they are eating.[266]

McFrankenstein Nuggets

Did you know that McDonald's Chicken McNuggets are only 50 percent chicken? The rest is a concoction of fattening corn derivatives, sugars, and completely synthetic/unhealthy chemicals including:

Dimethyl polysiloxane: a silicone-based anti-foaming polymer that is also used to make caulking, lubricating oils, and heat-resistant tiles.

Tertiary butylhydroquinone (TBHQ): a chemical preservative so deadly that eating just five grams can kill a human. It's a commonly used ingredient in varnishes, lacquers, pesticide products, as well as cosmetics and perfumes. A number of studies have shown that prolonged exposure to high doses of TBHQ may be carcinogenic, especially for stomach tumors.[267] [268] This is a common ingredient in chicken nuggets and fast food fried chicken.

Sodium aluminum phosphate: a chemical used in food processing that is synthetically produced from aluminum. Yes, that is the same stuff that is used to line cans of paint!

Not So Fast . . . "Food"

Whoever snuck the "S" in FAST FOOD was a clever marketer. The chemicals that fast food restaurants use have been linked to many health ailments including obesity. A group of teenagers sued McDonald's restaurant chain, claiming the food sold by McDonald's contained ingredients that caused their obesity. Although the case was dismissed in 2003, the plaintiffs appealed to the United States Court of Appeals for the Second Circuit, and in 2005, the district court's dismissal was reversed.[269] Robert Sweet, the federal judge who heard the case, agreed with the teenage plaintiffs and said, "Chicken McNuggets, rather than being merely chicken fried in a pan, are a McFrankenstein creation of various elements not utilized by the home cook." *Time* magazine reported that Judge Sweet "questioned whether customers understood the risks of eating McDonald's chicken over regular chicken."[270]

It's not just McDonald's chicken we need to be concerned about. Research published in *Nutrition and Cancer*, an international journal, revealed that consumers are being exposed to a known human carcinogen PhIP when they consume grilled chicken from Chick-fil-A, Chili's, T.G.I. Friday's, Outback Steakhouse, Burger King, Applebee's, and McDonald's.[271] One hundred samples from these popular chain restaurants were analyzed by an independent laboratory and PhIP was discovered in every sample. PhIP is one of a group of carcinogenic compounds called heterocyclic amines (HCAs), and it is a known mutagen that can cause DNA damage, which can lead to cancer. PhIP is formed in meat, especially chicken, that is chargrilled, pan-fried, and barbecued to high degrees. It's been linked to breast, colon, and prostate can-cers.[272] Even small amounts can increase a person's risk of developing cancer.

In January 2008, after results were made public, the Physicians Com-mittee for Responsible Medicine (PCRM) filed suit against these restaurants for knowingly exposing their customers to PhIP without warning them of its risks. In the press release, PCRM president Neal Barnard, M.D., stated, "Health-conscious Americans have long steered away from fried chicken, but they have no idea that grilled chicken may be as bad or worse."[273]

According to California law, if a high level of a known carcinogen, such as arsenic, is found inside food sold to consumers, a warning must be clearly posted. On August 15, 2012, Judge Jane L. Johnson ruled on the PCRM's lawsuit against these restaurants. She agreed that PhIP is considered a car-cinogen; however, she ruled that because of a California statute that said parties must gather evidence that a law has been violated before filing suit, the PCRM's claim was invalid. As part of the judge's ruling, an early consent judgment, McDonald's, Chick-fil-A, and Outback had agreed to disclose that some of their products contain chemicals known to cause cancer.[274]

To lower your risk of consuming high levels of PhIP at restaurants or when cooking chicken at home, avoid chargrilled, pan-fried, and BBQ chicken. Instead, go for boiled, steamed, stewed, or microwave-cooked chicken. Research shows that chicken cooked at levels around 212 degrees Fahrenheit significantly lowers risk of PhIP exposure.[275] [276] If you prefer grilled chicken, cooking until the meat is medium to medium rare is much safer than chicken that is cooked to well done.

Your Guide to Healthy Poultry

Looking for the healthiest birds for you and your family to enjoy is like learning a new language. The more you pay attention, the more you will notice different phrases and descriptions on packaging. One thing is for sure, not all words are equal. The following is a cheat sheet pertaining to chicken, turkey, and eggs to keep you from being a chicken when it comes to digging for your healthiest, most delicious poultry alternatives.

Industrial (Factory Farm)

This is the standard commercial chicken operation, located in a warehouse-like barn with a concrete floor. These factory-confined birds live in extremely crowded conditions and typically have less than half a square foot of floor space each. Industrial-raised birds have no exposure to fresh air or sunlight and often share their cage with hundreds of other birds. The cages are filled with excrement and feces splattered everywhere. To protect their personal space, it's common for the birds to peck at each other with their sharp beaks, which creates oozing and bloody wounds that are a haven for infections that require antibiotics. To keep this from happening, many farmers cut off the bird's beaks, which ends up killing some of them during the process.

Factory farms are profit driven, and their poultry is fed the cheapest food available to fatten up the chickens, with no regard to their health or the health of consumers that eat their products. A factory-farm–raised chicken eats feed that can contain pieces of meat from animals that have died and blood from other chickens that have been pecked by the sharp beaks. It also contains feathers, skin, hair, feces, plastics, antibiotics, unhealthy grain, and other animal waste.[277] Factory farmers induce molting/starvation. This is the practice of artificially provoking a complete flock of hens to molt simultaneously by not allowing them to eat for up to two weeks. After a molt, the hen's production rate usually peaks and so does the profitability for the farmers.

Cage Free

Ahhh, cage free. It sounds so nice! It conjures the image of chickens roaming around in the grass and not confined to the prison of a cage. Unfortunately, this is far from the truth. The term "cage free" is meaningless and intentionally misleading. This term is only relevant for egg-laying hens. Turkeys and chickens raised for meat are not and never have been raised in cages. Seeing "cage free" on a label is simply a way for the poultry industry to profit from consumers' ignorance. Even though they are not kept in cages, they are crammed into tight quarters with no room to walk around. They have little to no access to outdoors and are left standing in their own poop. Forced molting and beak cutting is permitted. They are not subjected to any third-party auditing.

Vegetarian Fed

When you see "vegetarian fed" on the label, you immediately think the chickens are healthy because they eat veggies. Not so. Nature never intended for chickens to eat vegetables. In a wild setting, they instinctively eat insects, bugs, worms, seeds, and grass—not corn and soybeans. Vegetarian-fed poultry means they are being raised on industrialized, genetically modified feed. The birds are rarely allowed outside. Forced molting and beak cutting is practiced. There is no mandated third-party auditing.

Humanely Raised Certified

The term "humanely raised certified" sounds great, doesn't it? That title alone sells the chicken. Unfortunately, humanely raised is meaningless and intentionally misleading to sell consumers more poultry. This label is issued by the National Chicken Council, a private industry group and not a welfare verifier. How "humane" does this sound? Chickens and turkeys can be confined to windowless sheds with thousands of other birds confined to a space about the size of a legal-size sheet of paper. It is not required that the birds have any access to fresh air or sunshine. Forced molting through starvation is prohibited, but beak cutting is allowed. Compliance is verified through third-party auditing by the American Humane Association.

Process Verified

The USDA gives "humanely raised" certification to companies enrolled in its Process Verified Program (PVP). This is totally meaningless and misleading. When poultry producers use this term on their packaging, it gives the customers false comfort that the USDA has federally certified them for using humane and animal welfare practices. In reality, no federal definition exists to define the term *humane*. So, the USDA merely verifies that the poultry producer is following its own arbitrary standards. Sadly, this means industrial producers can just submit "humane" practices to the USDA and display their "Process Verified" and "humanely raised" seals on their packages.

Free Range

"Free-range," also called "free roaming," conjures up images of feathered friends napping in the sunshine between snacks of grass and bugs. It's supposed to make you think happy thoughts—that's how marketing works. Unfortunately that's not reality. Anyone can use the label "free range" so long as their chickens have *access* to a door to the outside for, say five minutes a day, even if they never actually make it outside. And what exactly does "outside" mean? There are no criteria for the amount of space given to these birds. It could end up being a tiny cement platform with no roof, connected by a small doggie-door type exit. Free-range chickens are far from being "free," and these birds can be crammed together with twenty thousand birds inside a facility. There is no third-party auditing, and the USDA relies upon "producer testimonials" to support the accuracy of their free-roaming claims. Removing beaks and molting is performed.

Pasture Raised

Poultry that is pasture raised means the birds are free to roam around in the grass as they please and eat the bugs, worms, and grain they are intended to eat. True pasture-raised birds are kept outside (as the season and daylight hours permit), utilizing a movable or stationary house for shelter. Chicken meat from these birds may cost a little bit more money, but from a nutrient standpoint, you are getting way more chick for your buck! Pastured chicken and eggs also taste better and have more flavor. Because they are grass-fed, pasture-raised chicken has 21 percent less total fat, 30 percent less saturated fat, and 28 percent fewer calories than their factory-farmed counterparts.[278] Pasture-raised hens produce healthier eggs with brighter, more orange-colored yolks than conventional eggs. Their eggs have 10 percent less fat, 40 percent more vitamin A, 70 percent more beta carotene, and 400 percent more omega-3s.[279] While forced molting through starvation is prohibited, beak cutting is allowed but not necessary because the birds are not so confined and don't have the need to peck at each other. To find pasture-raised chicken and eggs, stores, and restaurants in your area visit: www.eatwellguide.org.

USDA-Certified Organic Chicken

It's important to point out that buying free-range and pasture-raised poultry doesn't guarantee the birds will have no pesticides, antibiotics, or additives. If you want the healthiest choice for your poultry, always look for "Pasture Raised; USDA-Certified Organic" on the label. The word *organic* is so overused and cannot be relied on unless it's *certified* organic by the USDA. The USDA mandates strict guidelines and conditions under which animals' feed must be composed exclusively of certified organic grains—without any animal byproducts, protein supplements, growth hormones, tranquilizers, antibiotics, pesticides, or herbicides used in the soil or feed. Birds must also be provided with pure chlorine-free and fluorine-free spring water. Molting cannot be *induced*, and beaks are not cut.

Beware of terms such as certified "Amish," "All natural," and "Farm fresh." The USDA has not provided official definitions or guidelines for such phrases, and they are used at will by mass producers of chickens. [280] Also be leery when you see "voted best chicken" on the label. There are no government or state poultry elections where the population votes for the best chicken. For all you know, the owner's wife voted it the best chicken.

Eggs—Deviled or Angel?

I treat a lot of champion bodybuilders at my office, and all of them share two things in common: they are in great shape and religiously eat a diet designed to make them lean and fit! I too delved into bodybuilding for several years, living and breathing a muscle-enhancing diet—or so I thought. I had always been told not to eat the egg yolk when bodybuilding because it would increase fat and decrease muscle definition. One of the most exciting days for me was meeting eight-time Mr. Olympia, Lee Haney. I got to pick his brain on diet and nutrition and received some insider tips on weight training. During our talk, he told me he ate a dozen eggs per day. Not per week . . . *per day!* I asked him if he removed the yolk on every egg to avoid all the extra fat. He replied, "I remove none of the yolks. I eat the entire egg." I asked him if he was concerned about his cholesterol and heart disease. He told me, "When God created the egg, he did not separate it. Taking away the yellow and just eating the white part makes no sense. How can chicken be one of the healthiest foods and something be wrong with the eggs they make?"

Even today, two decades after my chat with Mr. Haney, people diagnosed with high blood pressure or high cholesterol are still being told by their medical doctors to avoid eggs or to convert to egg whites. But Mr. Olympia, Mr. Twelve Eggs a Day, Mr. "120 Cholesterol" didn't have any health problems, and he sure had great muscle definition! The more I researched, the more I concluded that this egg scare was merely propaganda, and I felt *egg*stremely stupid for removing the yolk.

The yellow part of the egg contains lecithin and choline, which are lipotropics—*fat burners*—making the entire egg great for increasing lean muscle. Lee Haney knew what he was talking about. Let's examine some of the science and common sense and unscramble the dietary facts and myths about the egg.

There is archaeological evidence for egg consumption dating back to the Neolithic age. Jungle fowl was domesticated in India by 3200 BC. Records from China and Egypt show that birds were domesticated and lay eggs for human consumption around 1400 BC. The first domesticated fowl reached North America with the second voyage of Columbus in 1493.[281] All right, so your great-great-great-great-great-grandmother ate them, but does that mean eggs are healthy? Actually, the answer is "Yes!"

Eggs are a wonderful source of protein and healthy fat (polyunsaturated and monounsaturated). One egg contains 6 grams of high-quality protein, as well as all nine essential amino acids, and is one of the few foods that contain naturally occurring vitamin D. Eggs have been shown to benefit the eyes due to their carotenoid content, specifically the nutrients lutein and zeaxanthin, and prevent macular degeneration and cataracts. Both nutrients are more readily available to our bodies from eggs than from other sources.[282]

In 1961, the American Heart Association (AHA) guidelines recommended reducing total fat, saturated fat, cholesterol, and increasing intake of polyunsaturated fat. By the 1970s, the AHA's dietary recommendations advised the public to avoid the consumption of eggs. The Inter-Society Commission for Heart Disease Resources stated that ingestion of two eggs a day will seriously hamper dietary programs aimed at reducing serum cholesterol and "the public should be encouraged to avoid egg yolk consumption."[283]

In 1973, the American Heart Association changed its recommendations, limiting dietary cholesterol to no more than 300 milligrams per day and said that individuals should eat no more than three egg yolks per week.[284] Again, this was based on the *assumption* that eggs, being high in cholesterol, also increase heart-disease risk. However, at the time when these recommendations were formulated, there was no empirical evidence to support these claims. For decades people have avoided eggs, just as these respected organizations suggested. It was common knowledge that eggs contain cholesterol and, therefore, it was *assumed* they would cause an increase of blood cholesterol in humans. I'll give them that. It is logical to think that if a food contains cholesterol, it could increase our blood cholesterol, but logic is not the same as *proof*. For many, these anti-egg speculations continued, even though they were not based on any scientific evidence.

Then came some good news: eggs are okay to eat every day as long as you remove the yolk. Restaurant chains all over the nation carried "cholesterol-free" alternatives like egg white omelets, Egg Beaters, and the like. Actually egg yolks contain lecithin, which markedly *inhibits* cholesterol absorption.[285] Research also shows that the lecithin in egg yolks is very effective at *preventing* high cholesterol buildup in the blood vessels.[286] The yolk of an egg contains B12, which lowers homocysteine levels; this is great news because high levels lead to cardiovascular disease and stroke.

According to a fourteen-year study conducted by the Harvard School of Public Health, there is no significant link between egg consumption and heart disease. In fact, regular consumption of eggs may help prevent blood clots, stroke, and heart attacks.[287] One study found that people who ate two eggs, while on a calorie-restricted diet, lost weight and reduced their cholesterol levels.[288] Still not convinced? A collaborated study from the Wake Forest School of Medicine and the Center on Aging reported that egg consumption is not associated with higher cholesterol levels and the idea that egg consumption is a risk factor for coronary disease is a myth.[289] If you need to reduce your cholesterol level, don't give up the eggs. Instead, cut down saturated fats like beef, processed meats, fattening dairy products, cakes, biscuits, and pastries.

Your Guide to Healthy Eggs

Just as a factory-produced chicken can contain antibiotics, pesticides, additives, arsenic, and other carcinogenic fillers, so can the eggs it produces. Pasture-raised, USDA-certified organic eggs are the way to go. The Cornucopia Institute (www.cornucopia.org) rates egg manufacturers based on twenty-two criteria that are important for organic consumers. Their "egg scorecard" showcases ethical family farms and their brands, and it allows anyone to see which brands of eggs are produced using the best organic farming practices and ethics. This handy tool rates name-brand and even private-label eggs. Pasture-raised hens produce eggs with bright orange yolks. If the egg yolk is a dull, pale yellow color, it's a sure sign that the egg is from a caged hen that has not been allowed to forage as nature intended.

Discoveries: The only negative research on chicken comes from industrialized, commercialized chickens with added chemicals, hormones, antibiotics, coloring, food additives, contaminants, pesticides, appetite stimulants, flavorings, arsenic, insecticides, and bacteria! Add to the mix the preservatives and the chlorine from the cooling baths, and you can see how man has turned healthy chicken into a toxic meal. However, if you carefully choose your chicken and eat pasture-raised, certified-organic varieties, the safety and health attributes for eating chicken are backed by science. Eggs offer a wonderful source of nutrients, protein, and healthy polyunsaturated and monounsaturated fats (the good kind). Evidence in the literature shows eggs can help people lose weight and lower their cholesterol levels.

Instincts: When looking at chicken and deciphering if we should eat it, poultry does not contain Neu5Gc, a sugar found in cow's meat that causes inflammation and lowers our immune response. Chicken doesn't *increase* your risk of high cholesterol, heart disease, or stroke; it actually has the *opposite* effect. And when it comes to eggs, once you debunk their bad reputation for causing high cholesterol, there are only positive health attributes when eating pasture-raised, certified-organic eggs.

God: When you look at the anatomy of the human body, saliva, stomach pH, and the colon, humans can readily digest and assimilate USDA-Certified Organic chicken.

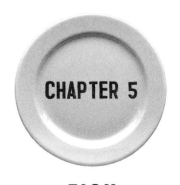

CHAPTER 5

FISH
IS THERE A CATCH?

"Give a man a fish and you feed him for a day;
teach a man to fish and you feed him for a lifetime."
—Maimonides

I remember the first time I caught my own fish. The pull of the line, followed by the bend of the pole, signaled my success to my jubilant father, who shouted, "You got one, David! Reel him in!" What felt like a half hour of fighting the mighty fish, was, in reality, only a few minutes, but the experience would last a lifetime. Once my ten-year-old hand reeled in that red snapper, I was hooked—not just on fishing but also on the scrumptious taste of the meal that I helped my dad clean and cook on the grill.

When it comes to fish as food, it's hard to deny all of the really good news about it. It's incredible for your brain, bones, heart, skin, mood, and eyes—just to name a few things. When contemplating the quote that opens this chapter, I have to agree, we should all eat a lot of fish and for a lifetime. To say fish is a super food would be an understatement. However, the fact that it is one of the greatest edible sources of essential vitamins and nutrients is precisely why it is critical to protect this mighty food group from practices that diminish its benefits. Unfortunately not everyone is on board with this mission. Believe it or not, there are some sinister things happening in the catching, farming, and production of fish that makes it so that once the food reaches your dinner plate, you might as well be eating a dish full of artificial colorings and bug spray. But before we look at which species get tainted and which ones get painted, let's look at how eating fish keeps you up to your gills in nutritional greatness.

The Fatty Fish

If we eat micronutrient-rich vegetables, we become micronutrient-rich. Likewise, eat protein, get protein. Eat sugar, increase our blood sugar. So it would be safe to say that eating fat, well . . . makes you fat. Not so. To confuse the issue even further, not all fats are created equal. We have heard that there are good and bad fats—unsaturated and saturated, respectively. Fish happens to be high in good unsaturated fat, compared to most other protein foods. Without good fats in our diet, we would die. These healthy unsaturated fats play a major role in fighting fatigue, regulating mood and weight, and enhancing memory. Saturated fat, on the other hand, is thicker, and more viscous than unsaturated fat, acting like goo muddying up your blood stream.

Fish are known for containing the most health enhancing fatty acids of all—omega-3 fatty acids, which are critical to the development and overall function of the brain. Our body doesn't produce these fatty acids on its own, so it must absorb them through food.

Omega-3 Fatty Acids

Omega-3 fatty acids are found in every kind of fish, but are especially high in fatty fish such as salmon, trout, sardines, halibut, herring, canned mackerel, and canned light tuna. The benefits available to you when you consume omega-3 include that it:

- Helps maintain a healthy heart by lowering blood pressure and reducing the risk of sudden death, heart attack, abnormal heart rhythms, and strokes
- Aids in healthy brain function and infant development of vision and nerves during pregnancy
- May decrease the risk of depression, attention-deficit/hyperactivity disorder (ADHD), Alzheimer's disease, dementia, and diabetes
- May prevent inflammation and reduce the risk of arthritis.

According to the U.S. Department of Agriculture, omega-3 fatty acids protect against fatty liver disease, the most common form of liver disease.[290] Fatty liver is a buildup of unhealthy fats, called triglycerides, in the liver, which over a period of time can lead to inflammation, hepatitis, fibrosis, cirrhosis, and cancer. Eating fish that contains healthy fats, especially the fish mentioned above, can help balance triglyceride levels in the body. Because eating fish helps discourage the buildup of plaque in blood vessels, it also helps decrease the risk of stroke and cardiovascular disease. A Harvard study shows that eating two portions of fatty fish a week could cut the risk of death from heart disease by 36 percent. Eating 1 to 2 servings of fatty fish per week reduces total mortality by 17 percent.[291]

Can You DIG This?

Fish offers a great source of protein and vitamin B2 (riboflavin). According to the *European Journal of Neurology*, riboflavin may prevent migraines.[292] Fish is high in vitamin B3 (niacin), which assists in the functioning of the digestive system, nerves, and the health of skin. Fish contains calcium and phosphorus and offers a great source of minerals, including iron, zinc, iodine, magnesium, and potassium. Fish is one of the very few foods that contain vitamin B12, critical to building DNA and RNA, the building blocks of the human body. B12 is also helpful for maintaining the skin, nails, eyes, mouths, lips, and tongue. It is important for normal vision and to prevent cataracts.[293] Fish offers a much better source of vitamins D and A than beef, pork, and chicken. Eating fish enhances the immune system and aids in the prevention of cancer.

Additionally, if you have a short fuse, get upset, are easily angered, or are compelled to hold up your middle finger, honk your horn, and scream the "F" word when someone cuts you off, you might need to add more of the other "F" word—fish! EPA (eicosapentaenoic acid) and DHA (docosahexaenoic acid) are two classes of fatty acids found in fish and have been shown to effectively defuse anger and decrease hostility.[294] When we examine different areas around the world, we find significantly higher rates of hostility where fish consumption is low, compared to regions where fish intake is high. Significantly lower omega-3s in red blood cells are seen in people with hostile or aggressive behaviors compared with their more amiable counterparts. Also it has been shown that male violent offenders have lower DHA in their red blood cells than non-violent men.[295]

The Ultimate Brain Food

If anyone has ever called you "fat head," you were actually paid a compliment. The brain is largely composed of fats, and it is these fats, along with water, which compose most of the brain cells and tissue surrounding the nerves. The anti-fat messages we hear as part of a heart-healthy diet don't apply to the human brain. Research shows that people with the highest fish consumption have the fattest (smartest) heads! When good fats build up in the brain, concentration and memory improve.

Fish lowers the risk of Alzheimer's disease, according to a University of Pittsburgh Medical Center study which analyzed brain scans of 260 healthy elderly volunteers over a ten-year period. Of the participants, those who regularly ate baked or broiled fish had a lower risk of developing Alzheimer's disease. Compared with non-fish-eaters, those eating fish at least once a week showed less brain cell loss in the hippocampus and frontal cortex regions of the brain, which are responsible for regulating memory. Fish eaters also showed stronger short-term memory, which allowed them to perform tasks more efficiently. People who consumed fish one to four times a week were significantly less likely to develop Alzheimer's disease or mild cognitive impairment over the five years following their brain scans, compared with those who didn't eat fish.[296]

As we age, our brain naturally shrinks, but fish helps decrease this brain shrinkage. Because one of the symptoms of Alzheimer's is a vast amount of brain cell shrinkage, omega-3 can preserve the function of brain cells. In addition to facilitating memory and cognition, omega-3 plays an important role in brain chemistry. A shortage can contribute to psychiatric illnesses, in particular depression—the most common form of mental illness. Research has found that depression is least common in countries where people eat the most fish, such as Japan, Iceland, and Korea, compared to countries with low fish consumption (and the highest rates of depression), including the United States, Canada, and West Germany.

As people have consumed more highly processed foods over the last one hundred years, omega-3 consumption in this country has drastically decreased, while rates of depressive illnesses have proportionately increased. *The National Institute of Mental Health* estimates that about 4 percent of adolescents suffer from serious clinical depression, which can lead to suicidal tendencies.[297] People who consume fish twice a week have a 37 percent lower risk of being depressed and a 43 percent lower risk of suicidal tendencies.[298] Autopsies conducted on people who have committed suicide have shown a lower fatty acid composition in their brains,[299] and those suffering from depression have lower levels of omega-3 fatty acids in their systems.[300] Although findings are still preliminary, studies have linked depression to inflammation in the brain. Perhaps it's the anti-inflammatory effect of omega-3s that helps with depression?

Fish Combats Inflammation

On my syndicated radio show, I have interviewed hundreds of scientists, doctors, authors, and health advocates. While most of them have opinions as different as night and day, there is one thing that many experts agree on—inflammation is linked to many chronic diseases, including:

- acid reflux
- allergies
- Alzheimer's disease
- arthritis
- bronchitis
- cancer
- chronic pain
- depression
- diabetes
- gingivitis
- heart disease
- high blood pressure
- osteoporosis
- skin conditions
- susceptibility to bacterial, fungal, and viral infections
- urinary tract infections
- wrinkles
- yeast infections

How can so many diseases be associated with inflammation? In a nutshell, the process of inflammation is the body's response to stress, or a lack of ease (dis ease). Any word followed with "itis" means inflammation. I remember my father, a medical doctor, telling me that when a patient sees his doctor about his symptoms, to reach a diagnosis, the doctor usually just adds -*itis* after the area of complaint. What a profound statement! Below are just a few examples of how true this is:

Table 5.1

Presenting Condition	Diagnosis
appendix pain	append*icitis*
sinus infection	sinu*sitis*
painful joint	arthr*itis* (*arthro* means "joint")
painful tendon	tendon*itis*
painful bursa	burs*itis*
persistent cough	bronch*itis* (bronchi are the lungs)
liver disease	hepat*itis* (hepatic is the liver)
acidic stomach	gastr*itis* (gastric is the lining of the stomach)
sore throat	tonsil*itis*
heart disease	card*itis* (cardium is the heart)
prostate disease	prost*itis*

Many diseases are simply inflammation affecting the blood, bones, organs, joints, or soft tissue. The longer inflammation remains in the body, the more life threatening it becomes.

The *American Journal of Clinical Nutrition* reported that fish might help reduce the need for anti-inflammatory medications. Because of the high levels of omega-3 fatty acids in fish, people taking nonsteroidal anti-inflammatory drugs (NSAIDs) are able to reduce their dosage or discontinue them completely.[301] An elevated C-reactive protein (CRP) level in the blood is a strong indicator of inflammation and infection in the body. CRP is a protein that develops in a wide range of acute and chronic inflammatory conditions like bacterial, viral, or fungal infections; rheumatic and other inflammatory diseases; malignancy; and tissue injury or necrosis. Several studies have shown a link between eating fish and reduced CRP levels.

The Japanese, who have a higher overall intake of fish, have lower CRP concentrations than Western populations. A team from Tohoku University surveyed 401 men and 570 women aged seventy years and older, living in Tsurugaya, Japan. Fish intake and CRP concentrations were measured by testing blood plasma samples. Analysis showed that increasing intake of overall omega-3 fatty acids from fish was significantly linked to a reduction of elevated CRP by 56 percent![302]

Another study on the inflammation-reducing properties of fish was conducted in Athens, Greece. Data on 1,514 men and 1,528 women aged eighteen to eighty-nine was gathered on the benefits of a Mediterranean diet on heart health. Those who ate the most fish (10.5 ounces per week or more) had a 33 percent lower level of CRP. They also had a 33 percent lower level of interleukin-6, another inflammatory marker found in plasma, and 28 percent less serum amyloid A, another blood protein that is increased by inflammation. This may explain why people who eat fish tend to have lower rates of heart disease and strokes.[303] Similar results were found in a study reported in *Hormone and Metabolic Research*. Scientists at Kronos Longevity Research Institute discovered that healthy adults adhering to a diet rich in omega-3s (fish) for eight weeks experienced decreases in CRP levels.[304]

Another study published by the *Journal of Nutrition* followed more than three hundred men and women for six years. At the beginning of the study, each participant's food intake was estimated, and the levels of circulating biomarkers for inflammation were measured. After six years, the biomarkers were measured again and compared to the baseline. The changes were then compared to the consumption of different food groups, namely fish, dairy products, fruits, vegetables, and alcohol. Their findings showed fish consumption was associated with lower levels of biomarkers for inflammation. Surprisingly, consumption of fruits, vegetables, dairy, and alcohol were not associated with any changes in biomarkers for systemic inflammation. Fish consumption contributed to 40 percent of the decreased inflammation.[305]

Polluted Waters?

Eating fish seems to offer a plethora of health benefits for humans, so what's the catch? Is there a downside? When I ask my patients if they eat fish, the majority tell me they eat very little, and many say they have boycotted the food group altogether. When I ask why, they always give me the same two reasons: water pollution and mercury poisoning. First let's address the issue of pollution.

Seventy percent of the earth's surface consists of uninhabited water. Pollution takes place on land, where humans live. Emissions from industries and crop dusting, fumigating homes, household cleaning products, painting supplies, insect/pest killers, factories, trucks, trains, cars, and other environmental pollutants—all of these put harmful chemicals into the air and ground. We breathe this pollution. It ends up in the soil and on plants, fruits, and vegetables, and it's ingested by the cows, pigs, and chickens we eat. Why, then, do people put fish on this high pollution pedestal? Think about it. Fish live in 326 million trillion gallons of water. The ocean is 10,994 meters deep (roughly 7 miles). To put that into perspective, the highest a commercial airline will fly is 6.7 miles.[306] So if you've ever looked out of an airplane window while on a flight, that's a good sense of how incredibly deep down the ocean goes. Considering the tremendous dilution factor coupled with self-sufficient micro-organisms that help clean the waters, if polluted water is your reason for not eating fish, why do you eat food from polluted land?[307]

The Great Mercury Fish Farce

In the months leading up to January 1, 2000, I realized just how powerful the media is, recognizing firsthand its ability to instill fear into everyone. As we all watched on television, heard on the radio, read in magazines and every major newspaper in the nation, Y2K was approaching—"the end of the world!" The Y2K scare was based on the fact that computers had neglected to account for the new four-digit year "2000," and only read two-digit years like "99," which stood for 1999.

Because the stock market, banking institutes, and even the military depend on computers to function, the media scared people into believing that the New Year could be our last year! In preparation for this apocalypse, Americans purchased a year's worth of canned foods, dehydrated food, and jugs of water. One of my patients who owns a waterbed store told me he had completely sold out of beds. People were buying the beds not for sleeping purposes but because they hold three hundred gallons of water that could be used to drink. Yep, people were prepared to drink their beds! Long lines formed at stores as the nation spent billions of dollars on generators, flashlights, batteries and gasoline, and stockpiled propane. It was predicted that ATMs and banks would no longer be functional after the stroke of midnight, and millions of people withdrew money from their accounts. They said all the software systems used by grocery stores, phone, and electric and cable companies would cease to function. People purchased guns to protect their families from looting and riots that would surely take place.

I remember watching "Dick Clark's New Year's Rockin' Eve" that night and vividly recall the countdown to the year 2000. I must admit that I, too, was scared. I had so much more I wanted to accomplish in life. So many goals I had not achieved. I was just too young to die! I called my mother to say a final "goodbye," just in case the phones never worked again and to thank her for taking such good care of me as a child. As if I were experiencing a head-on car accident in slow motion, the ball on Time's Square began to drop slowly along with the countdown to doomsday: 5-4-3-2-1 . . . *Happy New Year!*

I held my breath in preparation for the darkness. But then I realized that my electricity was still on. My phone was working. My computer was still working. I didn't hear any gunfire in my neighborhood. A few minutes later, my phone rang. It was my friend from Florida wishing me a happy new year. We joked about what we were going to do with all the dehydrated food we had purchased. It was then that I realized the power that the media has to invoke fear into all of us.

The media also has a profound influence on our decisions regarding what we should eat and what to avoid. For decades, television networks, magazines, and newspapers have scared us into believing that we should avoid eating too much fish because it contains dangerous and life threatening levels of mercury. This might be an appropriate moment to recall my favorite Benjamin Franklin quote, which states: "Believe none of what you hear and half of what you see."

Mercury is a naturally occurring element found in the soil, air, water, and food. It can be found in metal form, as mercury salts, or as organic mercury compounds. Mercury enters the environment as a result of the normal breakdown of minerals in rocks and soil through exposure to wind and rain. In addition to a natural accumulation, mercury is also released into the soil or water from the application of agricultural fertilizers and industrial wastewater disposal.

We hear all about the dangers of mercury in fish, but cattle products also contain mercury, and so do mushrooms and various other crops in agriculture.[308] High fructose corn syrup (HFCS), a common sweetener used in fruit juices, cereals, salad dressings, and condiments, has been found to contain mercury. In a study published by *Environmental Health*, researchers found mercury in nine of twenty samples of commercial HFCS. Another study conducted by the Institute for Agriculture and Trade Policy (IATP) found that nearly one in three of fifty-five brand-name foods contained mercury.[309]

Most sea vegetables contain the trace mineral mercury, and it's also found at the bottom of streams, rivers, and oceans. Nearly all fish and shellfish contain traces of mercury. The FDA and Environmental Protection Agency (EPA) have advised young children and women who may become pregnant, are pregnant, or nursing, to eat fish that are lower in mercury content. Eating fish that is higher in mercury is believed to cause a potential health risk to an unborn baby or young child's developing nervous system. These risks are dependent on just how much fish is eaten and the levels of mercury they contain. In 2001, guidelines were published spelling out which species of fish/shellfish have the lowest and highest levels of mercury and how many servings of each are considered safe. The FDA recommended the following:

Safest Fish and Shellfish with the Lowest Levels of Mercury		
Anchovies	Herring	Sardine
Butterfish	Mackerel (N. Atlantic, Chub)	Scallop
Catfish		Shad (American)
Clam	Mullet	Shrimp
Crab (domestic)	Oyster	Sole (Pacific)
Crawfish/Crayfish	Perch (ocean)	Squid (Calamari)
Croaker (Atlantic)	Plaice	Tilapia
Flounder	Pollock	Trout (freshwater)
Haddock (Atlantic)	Salmon (canned)	Whitefish
Hake	Salmon (fresh)	Whiting

Fish and Shellfish with Moderate Levels of Mercury (Eat only two times per week.)		
Bass (striped, black)	Jacksmelt	Skate
Carp	Lobster	Snapper
Cod (Alaskan)	Mahi Mahi	Tuna (canned chunk light)
Croaker (White Pacific)	Monkfish	Tuna (Skipjack)
Halibut (Atlantic)	Perch (freshwater)	Weakfish (Sea Trout)
Halibut (Pacific)	Sablefish	

Fish with High Levels of Mercury (Eat only three servings or less per month.)		
Bluefish	Sea Bass (Chilean)	Tuna (Yellowfin)
Mackerel (Spanish, Gulf)	Tuna (canned Albacore)	

Fish with the Highest Levels of Mercury (Pregnant or nursing females and children are advised to avoid eating.)		
Mackerel (King)	Shark	Tuna (Bigeye, Ahi)
Marlin	Swordfish	
Orange Roughy	Tilefish	

The larger-size fish, and those that live longer, tend to accumulate the most mercury throughout their lives. The mercury level in fish is measured in parts per million (PPM). The fish with the highest levels of mercury contain around 0.6 parts per million. That's only 0.00006 percent of mercury, an extremely diluted concentration. Below are comparisons to provide an example of just how low these concentrations are. Examples of 0.6 parts per million include:

- one motorcycle in bumper-to-bumper traffic from New York to Los Angeles
- one inch in 32 miles
- one minute in four years
- one ounce in 64 tons
- one penny in $20,000.00
- one banana peel in Dodger Stadium

The truth is, people who live in fear of eating fish because of the "dangerous" mercury levels have been manipulated by the media. First, let me state for the record, mercury is a toxic poison! If you are exposed to large enough amounts of it, you can develop debilitating damage to the brain, kidney, and lungs.[310] It can cause vision, hearing, and speech loss and lack of coordination. This depends on the dosage and duration of exposure. For the majority of people, there is absolutely no health concern from ingesting mercury from fish. In fact, there exists no scientific proof that the minuscule amount of naturally accumulating mercury adults ingest from eating fish can cause any of these health concerns. On the contrary, there does exist evidence showing a dangerous source of mercury that Americans do put into their mouths every day that doesn't seem to get as much media attention—dental fillings!

The mercury in amalgam fillings, called elemental mercury, releases small amounts of mercury vapor, a substance that at high levels can be toxic to the brain and kidneys. These remain a permanent part of the mouth and cause a constant exposure to mercury. The International Academy of Oral Medicine and Toxicology issued a report titled, "The Scientific Case Against Amalgam." The analysis showed that the body absorbed as much as 27 PPM of mercury per day. The World Health Organization states that fillings produce the majority of human exposure to mercury on the planet.[311]

The FDA has taken the stance that the amount of mercury people get from fillings is not large enough to cause any health concerns.[312] Yes, you read that right! They list fish at "high" levels of mercury when it contains only 0.6 PPM for one meal, yet within twenty-four hours, dental amalgams emit 27 PPM of mercury that is absorbed into the bloodstream, which the FDA considers safe. For a person to ingest the same amount of mercury contained in amalgam fillings from eating Spanish mackerel, which the FDA has listed as a "high mercury concern," they would have to eat forty-two 6-ounce servings per week! Amalgam fillings expose people to a *million times* more mercury than the safer form of mercury found in fish. Holy mackerel!

No one eats fish for breakfast, lunch, and dinner every single day of their lives. If you have amalgam fillings in your mouth, they release mercury vapors every minute of every hour of every day, 365 days a year.

Even though they are called "silver," the truth is they have twice as much mercury as silver. Consumers for Dental Choice (www.ToxicTeeth.org) stated:

> The American Dental Association is basically a gigantic
> fraud agent when it comes to amalgam because for years
> they promoted amalgam as *silver* fillings and they're not.
> It's a gigantic consumer fraud perpetuated by thousands of
> dentists in the United States who use the word *silver* fillings
> when by far the most prevalent material is mercury.[313]

The FDA defends its stance that the fillings are "silver fillings" because they are colored silver. This is total deception! These "silver" fillings release mercury into the blood stream from any kind of stimulation. This happens when you eat, drink, chew gum, brush your teeth, and grind your teeth. These mercury vapors from the amalgams travel through cell membranes in your mouth, across your blood-brain barrier, and into your central nervous system. From there, it can lead to neurological damage. I asked my holistic dentist, also an avid fisherman, for his views on the topic. He replied, "Having amalgam fillings in your mouth is like being hooked up to an IV that is constantly injecting mercury into your blood. Dentists using mercury in oral health care is malpractice!"

There is a large body of scientific literature showing that mercury from amalgams spread throughout the body to your bones, muscles, and organs. Several autopsy studies showed a correlation between the mercury concentration in various tissues and organs of human cadavers and the number of amalgam fillings present. Blood levels of mercury in the body correspond to amalgam exposure, but mercury in urine, blood, and feces declines after amalgams are removed.[314]

Autopsy samples from human stillbirths and early postnatal deaths have been studied to show that mercury concentration in the infants' kidneys, liver, and cerebral cortex correlated significantly with the amount of amalgam fillings in the mother's mouth. Two labs also found that mercury concentration in human breast milk correlated significantly with the mother's amalgam fillings.[315]

The first thing many OB-GYN doctors tell their pregnant patients is to limit eating fish because it contains mercury. Rarely in this discussion will the pregnant patient be told of the dangerous effects that her amalgam fillings may have on her unborn child. This is puzzling to me considering there is no evidence that eating wild-caught fish leads to a dangerous buildup of mercury in the body.

Consumers for Dental Choice sued the FDA over the issue of mercury fillings. A court settlement required the FDA to remove from their website that mercury fillings were considered "safe" and in its place publish the following statement: "Dental amalgams contain mercury, which may have neurotoxic effects on the nervous systems of developing children and fetuses."[316] That required statement mysteriously disappeared from the FDA's website a couple months later. Also removed was a "question and answer" page, which discussed the health risk of mercury fillings. But what did not disappear is the FDA's press release stating that "the levels of mercury released by dental amalgam fillings are not high enough to cause harm in patients."[317]

Being a seafood lover, I eat fish at least two times per week but, just for giggles, let's explore cultures that eat massive amounts of fish *every day*. A twelve-year study conducted in the Seychelles Islands found *no negative health effects* from dietary exposure to mercury through heavy fish consumption.[318] This culture eats more than a dozen fish meals *every week*, and the mercury levels taken and measured from these island natives are approximately ten times higher than those measured in the United States; however, none of the studied natives has ever suffered any ill effects from the mercury in fish.

The *American Journal of Preventive Medicine* published research from Harvard that puts the risk people are subjected to from fish-borne mercury in its proper perspective. Dr. Joshua Cohen, the study's lead author, summed up the issue for *MedScape Medical News*: "We're talking about a very subtle effect of mercury . . . changes that would be too small to measure in individuals."[319]

We are also told that children are the most at risk for mercury poisoning. Actually, that's not true. A 2004 study of children in Bristol, England, showed that offspring of pregnant women who consumed high amounts of fish during pregnancy scored higher on mental development tests. That same study found "no adverse developmental effects associated with mercury." Measurements of the amounts of mercury in umbilical cords of 1,054 infants were conducted. The amount of mercury detected was miniscule and not associated with any negative neurodevelopment.[320] In 2016, the *American Journal of Epidemiology* published a study on the maternal consumption of fish during pregnancy and the phsycological development of the child. They found positive association between fish consumption and neurological development, motor development, verbal intelligence, perception, social behavior, and attention, along with a decline in hyperactivity.[321]

Children of mothers eating fish during pregnancy, and during their infant's postnatal phase, have also shown higher mean developmental scores. Moderate fish intake during pregnancy and infancy can actually benefit development. Language comprehension scores, based on the MacArthur Communicative Development Inventories, of children eight to thirty months old whose mothers consumed fish four or more times per week during pregnancy were higher compared to those whose mothers that did not consume fish.[322]

Researchers from the National Institute of Environmental Health Sciences examined the effects of prenatal mercury exposure in a group of women living in Manhattan at the time of the World Trade Center disaster. The women who ate more seafood did have higher levels of mercury in their umbilical cord blood, but that did not translate into worse outcomes for their children. On the contrary, consumption of seafood during pregnancy was found to have significant benefits in motor development and verbal and total IQ.[323]

Are there *any* studies showing maternal consumption of fish can lead to negative health consequences? I did find a study conducted at the Faroe Islands, located approximately halfway between Norway and Iceland.[324] This study examined the neurological and developmental effects of maternal consumption of pilot whale meat, which is the primary seafood consumed by pregnant women in this region. Clinical examination and neurophysiological testing did not reveal any clear-cut mercury-related abnormalities. However, a slight lack of attention and memory were noticed in children. What this study failed to mention is that whale meat is one of the few species of seafood that contains more mercury than selenium. Selenium, naturally found in fish, counteracts any questionable adverse effects of mercury exposure. [325] [326] In fact, mercury cannot cause harm unless it occurs in extremely high enough amounts to inhibit selenium-dependent enzymes (selenoenzymes) which naturally protect the cells of the brain. In other words, if fish contains more selenium than mercury, it cancels out the mercury that is absorbed by the body.

Below is a selenium-mercury chart from the Western Pacific Regional Fishery Management Council, which includes fifteen Pacific species of fish, including four major tuna types, swordfish, mako shark, wahoo, and other species. As you can see, all but the mako shark are higher in selenium than mercury, with swordfish having equivalent selenium and mercury levels.

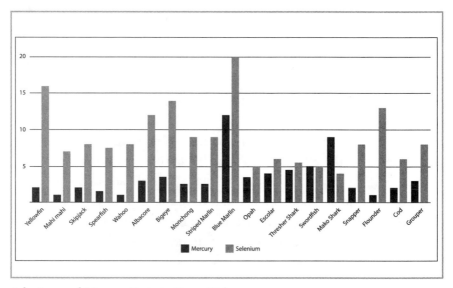

Selenium and Mercury Ratio in Ocean Fish
Source: *Western Pacific Regional Fishery Management Council (www.wpcouncil.org)*

So where did this fear of mercury come from? There have been a handful of documented cases in history of people who have been poisoned by mercury in their food. In Iraq from 1971 to 1972, grain that was treated with a mercury-containing fungicide led to six thousand hospitalizations and five hundred deaths. The mercury levels measured in mothers from this region were as high as 674 PPM.[327] By comparison, the highest mercury concentrations found among American women of childbearing age was only 1.4 PPM. Iraqi women had mercury levels *more than four hundred times higher* than what typical American females experience from eating fish. During the 1950s, 111 people from Minamata City, Japan, were poisoned after they ate fish contaminated with mercury, thanks to a chemical factory releasing methylmercury in industrial wastewater. This highly toxic chemical bioaccumulated in fish in Minamata Bay and the Shiranui Sea, which, when eaten by the local population, resulted in mercury poisoning. The fish in Minamata Bay displayed high levels of Mercury (36 PPM) and hair analysis of inhabitants who ate the fish showed excessive mercury levels (705 PPM).[328] And, just like today, the Japanese ate far more fish than Americans do.

In a similar case in 1965, 120 residents of Niigata, Japan, were also poisoned by industrially contaminated fish. According to University of Rochester School of Medicine toxicologist, Dr. Thomas Clarkson, these Japanese poisonings are the *only* clinical cases anywhere in the scientific literature that document acute mercury poisoning from fish.[329] If others exist, they are far and few between.

FDA's Fishy Hypocrisy

People avoid fish because of the mercury fear but have no issues with getting a flu shot every year, using antiseptic ointments, nasal sprays, eye drops, spermicides, or even using diaper rash cream on their babies. All of these contain thimerosal, an antimicrobial and preservative. Thimerosal is 50 percent mercury by weight. This mercury kills organisms and prevents the growth of fungi. Most flu-shots recommended for routine administration to pregnant women and children in the United States contain an unsafe level of thimerosal. What? The FDA recommends that *pregnant females and children* be cautious about consuming fish because they contain mercury but injecting mercury directly into their blood stream is okay?

Approximately 140 drugs and vaccines used in the U.S. contain mercury.[330] Thimerosal is used in concentrations of 0.001 percent, which is 1 part per 100,000, to 0.01 percent, which is 1 part per 10,000. This massive amount is required to kill a broad spectrum of pathogens; however, the FDA considers a mercury level of 0.5 part per million in fish to be "high" and should be avoided? Below is a comparison showing just how much more mercury 1 part per ten thousand is compared to the 0.5 part per million found in fish labeled "high mercury risk." Consider that one part per ten thousand of mercury in thimerosal is equivalent to

- one ounce in 640 pounds (compared to 1 ounce in *64 tons* found in fish)
- one minute in one week (compared to one minute in *four years* found in fish)
- one inch in 845 feet (compared to one inch in *32 miles* found in fish)
- one cent in $100 (compared to one cent in *$20,000.00* found in fish)
- one entire section of seats at Dodger's Stadium (compared to *one banana peel* in Dodger's stadium found in fish)
- one hundred semitrucks in bumper-to-bumper traffic from New York to Los Angeles (compared to *one motorcycle* in the same traffic jam found in fish).

Enough examples? I think you get the idea. The amount of mercury found in thimerosal is massive compared to the miniscule amount found in fish labeled by the FDA as a "high risk." Thimerosal has been banned in many countries. In 1977, a Russian study found that people exposed to the mercury in thimerosal suffered brain damage. Studies on thimerosal poisoning also show kidney and neurological damage, lethargy, coma, and death.[331] As a result of these health concerns, Russia banned thimerosal from children's vaccines in 1980.

Austria, Denmark, Japan, Great Britain, and all the Scandinavian countries have also banned the preservative. But the good ole United States still keeps it on the market. Under the FDA Modernization Act (FDAMA) of 1997, the FDA conducted a comprehensive review of the use of thimerosal in childhood vaccines. This review found "no evidence of harm from the use of thimerosal as a vaccine preservative, other than local hypersensitivity reactions."[332]

On July 9, 1999, the American Academy of Pediatrics joined the U.S. Public Health Service in issuing a joint statement recommending the removal of all thimerosal. The FDA's reply was that they "will work with vaccine manufacturers to reduce or eliminate thimerosal from vaccines."[333] Fast forward to today, thimerosal still exists in some of our vaccines. Approximately 75 percent of the flu vaccines recommended to be given to children as young as six months contain thimerosal.

The mercury in childhood vaccinations has been linked to a rising increase of autism, whereas fish has been shown to help aid in brain function. Autism is a developmental disorder that appears in the first three years of life and affects the brain's normal development of social and communication skills. Autism was once considered a rare disease that affected an estimated 1 in 10,000 individuals in the United States. Autism has grown at an annual rate of 10 to 17 percent since the late 1980s. Some scientists have estimated the number of cases of autism has increased fifteen-fold—1,500 percent—since 1991, which just so happens to correlate with childhood vaccination increase during this time frame. Prior to 1991, 1 in every 2,500 children was diagnosed with autism, and after that year, 1 in 166 children have the disease.[334] A U.S. study found that children who received vaccines containing thimerosal are more than twice as likely to develop autism as children who did not.[335] Many other experts believe the high rates of autism today are due to increased diagnosis and reporting and changing definitions of autism; from that viewpoint there is no association between vaccines and autism.[336]

Due to the ongoing ridicule the FDA was receiving regarding its stance that mercury in dental fillings and mercury in vaccines are safe, in 2008 they revised their initial warnings about mercury in fish. The FDA stated that eating mercury-contaminated fish no longer posed a health threat to children, pregnant women, nursing mothers, and infants.[337] Why would they make a completely opposing recommendation? Because it was getting too difficult for the FDA to say dental fillings and vaccines contain a safe level of mercury when, out of the other side of its mouth, they were stating that the level of mercury in fish is dangerous. Who do you think makes the FDA more money, the fish industry or the pharmaceutical industry? Looks like they've been *caught* . . . hook, line, and sinker!

In 2014, the FDA quietly revised their recommendations, stating that pregnant woman should avoid just four types of fish: tilefish, shark, swordfish, and king mackerel. This updated advisory document no longer focused on the amount of mercury exposure considered "unsafe"; instead, it was about general risk reduction.[338]

Can You DIG This?

In the chapters about beef and chicken, we explored how the use of hormones, antibiotics, and pesticides has markedly increased over the past hundred years. When looking at the amount of mercury found in fish, the opposite holds true. The mercury levels in fish have remained the same, and may have even *decreased*, during the past 100 years.

Researchers from Duke University and the Los Angeles County Natural History Museum compared twenty-one specimens of Atlantic Ocean blue hake preserved during the 1880s with sixty-six similar fish caught in the 1970s. They found no change at all in the concentrations of mercury. Princeton scientists compared samples of yellow fin tuna from 1971 with samples caught in 1998. To their surprise, they actually found a *decline* in mercury levels. The Smithsonian Institution tested tuna fish samples that had been archived between 1878 and 1909, and these were compared with similar fish tissue from 1971 and 1993. They found significantly *less* mercury in the more recently caught fish. In some cases, the difference was more than 50 percent.[339]

The media warns us, "The level of mercury in the Pacific Ocean is on the rise and projected to increase by 50 percent by 2050!"[340] However, Alaska's Public Health Department shows quite the opposite is true. When the hair of eight 550-year-old Alaskan mummies was tested for mercury, the results showed levels averaging *twice* the blood-mercury concentration of today's Alaskans.[341]

Farmed and Dangerous!

The picket fence, the silo, the green grass; nothing says wholesome like "farm fresh." This image is splashed on labels at the grocery store as *the* symbol of wholesomeness. From veggies to fruits to the grain we eat, food is perceived as healthy as long as it is fresh off the farm. Not so when it comes to fish. Farmed fish are commercially raised in cages or tanks. The most common farm-raised fish are salmon, carp, tilapia, European sea bass, catfish, and cod. Because these farmed fish live in confinement, they get no exercise, nor do they ever see the wild. They are packed so tightly, they rub against the sides of their cages as well as one another, causing damage to their fins and tails, which leads to infection. Similar to what happens when chickens are caged, this creates the need for antibiotics.

The most commonly farmed fish is the Atlantic salmon. This is also the second-most-popularly eaten fish in America, behind tuna. Ninety percent of the salmon sold in the United States is farm raised.[342] [343] Farmed-raised fish have two to three times fewer omega-3s than their wild counterparts. Meanwhile, the fat content of farmed fish ranges between 11 percent and 20 percent versus 7 percent for wild.[344]

Farmed salmon contains polychlorinated biphenyls (PCBs). PCBs used to be widely used as electric and cooling fluid. Because of its carcinogenic effects and classification as an organic pollutant, PCB production was banned by the United States Congress in 1979 and by the Stockholm Convention on Persistent Organic Pollutants in 2001.[345]

How do PCBs still show up in farm-raised salmon today? In order to feed farmed salmon, which are carnivores, producers have to harvest other wild fish, and quite often, these fish come from areas high in PCBs, like the North Sea, in which they feed off of smaller organisms that have been PCB contaminated. Consumption of salmon that have eaten PCB has been linked to increased risk of cancer.[346] Cornell University showed concentrations of PCBs are significantly higher in farmed than wild-caught salmon.[347] The reason for this is because farmed salmon contains more fat than wild salmon, and PCB accumulation settles in the fat. If you weren't allowed to exercise and confined to a tiny cage your entire life, wouldn't you gain more fat than someone who was able to run around the block all day?

Farm-raised salmon are also fed corn to fatten them up even more. Salmon don't eat corn; it's not part of their natural food chain. Salmon from the wild have less fat than those that are farmed raised. Salmon are very strong fish and are able to swim upstream against rugged waters. Just like a professional marathon swimmer would have less fat on his body, so do wild-caught salmon. Professional swimmers generally have the lowest percentage of body fat compared to any other type of athlete. Because PCBs grow in fat tissue, stoic, obese farm-raised salmon are a haven for these toxic chemicals.

The Environmental Working Group (EWG) in 2003 released results of the most extensive tests to date of cancer-causing PCB levels in farmed salmon consumed in the United States. EWG bought the salmon from local grocery stores and found 70 percent were contaminated with so much PCB that they seriously raise cancer-risk concerns, in accordance with standards set by U.S. health agencies. Farm-raised salmon has forty times more PCBs than any other food on the market.[348] There are also other toxins found in farm-raised salmon, including toxaphene (a banned insecticide linked to cancer) and dieldrin (linked to Parkinson's disease, breast cancer, and reproductive- and nervous-system damage), both of which were abundant in farm-raised salmon. Consumption of farmed salmon at relatively low frequencies results in elevated exposure to highly toxic compounds with commensurate elevation in estimates of health risk.[349]

Tainted, Painted Meat

Wild salmon are deep reddish orange on the inside. What most people don't realize is that salmon get their color from what they eat. Wild salmon eat krill, tiny shrimplike crustaceans that contain carotenoids, which are naturally occurring orange pigments. Farm-raised salmon eat feed that is made of corn, soy, other fish, poultry litter, and hydrolyzed chicken feathers. Because of this unnatural diet, farmed salmon meat doesn't turn its natural orange-to-red color but, rather, a less-appetizing light gray. Studies have shown that consumers won't buy gray-colored salmon, so in order to make these artificially grown fish look natural, farmers use chemicals called canthaxanthin and astaxanthin to dye their insides to make for a more pleasing aesthetic.

Several major chemical companies produce these "internal paints," the largest being Swiss chemical giant, Hoffmann La Roche. This is the same pharmaceutical giant that produces tranquilizers like Valium and Rohypnol (aka the "date rape" drug). To help the farmer decide exactly what tint of pink they want to paint the fish's insides, the salesman will bring a SalmoFan. This is a color selection fan similar to one you would find at a paint store when deciding what color you want to paint your bathroom walls. Scientists have found a link between a high canthaxanthin intake and damage to the human retina, prompting the European Union to ban canthaxanthin for direct human consumption, due to its potential for vision damage.[350]

Pesticides and Antibiotics

Farm-raised fish are fed land ingredients like soy and corn, and that means they are also eating the pesticides used in the process of harvesting them. When these chemicals are ingested by fish, they end up in their meat, which is then consumed by humans. Scientists have tested the flesh of farm-raised fish using a highly analytical system that detects the accumulation of pesticide residue. The more fat-soluble a substance is, the higher the probability of the pesticide accumulating in fish."[351] Farm-raised fish are FAT-raised fish! Pesticides are among many toxins found to be up to ten times greater in farmed salmon than in wild Pacific salmon.[352] An international survey revealed that eleven compounds representing five pesticide types are currently being used on commercial salmon farms for sea lice control.[353]

The most widely used compounds are called dichlorvos, azamethiphos, and cypermethrin. Sadly all of these compounds have been associated with health risks in humans. Dichlorvos shows up in fish meat and is considered toxic. A study by the National Toxicology Program reported that dichlorvos increases the incidence of tumors of the pancreas, mammary glands, and stomach in animals.[354] We've discussed antibiotic use in cattle and poultry, and these same issues apply within the farm-raised fish industry. With the combination of exposure to disease and the ability of disease pathogens to multiply quickly in the high-density conditions common to confined cages, antibiotic use is a common practice in the salmon-farming industry. Farmed salmon get antibiotics into their system through medicated food. And in this industry, too, the drugs used for farm-raised fish are also used to treat human diseases. The frequent use of antibiotics in aquaculture and other industries poses a risk to human health by allowing disease microbes to become resistant to antibiotic treatments, making it more difficult to treat human disease.

From Label to Liable

I love the famous line used by Tom Hanks in the movie *Forrest Gump* when Forrest says, "Life is like a box of chocolates; you never know what you're going to get." Unfortunately, this holds true when relying on fish labels. Sometimes you have to play detective instead of relying on what you read. In 2005, Alaska passed legislation requiring that any farm-raised fish sold in the state be labeled as such.[355] In 2006, a *Consumer Reports* investigation revealed that a considerable amount of salmon sold on the market labeled as "wild-caught" is actually farm raised. They bought twenty-three supposedly "wild" salmon fillets, and lab tests revealed that only ten of the twenty-three fillets were from wild-caught salmon.[356] If a label on salmon states, "Fresh Atlantic Salmon," the manufacturer is trying to deceive you.

That means it's farm-raised salmon. There are no commercial fisheries left for Wild Atlantic Salmon.[357] If the term "wild-caught" is used correctly, it means the salmon is Alaskan, Norwegian, or Tasmanian.

In 2005, the *New York Times* published another investigative report on consumers being conned into believing they were buying wild-caught salmon. Their tests revealed that six of the eight "wild-caught" fish were really farmed raised.[358] They also concluded that salmon label deception is more frequent when wild fish go out of season. Fast forward six years to December 2011, when *Consumer Reports* published findings on fish label accuracy, and discovered something very fishy was still going on! They analyzed 190 fish purchased at retail stores and restaurants in New York, New Jersey, and Connecticut. DNA testing was used for genetic sampling and researchers compared the genetic sequences against standardized gene fragments that identify its species, similar to what criminal investigators use. They concluded that "king salmon" and "sockeye salmon" fillets were actually coho, generally the least expensive of the three salmon species.[359] Below are some of their additional findings:

- Eighteen percent of samples tested didn't match the names on place cards, labels, or menus. Fish were incorrectly passed off as catfish, grey sole, grouper, halibut, king salmon, lemon sole, red snapper, sockeye salmon, and yellow fin tuna.
- Four percent were incompletely labeled or misidentified by employees.
- All ten of the "lemon soles" and twelve of the twenty-two "red snappers" purchased weren't the claimed species. One sample, labeled as grouper, was actually tilefish.

The FDA has spent very little time looking for seafood fraud in recent years. Eighty-six percent of the seafood that Americans consumed in 2011 was imported, mainly from China, Canada, Indonesia, Ecuador, Thailand, and Vietnam. FDA officials physically examined only about 2 percent of imported seafood from 2003 to 2008. Only 0.05 percent was checked for seafood fraud (mislabeled, substituted, or short-weighted items).[360] In 2015, the conservation group Oceana had researchers collect 82 samples of salmon labeled "wild" from restaurants and grocery stores in Chicago, New York, Washington, D.C., and Virginia. Using DNA analysis, they found almost half the salmon, 43 percent, was mislabeled—and 69 percent of that mislabeling was farmed Atlantic salmon being sold as wild.[361]

Sadly, label laws have not changed. It's important for you to look at labels as a preliminary gauge point but not to rely on them for total accuracy. Most restaurants and grocery stores don't try to hide the fact that their fish are farm-raised. Many proudly boast this fact. Remember, the word *farm* on anything sells more product, and most people don't associate this four-letter word as being a negative. During one of my health segments on Lifetime television, I did a feature on farm-raised fish and I shared photos on how to recognize if a fish is farm raised or wild caught. You can see that segment on my website: DrDavidFriedman.com.

Fish Oil in a Bottle

Fish oil supplements are touted for their seemingly miraculous health benefits because they contain omega-3 fatty acids. But just like their farmed-fish counterparts, many fish-oil supplements contain undisclosed and unnecessarily high levels of PCB contamination. This is so much so that a lawsuit in California names eight of the largest fish-oil producers and retailers in the country as having PCBs, including CVS, General Nutrition Center (GNC), Rite Aid, Pharmavite LLC (Nature Made brand); Solgar, Inc.; and TwinLab Corp.[362]

In addition to the cancerous PCBs, another issue of concern is the instability of fish oil. From fish extraction to the time it gets placed in the bottle, fish oil is exposed to oxygen, light, and heat, all of which cause the oil to oxidize and break down. This causes the fish oil to go rancid. When fish oil rots, it can put consumers at risk of *getting* heart disease and other chronic diseases, instead of *preventing* them. In humans, oxidized fats raise the risk of hardening of the arteries and blood clots, even at the low levels found in fish oil capsules. By increasing the activity of free radicals—the substances that promote inflammation within the body—oxidized fats pose a chronic threat to human health.[363] Fish oil begins to rot within days of extraction, even though labels often say it's safe to use it for three or four years.[364]

An easy way of telling whether or not your fish oil supplement is rancid is to cut your gel cap in half and put the oil on a piece of paper. If it looks creamy, yellow, or has a brownish tint, it's rancid. Good pharmaceutical-grade fish oil is clear like water. Also, rancid fish oil smells and gives you "fish smelling burps." These supplements should be sold next to Listerine. Also, taste the oil. It should taste fresh and mildly fishy. Look at the label and choose brands that include d-gamma and d-delta forms of tocopherols (vitamin E) to prevent harmful oxidation and rancidity.

Dr. Barry Sears (author of *The Omega Rx Zone*) is one of the nation's leading authorities on the health benefits of omega fatty acids. He says that a lot of fish oil supplements people buy today aren't that far removed from being "the sewer of the sea." He shared with my listeners that the majority of fish oil supplements contain dangerous toxins and cancer-causing chemicals, and he recommends performing the following experiment: "Break open about four or five fish oil gel caps, put them in a shot glass, and put the shot glass in the freezer. Come back five hours later with a toothpick. If you can put the toothpick through the fish oil, meaning it's not frozen, it's probably okay. If you can't, it's sewage of the sea. That means it's rich in things like PCBs, which are similar to a roach motel: when they check into your body, they don't check out. They contain neurotoxins, carcinogens, and endocrine disrupters."[365]

Although taking a pure, high-quality fish oil supplement definitely has health benefits, I personally have never taken fish oil in a pill. If you don't get enough omega-3s from *eating fish* and want to take a supplement, why not get your omega-3s from the same place that fish do? Krill. These are small shrimp or prawn-like creatures that contain the omega-3 fatty acids that fish eat. Salmon eat krill, which gives them their omega-3s and their rich reddish orange color. Krill also feed the world's most mammoth animals—the great whales. Toothless great whales devour large quantities of krill to receive the nutrients they need to fuel their massive bodies. Many other animals depend on krill for their nutritional needs, including seals, penguins, sea birds, squid, and fish. Krill is considered the most necessary and renewable food resource on the planet. Together with plankton, krill make up the largest biomass on Earth.

Krill contain a high level of antioxidants, which help keep the omega-3 oils from oxidizing. Because krill are at the bottom of the food chain, mercury and PCBs are not an issue. The omega-3 fatty acids from krill are absorbed better and released into the human bloodstream at a more efficient rate compared to fish oil.[366] You can purchase krill-oil supplements at most major health food stores.

Can You DIG This?

Pretty in Pink

Lots of other fish eat krill, so how come salmon is pink while others are not? Scientists are not 100 percent sure about this, but they believe there is a genetic component in salmon that causes their meat to turn orange-red when they eat krill. The same thing happens to crabs and lobsters.

If you're a vegetarian, the best source for your omega-3 fatty acid is flaxseed oil. Besides being a great source of omega-3s, flax oil is a good source of healthy linoleic acid (LA), another essential fatty acid referred to as omega-6. Sunflower, safflower, and sesame oil offer a good source of LA but do not contain any omega-3 fatty acids. Of all of the omega fatty acids, my personal favorite vegetarian source is called sea buckthorn berries. Sea buckthorn, despite its name, is not an ocean plant. The sea buckthorn is a plant that grows in high-salt conditions, both along the ocean shoreline and in deserts, from Western Europe to Mongolia. These tart berries have powerful anti-inflammatory, cancer-prevention, cardiovascular, and liver-support properties.[367] Sea buckthorn berries are loaded with omega-3, -6, and -9 and contain the elusive omega-7, a rare and vital component for cellular support and healthy skin, hair, and nails.

10 Tips for Selecting Healthy Fish

1. **Choose wild salmon.** Farm-raised salmon sells year round, while wild salmon is generally available only from June through October. If you are on a budget, eat canned salmon. Farmed salmon doesn't can well so most salmon sold in a can are wild caught.
2. **Trim the fat from fish.** To reduce your exposure to PCBs, trim fat from fish before cooking. Fat is where these chemicals migrate. Also, choose broiling, baking, or grilling over frying, as these cooking methods allow the PCB in the fat to cook off the fish.
3. **Be wary of color.** Farm-raised salmon has been fed artificial coloring to fool you. Avoid light orange- or pink-colored salmon, especially when you see white stripes (fat) between the meat layers. Wild salmon contains minimal fat, and the color is a deeper, darker shade of red that is more consistent throughout. If you don't trust

your eyes, take the taste test: wild salmon tastes tangier without a metallic taste, and the meat has a firmer consistency.

4. **Buy fish that is refrigerated or properly iced.** The ice should be fresh and not melting. It should also be stored in a case or under some type of cover.

5. **Consider how fish are stored**. Fish should be arranged with the bellies down so that the melting ice drains away from the fish, thus reducing the chances of spoilage.

6. **Follow your nose.** Fish should smell fresh and mild, never fishy, sour, or ammonia-like.

7. **Look at the eyes.** A fish's eyes should be clear and bulge a little (except for a few naturally cloudy-eyed fish types, such as walleye pike).

8. **Check out their bodies.** Whole fish and filets should have firm, shiny flesh, and bright red gills free of slime. Dull flesh could mean the fish is old and starting to rot. Fish filets should display no darkening or drying around the edges. They should have no green or yellowish discoloration and should not appear dry or mushy in any areas.

9. **Test the meat.** Press on the flesh and quickly let go. If the meat is fresh, it will spring back. If the fish is not, it will leave an indentation that remains (similar to what memory foam does when pressed).

10. **Frozen fish.** Avoid fish with white, dehydrated areas—this is a sign of freezer burn. Examine the package for ice crystals that may form around the inside of the package or be concentrated in one area of the package. Both of these indicate a moisture loss from the fish flesh, and this is most likely the result of thawing and refreezing. The fish should be wrapped in a moisture-proof and vapor-proof material. Fish wrapped in plastic is generally better if the plastic is vacuum-packed rather than over-wrapped. High-quality frozen fish will have very little or no odor.

 Discoveries: Eating wild-caught fish offers a great source of protein and omega-3 fatty acids. Science shows fish consumption helps maintain a healthy heart by lowering blood pressure and reducing the risk of heart attack, abnormal heart rhythms, and strokes. Fish aids in healthy brain function and helps reduce depression, Alzheimer's disease, and diabetes.

Almost all diseases have been linked to inflammation as the root cause. Fish is nature's "anti-inflammatory" answer to overall good health and longevity.

Instincts: Once you debunk the over-hyped "mercury farce" science and common sense supports the importance of eating fish. Wild-caught fish plays a vital role in a healthy diet.

God: Our body readily absorbs and utilizes all the health-enhancing nutrients found in fish. Fish supplies us with vital omega-3 fatty acids, which reduce inflammation in the body (the cause of *dis-ease*) and keeps our brains functioning at an optimal level.

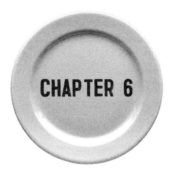

CHAPTER 6

PORK
THIS LITTLE PIGGY WENT TO MARKET

"I am fond of pigs. Dogs look up to us.
Cats look down on us. Pigs treat us as equals."
—Winston Churchill

For thousands of years society has considered pigs synonymous with negativity. Pigs are associated with greed ("as greedy as a pig"), gluttony ("pig out"), and of course, to dirtiness ("live like a pig"). People who believe they are superior to any other race, party, or sex are considered "chauvinistic pigs!" The word *pig* is widely used by many revolutionary and radical organizations to describe any supporter of the status quo, including police officers, industrialists, capitalists, and soldiers. If someone says to another, "In a pig's eye," this means the person is accusing the other of lying. "A pigsty" means living in filth. And let's not forget the most commonly used phrase, "sweating like a pig." Why are there so many unfavorable idioms for the pig? An even bigger question is this: since these animals have been deemed so despicable, should we be eating their meat?

The Pig: A Superior Animal

In George Orwell's allegorical novel, *Animal Farm*, he wrote, "All animals are equal, but some animals are more equal than others." When it comes to pigs, he was quite right. Pigs are one of the most intelligent animals on the planet. Inquisitive and possessing remarkable learning and problem-solving abilities, pigs are able to operate levers and press buttons to obtain food and water.[368] If pigs are too hot or too cold, they are able to adjust thermostats to their liking.[369] Just like a street-smart convict plotting an escape from prison, pigs have been observed working in collaboration to free themselves from their pens.[370]

Pigs have similar learning skills as primates. Penn State University conducted research showing pigs can be taught to maneuver a modified joystick and cursor on a video monitor. When researchers set out to test the memory and cognitive skills of pigs, they were astounded to learn that pigs were able to distinguish between drawings they had seen before when they were mixed with drawings they were seeing for the first time. The pigs mastered these tasks just as quickly as chimpanzees.[371] Pigs also possess a degree of theory of mind, which is the ability to interpret the intentions of others' behavior.[372] [373]

Pigs have an IQ higher than dogs and are considered by animal experts to be more trainable than dogs and cats. Domesticated pigs can be trained to use a litter box, just like a cat. Pigs can even learn how to use the toilet and flush it afterward!

I remember watching the TV show *Lassie* as a child and seeing the collie run for help and lead rescuers to his master, who was trapped in the forest with a sprained ankle. Meet LuLu, a Vietnamese pot-bellied pig who actually makes Lassie's rescue missions lame in comparison. JoAnn Altsman, of Beaver Falls, Pennsylvania, didn't twist her ankle, but she had a massive heart attack. LuLu, her pet pig, started to cry when she heard the distress calls coming from the bedroom. Knowing time was of the essence, LuLu pulled herself together, found her way out of the house, pushed open the gate in the yard, and ran to the road . . . well, waddled to the road. LuLu gave new meaning to the phrase "hogging the road" as she waited until a car approached and lay down in front of it. This superhero pig led a motorist to JoAnn's rescue, just in time. Thanks to a pig, JoAnn underwent emergency heart surgery, which saved her life. Had fifteen more minutes elapsed, doctors told her, she likely would have died. Interestingly, Altsman's American Eskimo dog was no Lassie. He did nothing but bark during her cries for help.[374]

Okay, so pigs are smart, but they're still disgusting and filthy animals. Or are they? Actually pigs are naturally hygienic. Unlike most animals, pigs designate discrete sites for defecating and urinating far away from their sleeping and feeding areas.[375] [376] When given the room and freedom to decide, pigs will choose to be clean and tidy. The reason pigs in captivity smell bad is because they are confined to small spaces and surrounded by their fecal matter.

Additionally, the popular term "sweating like a pig" couldn't be farther from the truth. Pigs have very few sweat glands, and because of this, they are prone to heat stress. To keep this from happening, they take frequent baths in water, which is necessary to maintain their temperature. If water is not available, they wallow in the mud. What's so terrible about that? Even humans savor mud baths and are willing to pay a fortune for the privilege of having mud poured all over them at spas. Additionally, pigs in their natural environment have rubbing sites, usually trees, which they use to aid in grooming and staying clean.[377]

Can You DIG This?

When humans sweat, toxins are released from the body. Because pigs don't sweat, they are more likely to keep toxins and infectious agents inside, which can be ingested by humans. A pig is one of the only animals that cannot be killed by snake venom. After being bitten, the poison is stored in the fat under the pig's skin and gets ingested by anything that subsequently eats that pig. If you choose to eat pork, cut the fat off before cooking in order to reduce the risk of eating toxins that have been trapped inside the pig's fat.

Problematic Pork Preparation

When looking at pork as food, there are two forms, distinguished by their preparation: cured and fresh. Cured pork, such as bacon or ham, is treated with salt, nitrates, and sugar for preservation. Fresh pork, on the other hand, receives minimal processing, if any, and includes chops, ribs, and roast. Sausage with ground pork encased in a film made from pig intestines is not cured.

Curing

Curing means "to alter something by a chemical or physical process" and the most common element used is salt. This process became popular in the days before refrigerators because it provided a way to prevent the meat from rotting. Curing also gives the meat a "tangy" flavor, which is why it's still used today. When curing with salt, the sodium content of the meat is the biggest concern. Just one single serving of salt-cured ham can contain 50 percent of the recommended sodium intake for an entire day.[378]

Sodium nitrate is a type of salt that is used as a food preservative. When used in cured ham and bacon, it can lead to bloating, hypertension, inflammation, cell damage, and joint problems, just to name a few things.[379] To subdue the salty taste, manufacturers add sugar or molasses to the meat. Then come the nitrites, which gives ham its characteristic pink color and kills bacteria like clostridium botulinum, which can cause botulism in humans. The main concern about the use of sodium nitrates in cured meat is that when meat is cooked, the high temperatures cause sodium nitrates to combine with amines (a derivative of ammonia), which is naturally present in meat, to form carcinogenic compounds called nitrosamines.[380] Case-controlled studies show that nitrosamines can trigger migraine headaches and cause increased risk of bladder, esophagus, stomach, brain, and gastric cancer risk.[381] [382] [383]

A 2007 study by Columbia University shows a connection between eating cured meats and chronic obstructive pulmonary disease.[384] *Public Health Nutrition* found a substantially increased incidence of brain cancer in children whose mothers ate a large amount of cured meats while pregnant.[385]

There is simply no denying it: eating cured pork creates a health risk. In fact, diseases caused from cured meats date back to the 1920s. Since then there has been a 69 percent decrease in U.S. meat-curing practices, which may be linked to a marked decline in gastric cancer mortality.[386] The USDA actually tried to ban sodium nitrite in the 1970s but was preempted by the meat-processing industry, which relies on the ingredient as a color fixer to make foods have that visually appealing pink look to them. Who cares if it causes cancer, just as long as the ham at the grocery store looks pretty. Because it has been confirmed that ascorbic acid (vitamin C), an antioxidant, inhibits nitrosamine formation when the meat is cooked,[387] manufacturers in the United States are required to add ascorbic acid to meats. In chapter 9, we'll explore the origins of this questionable synthetic chemical.

Smoked

In addition to salt-curing, another method of preparation is hanging meat over an open fire, which gives the meat or fish, like ham and salmon, a rich "smoky" flavor. Meats smoked over an open fire, however, are exposed to tar and a-benzopyrene—carcinogenic chemicals in the smoke. Benzopyrenes are problematic because they attach to and disrupt human DNA.

To avoid such carcinogens, pork is often treated with an artificial smoke flavoring called "liquid smoke," whereby smoke's vapor is condensed into a liquid. But this attempt to avoid dangerous chemicals in real smoke isn't much help. The European Food Safety Authority (EFSA) warns about the dangers of artificial smoke flavorings, claiming these products may cause adverse health effects, namely changes in the liver and kidneys.[388]

One of the smoke flavorings tested on animals was called Primary Product FF-B, which the EFSA panel on food additives concluded can be regarded as genotoxic, i.e., damaging DNA in living cells. But because this evidence had been collected solely through animal testing, the panel could not establish its safety when added to food and consumed by humans. Another smoke flavoring additive called Primary Product AM 1 was described by the EFSA as being potentially toxic to humans.[389] Avoid products with "Hickory smoke flavor" and "Natural wood smoke" on the label.

Can You DIG This?

What's the moral of the story, thus far? It's probably easier to find a good rescue pig that can also do algebra and play video games with your ten-year-old than to digest the meat of a pig. I say this because, as already mentioned, pigs raised in factory farms live in perilous conditions that put them at risk, and therefore puts people in a precarious predicament when it comes to dinnertime.

Pigs have just one stomach, not four, like other grass-eating animals considered ruminants, such as cattle, sheep, buffalo, and goats. Like humans and dogs and cats, among other animals, pigs have one stomach, making them monogastric. Pigs usually digest what they eat in four hours, compared to a cow, which fully digests its food in twenty-four hours. Pigs are gluttonous creatures that never stop eating (which is where the phrase "to pig out" came from), and because of this massive volume of food, a pig's stomach acids become diluted, which enables all kinds of vermin to pass through without being destroyed.[390] Overeating allows bacteria, parasites, viruses, and toxins to more easily infuse into the pig's flesh. If the gluttonous pig is hungry enough, he will eat carcasses of dead animals. For this reason, grass-eating ruminants are not subject to the infection of flesh worms as pigs are.

Processed Piggy: The Hazards of Bacon and Sausage

Processed pork means just that: it's taken through a process that alters it from its original and natural state. This includes curing by smoking or salting, canning, or adding preservative chemicals. The two most-heavily processed pork products are bacon and sausage, which are two of the staples of the all-American breakfast.

Sausage

The name *sausage* is derived from Old French *saussiche*, from the Latin word *salsus*, which means "salted." There's definitely nothing "heart healthy" about sausage. It's filled with ground meat, usually pork, but sometimes beef or poultry. The casings of sausage are most often created from the intestines of the pig or cattle. Commercial manufacturers cannot use natural casings because they differ in diameter, texture, and length, making it difficult to uniformly package and sell sausage, and for that reason, synthetic casings are used. Sausage contains bits of pigs' lungs, so those who eat pork sausage are more susceptible to epidemics of influenza (a disease pigs and humans have in common).[391]

Sausage is the worst health offender in the category of processed meat. One slice of bacon contains 192 milligrams of sodium, while one link of smoked pork sausage contains 562 milligrams of sodium.[392] Sausage has been linked to causing leukemia. In fact, if a child were to eat two breakfast links of sausage once a week, his chances of getting leukemia would increase by 74 percent.[393] If adults were to eat one link of breakfast sausage every day, it would increase their chances of developing colon cancer by almost

20 percent. Processed meats (sausage, bacon, ham, cold cuts) have also been linked to increased risk for pancreas and bladder cancer.[394] [395] Baby Boomers, beware! A seven-year study of 190,000 people, ages forty-five to seventy-five, showed that those who ate the most processed meat had a 68 percent higher rate of pancreatic cancer. This analysis was reported in the *Journal of the National Cancer Institute* in 2005.[396]

In 2010, researchers from the Harvard School of Public Health found that eating processed meats, such as sausage preserved by smoking, curing, or salting, or with the addition of chemical preservatives, was associated with 42 percent higher risk of heart disease and a 19 percent higher risk of type 2 diabetes. This Harvard study reviewed twenty relevant medical studies involving more than 1.2 million people from ten countries in North America, Europe, Australia, and Asia.[397] We're not talking about studying a room full of sausage-eating people. Of course, these findings were belittled by the pork industry.

Bacon

Bacon is cut from the unhealthiest parts of the pig—the sides, belly, or back—and salt-cured and/or smoked. Bacon contains fat—plenty of it! In fact, almost 70 percent of bacon's calories come from fat, and 50 percent of that is saturated fat—the bad kind of fat that increases the risk of heart disease and stroke. Just one ounce of bacon contains 30 milligrams of cholesterol. This is a lethal combination because a food high in both saturated fat and dietary cholesterol is a heart attack in the making.

Can You DIG This?

Cancer is at an all-time high, and bacon and sausage consumption is part of the reason.[398] The American Institute for Cancer Research performed one of the most in-depth studies to date. Hundreds of cancer researchers took part in a five-year project, and they reviewed more than seven-thousand clinical studies that show a link between diet and cancer. Their conclusion:

"All people should immediately stop buying and eating processed meat products and all processed meat should be avoided for life."[399]

Processed meats like sausage and bacon, explains the report, are simply too dangerous for human consumption. That said, if you do continue to eat this part of the pig after reading this chapter, be prepared for two "C" words your doctor will more than likely be using in the future: "chemotherapy" and "CLEAR!" Why wait until you need chemotherapy or a defibrillator zapping your chest? Take action now to eliminate these meats from your diet.

Digesting the Pig's Diet

Every year in the United States, food poisoning makes 76 million people sick and kills 5,200. All of the major pathogens linked to foodborne illness and death annually are well-documented as being present in pigs or pork products, making pork a big contributor to foodborne illness.[400]

A pig's body contains many toxins, worms, and latent diseases. Veterinarians say that pigs are far more predisposed to these illnesses than other animals because pigs are scavengers and will eat anything and everything, including dead insects, worms, rotting carcasses, garbage, feces, and sometimes even other pigs. Pigs have internal parasites (worms), which devitalize pigs by robbing them of essential nutrients and injuring their vital organs. When humans ingest these infected pigs, it can cause many health concerns.

Worms

Pigs are major carriers of various worms, and when humans eat their meat, they are ultimately eating their worms. The two most common worms that affect humans are roundworms and tapeworms.

Roundworms produce thousands of eggs daily. The most common roundworm found in pigs is called *Trichinella spiralis*, or trichina worms. (The rat, another scavenger animal, also harbors these worms.) Eating raw or undercooked larvae-infected pork can cause a parasitic disease in humans known as trichinosis. The larvae are released, reach maturity, and replicate in the intestines. The parasites are then carried by the bloodstream from the gastrointestinal tract to various muscles.

Many people that have trichinosis will have no symptoms, and when they do, it resembles symptoms of many other illnesses: diarrhea, colitis, edema, fatigue, irregular fever, profuse sweating, muscle soreness, and pain.[401] These worms are not noticed during meat inspections, nor does salting or smoking kill them. The only way to destroy these parasites is to thoroughly cook the meat to 170 degrees Fahrenheit.

Tapeworms infect humans' digestive tracts when their larvae are ingested by consuming undercooked pork. Once inside the human digestive tract, a larva can grow into a very large adult tapeworm—approximately 30 feet, filling the entire intestines! The longest tapeworm ever removed from a human came out of a woman named Sally Mae Wallace on September 5, 1991. Doctors pulled 37 feet of pork tapeworm out of her body through her mouth![402]

Taenia solium is the most common type of tapeworm found in pigs. It is also the most dangerous. Once the development of multiple larvae in the organs takes place, they attach to the intestines, infecting them with a disease called cysticercosis. If not treated in time, the infection can be fatal. Approximately 50 million people worldwide are infected by *Taenia solium*, which kills fifty thousand people annually. Prevalence rates in the United States have shown that immigrants from Mexico, Central and South America, and Southeast Asia account for most of the domestic cases of cysticercosis.[403]

Tapeworms are usually asymptomatic. However, heavy infection often results in weight loss, dizziness, diarrhea, headaches, nausea, abdominal pain, constipation, chronic indigestion, and loss of appetite. They can grow to cause intestinal obstructions in humans that have to be surgically removed.

Can You DIG This?

Did Mozart die of worms? Wolfgang Amadeus Mozart was a prolific and influential composer of the classical era but died in 1791 at the age of thirty-five. Historians have posed many theories on the cause of his death, but evidence now shows one of the top composers of all time died from eating pig! After reviewing testimonials, medical records, biographies, and correspondences, evidence points to the cause of his death being trichinosis, a disease caused by the swine roundworm, *Trichinella spiralis*. Forty-four days before Mozart's illness began, he wrote his wife a letter: "What do I smell? … pork cutlets! Che Gusto [What a delicious taste]. I eat to your health."

Since the incubation period for trichinosis is up to fifty days, it seems that Mozart unwittingly documented the precise cause of his death—those delicious tasting pork chops! Trichinosis produces symptoms strikingly similar to what is known about Mozart's illness— extreme swelling (edema), vomiting, rashes, fever, and severe pain.[404]

Bacterial and Viral Infections

In addition to worms, pigs are susceptible to many other bacterial and viral infections.

Staphylococcus aureus (staph) is one of the most common and devastating bacterial infections affecting humans. It can cause a range of illnesses from minor skin infections, such as pimples, boils, cellulitis, folliculitis, carbuncles, and abscesses, to systemic life-threatening diseases such as pneumonia, meningitis, osteomyelitis, and endocarditis. More than thirty types of *Staphylococcus aureus* exist. This bacteria is salt tolerant, which means it can grow in salty foods like ham. Staph's toxins are resistant to heat and not easily destroyed by cooking. In 1993, one study showed that 50 percent of ham on the market was contaminated with staph.[405]

One of the most feared staph infections is called Methicillin-resistant *Staph aureus*, abbreviated MRSA, and often pronounced "*mer*-sa." MRSA strains are found in institutions, such as hospitals, and in meat products, such as pork. Pig farmers have a prevalence of MRSA nasal colonization 760 times greater than patients admitted to hospitals with no pig exposure.[406] The rate of MRSA colonization in both humans and swine on the farms is extremely high because once MRSA is introduced, it may spread quickly among both swine and their caretakers. MRSA is responsible for 185,000 cases of food poisoning, 94,000 serious infections, and more than 18,000 deaths in the United States.[407]

The Translational Genomics Research Institute showed that nearly half of the meat in U.S. grocery stores were contaminated with *Staph*, with more than half (52 percent) resistant to antibiotics.[408] On January 21, 2012, a study was published in the science journal *PLoS ONE*, which represented the largest sampling of raw meat products for MRSA contamination to date in the United States. The researchers collected 395 raw pork samples from thirty-six stores in Iowa, Minnesota, and New Jersey. Of these samples, twenty-six samples, or about 7 percent, carried MRSA.

"This study shows that the meat we buy in our grocery stores has a higher prevalence of staph than we originally thought," says lead study author Tara Smith, Ph.D., interim director of the University of Iowa Center for Emerging and Infectious Diseases and assistant professor of epidemiology.[409] Pig farms throughout the world have become breeding grounds for strains of MRSA. When analyzing pork farms in the states of Iowa and

Illinois, it was discovered that traces of this MRSA "superbug" were found inside the nostrils of 49 percent of pigs. Piglets had the highest rates of infection, and in fact, every single pig under the age of twelve weeks harbored MRSA colonies.[410]

MRSA is the most dangerous infection, because it is completely resistant to antibiotics. Ever notice on the label of hand sanitizers, "kills 99.99% of germs"? MRSA is in that 00.01 percent of germs not destroyed by hand sanitizers.[411] Investigators have postulated that this spread may be facilitated by a resistance to the antibiotic tetracycline, which is commonly used in swine farming.[412]

Salmonella is a bacteria that is transmitted by the fecal-oral route. The salmonella bacteria are shed in the feces of infected people and animals. Humans contract salmonella by eating food or drinking beverages that have been contaminated with the feces. More than 2,500 different strains of salmonella exist. Heat can destroy salmonella, but a particular strain found in pork, *Salmonella typhimurium*, is not easily destroyed by heating, salting, and smoking of the raw pork.[413]

Pork is a major cause of foodborne salmonellosis, which is considered the leading cause of death in developed countries due to foodborne bacterial pathogens. In Canada, it ranks sixth among all notifiable diseases, and second in bacterial foodborne illness, after campylobacteriosis (from red meat products).[414] In Europe, it has been estimated that the consumption of contaminated pork and its products may account for up to 23 percent of the total number of cases of human salmonellosis.[415] A study of pork in U.S. retail stores found 9.6 percent of samples were contaminated.[416] Commercial feed appears to be a source of *Salmonella* contamination in commercial swine production units, according to a paper in the November 2010 issue of the journal *Applied and Environmental Microbiology*. Samples collected from feed bins were tested prior to exposure to the barn environment, as well as fecal samples and environmental samples from the barns. Eighty percent matched the feed samples from the same barn and time period, suggesting that the feed was the contamination source.[417]

Most salmonella infections can be classified in the gastroenteritis category and symptoms include nausea, vomiting, abdominal pain, diarrhea, fever, chills, headache, and bloody stools. As with chicken, it's imperative when handling pork to wash hands prior to and after touching it. Also, after touching uncooked or undercooked pork, make sure to not touch any handles, garbage can lids, or faucets.

Yersinia enterocolitica, also known as *Y. enterocolitica*, is an infectious bacteria that is present in other foods but is most frequently caused by eating pork. It can grow even in refrigerated conditions. According to the Center for Disease Control (CDC), nearly all outbreaks in the United States have been traced to pork.[418] This organism is most commonly found in raw pork or pork products such as chitterlings (pig intestines). In humans, *Y. enterocolitica* infections can cause gastroenteritis, diarrhea, colitis, and arthritis and have been linked to an autoimmune disease called Graves-Basedow thyroiditis.[419] [420]

Liver Cirrhosis

The disease we've been told comes from drinking too much alcohol may also be associated with eating pork. This was the finding of an investigation from the 1980s on the relationship between "per capita" consumption of pork in sixteen countries looking at the mortality rates of liver cirrhosis. The focus was on countries where alcohol consumption was relatively low. As expected, countries where citizens drank the most alcohol showed a higher amount of cirrhosis, but there were countries where deaths from cirrhosis occurred where alcohol consumption was low. It was in these countries that scientists hypothesized that some other factor besides alcohol must be at work. There was also a marked correlation between pork consumption and cirrhosis mortality for these same countries. In the early stages of this degenerative disease, the liver becomes inflated by fat, a condition called "alcoholic fatty liver." If not treated early enough, the victim eventually dies from liver failure. When examining the relationship in terms of pork consumption multiplied by alcohol consumption, the results were staggering.

The Canadian group showed cirrhosis mortality was significantly associated with pork, not with alcohol consumption, presumably because Canadians collectively are not known to be heavy drinkers. In the Canadian provinces where alcohol consumption is highest, the death rate from cirrhosis was still directly related to "per capita" pork consumption and not to alcohol intake. Those that drank slightly more but ate less pork suffered less from cirrhosis deaths than people who have a higher pork intake.[421] [422] It's not certain as to why eating pork can cause cirrhosis; however, pork is high in sodium and fat, two of three items, along with alcohol, that should be excluded for patients suffering from cirrhosis.

The Health Benefits of Eating Pork Loin

Okay, if we ignore the worms, high salt, and saturated-fat content as well as the dangerous smoked flavoring, nitrates, nitrosamines, and the many idioms of negativity pigs have, are there *any* health benefits to eating pork? Actually there are. The key is eating the leanest part of the animal. Avoid the fattier cuts, such as ribs, blade, shoulder, sausage, and bacon. And stay away from the belly, which is a favorite of many. The leanest, less-fattening, and healthiest option is pork loin.

Pork loin (no more than 8 ounces), taken from organic pigs that are grass-fed or free-range, can be quite good for you. The loin part of the pig is often referred to as "the *other* white meat," because these cuts of pork qualify as a source of lean protein with fat-burning properties. Research published in the journal *Nutrients* studied 144 overweight people who ate a diet rich in fresh, lean pork. After three months, the group saw a significant reduction in waist size, BMI, and belly fat, with no reduction in muscle mass. They speculate that the amino acid profile of pork loin may contribute to greater fat burning.[423] If you want the leanest and most nutritious loin, go for the center portion, sold as the "center loin," with the second-best choice being tenderloin.

Nutritional Benefits of Pork Loin

Pork loin
- contains more B-vitamins (thiamin, niacin, B6, and B12) than many other types of meat. These vitamins play a role in a variety of body functions, including metabolism and energy production. There are very few foods that have as much riboflavin (B2) per serving as loin meat from pork.
- provides 65 percent of the recommended daily intake of thiamine (B1), twice that of beef and chicken.
- is lower in "saturated" fats than other parts of the pig. Saturated fats are linked to increasing the LDL (bad cholesterol) count.
- contains only 4 percent (4g per 100g) fat, is an excellent source of protein (21.8 percent per 100g), and supplies essential amino acids.

- contains zinc, which is essential for the healthy development and maintenance of the immune system and bone structure. Adequate zinc status improves resistance to infections, enhances bone formation in children and young adults, and protects against bone loss in older adults. Pork loin is an excellent source of zinc and contains healthy compounds such as cysteine and glutathione, which helps in the neutralization of free radicals.[424]

- contains phosphorus, which can aid in strengthening bones and teeth. One 3-ounce serving of pork loin provides 22 percent of the recommended daily intake of this vital nutrient.

- offers a great source of potassium, more than lamb, chicken, and beef. A pork loin chop contains about 693 milligrams of potassium. Potassium is a mineral necessary for many bodily functions including nerve sensations, muscle movement, and fluid balance. Potassium is linked with a number of health benefits, including lower blood pressure and reduced risk of stroke.

Tips for Making Your Pork as Healthy to Eat as Possible

1. **Choose organic pigs that are grass-fed or free-range.** A good choice is Prairie Pride Farm of Minnesota (prairiepridepork.com). People here sustainably raise Berkshire Pork without the use of antibiotics, growth hormones, animal by-products, or drugs. Prairie Pride grows its own non-GMO corn, offers "uncured" meat, and avoids the use of liquid smoke in their smoked products. You can order their products and have them shipped to you. Another pork option you may find at health food and select grocery stores is the brand Surry Farms (Surryfarms.com), which farm raises their pigs with no antibiotics, growth stimulants, hormones, or animal by-products.

2. **Look for the word *uncured* on the label.** This indicates the meat is free of added sodium and nitrates. Also, avoid processed meats, e.g., sausage, bacon, and cold cuts. Beware of the term "country" ham, which is native to the south, as it tends to be very high in sodium (four times the sodium content of "city ham").

3. **Avoid pork products with additives.** Reading the ingredients list on the package is critical. MSG, high-fructose corn syrup, preservatives, artificial flavor, hickory smoke, or artificial color are unhealthy additives.

4. **Choose only lean cuts.** Eating pig does offer *some* healthy nutrition, especially the leaner loin portions. Purchase tenderloin, center loin, fresh pork leg, or lean ham. Avoid fattier cuts, such as ribs, loin blade, shoulder, sausage, and bacon.

5. **Dispose of fat.** Since pigs don't sweat, toxins can build up in their fat. Cut off the visible fat prior to cooking to make your pork leaner and more healthful. When cooking, do not leave your pork sitting in a pool of fat. Pour the fat out or use a broiling pan in the oven to allow the fat to drip off and separate from the meat.

6. **Limit portion sizes.** Eat pork in moderation. If you choose to consume pork, limit this to 3 to 5 ounces (85 to 140 grams) per meal. Paying attention to portion sizes will reduce the amount of fat and cholesterol consumed. If this won't fill you up, try making kabobs or stir frying pork with vegetables.

7. **Cook at the appropriate temperature.** Pork is considered done (and safe to eat) when it reaches an average uniform internal temperature of 170 degrees Fahrenheit, hot enough to kill worms like *Trichinella spiralis*, the organism that causes trichinosis.

8. **Clean to avoid cross contamination.** Clean all utensils thoroughly with soap and hot water. Wash your wood or plastic cutting board with hot water, soap, and a bleach-and-water solution. For ultimate safety in preventing the transfer of microorganisms from meat to other foods, keep one cutting board exclusively for raw meats and a second one for everything else.

9. **Never cook pork in the microwave.** A pervasive myth is that microwaves cook from the inside out. The truth is, microwaves actually cook from the outside in, similar to other heating methods. When cooking pig, it's best to not to use the microwave. However, if that's your only option, rotate and flip the meat half way through the cooking cycle, and always make sure the center is fully cooked before eating. This applies to other meat products, as well.

Healthiest Pork Choices

Baked ham. If you are a ham fan and want to keep it as part of your diet, eat it baked. Prior to baking your ham, make linear slices on the meat and place a meat rack under it, to allow the excess fat to drip away. Always discard the fat that has dripped away, instead of using it to cook the meat. Remember: just like farm-raised salmon, it's the fat that you want to stay away from.

Turkey bacon and sausage. One of the best alternatives for pork bacon and sausage is a turkey option. These are healthier because they are lower in fat and cholesterol. Jennie-O Lean Turkey bacon and sausage are great choices and available at most grocery stores (jennieo.com).

Meat-free sausage and bacon. A delicious vegetarian alternative to pork sausage is called Field Roast Sausage (fieldroast.com). For a healthy meat-less bacon alternative go with Phoney Baloney's GMO-free coconut bacon (phoneybaloneys.com).

 Discovery: Science has proven that pork is a major known carrier of foodborne pathogens, including toxins and worms. Excessive quantities of histamine and imidazole compounds are also found in pig meat, which has been linked to inflammation in the human body and may contribute to diseases like heart disease, diabetes, and cancer.

Instinct: Pigs are scavengers and more predisposed to parasites and worms than other animals. They eat dead insects, rotting carcasses, feces, garbage, and sometimes even other pigs. Remember: *you are what your food ate.*

God: Pigs are so similar to humans, their body parts are used to heal human hernias, ulcers, wound care, plastic surgery, and to serve as heart valves. Pigs are also smart and caring animals—even more so than dogs ("man's best friend").

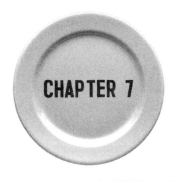

CHAPTER 7

A PLANT-BASED DIET
HEALTH FROM THE GROUND UP

"Nothing will benefit human health and increase
the chances for survival of life on Earth as
much as the evolution to a vegetarian diet."
—Albert Einstein

Adam and Eve might be famous for eating an apple, but their diet also consisted of grains, vegetables, seeds, nuts, and many other fruits. In the book of Genesis (1:29) God said, "I have given you every plant with seeds on the face of the earth and every tree that has fruit with seeds. This will be your food."

The Greek philosopher Hippocrates (460–360 BC), known as the "Father of Medicine," and for whom the Hippocratic oath is named, stated: "Let food be thy medicine." Hippocrates knew that medicine needed to line up with nature and the design of the body. God, "The Father of Creation," revealed to Ezekiel that plants are the medicine for the physical body. ". . . the fruit shall be for food, and the leaves for medicine" (Ezek. 47:12). The Apostle John confirms this in Revelation: "The leaves of the tree are for the healing of the nations" (Rev. 22:2). Notice something striking? The Father of Medicine and Father of Creation were on the same page.

Fast forward to our modern-day society, when the most brilliant scientists at Johns Hopkins University, Harvard University, Mayo Clinic, and Mount Sinai all agree—fruits and vegetables are vital to human life. They contain every vitamin, mineral, amino acid, and enzyme known to man, and those still unknown.

But today, with a trillion-dollar pharmaceutical industry, it is not uncommon to turn to drugs instead of food to cure that which ails us. We've been nothing short of brainwashed into believing drugs are the first responders to help our joints move smoothly, our bodies sleep soundly, our minds concentrate sharply, our hearts pump efficiently. Wherever we go, the friendly neighborhood pharmacist is able to give us a pill to thin our blood, thicken our hair, lower our cholesterol, and increase libido. Is this modern medicine to the rescue or modern capitalism at work? What's gone wrong? For that answer, we must follow the money.

The War on Fruits and Veggies

Annual global spending on prescription drugs has surpassed $1.1 trillion.[425] To put that number into perspective, in 2016, consider that the personal care product industry (makeup, soaps, perfumes, nail polish, shampoos, hair color, toothpaste, and deodorants) had worldwide annual sales of $260 billion.[426] According to the International Federation of Health Plans, the United States pays more money for drugs, physician visits, scans, and surgeries than any other country in the world.[427] Do you think Big Pharma execs, *their* politicians, scientists, doctors, insurance companies, and the American Medical Association want you preventing or curing diseases with a bag of apples and a bushel of broccoli? Imagine the hundreds of billions that Big Pharma and company would lose if it were common knowledge that disease could be prevented, treated, and cured with a healthful diet, especially one filled primarily with fruits and vegetables. We can, with just the information in this book, build our personal wealth from within, instead of lining the pockets of those who financially benefit from our aches, pains, and illnesses.

After analyzing the rising trend of diseases afflicting our nation, former surgeon general of the United States, C. Everett Koop, concluded, "Sixty-seven percent of all diseases are diet related." The 1988, C. Everett Koop's *Surgeon General's Report on Nutrition and Health* stated that diet is a contributing factor for high blood pressure, obesity, dental diseases, osteoporosis, gastrointestinal diseases, and a major cause of death in America.[428] Marion Nestle, former director of nutrition policy for the U.S. Department of Health and Human Services and managing editor of the *Surgeon General's Report on Nutrition and Health*, stated: "There is no question that largely vegetarian diets are as healthy as you can get. The evidence is so strong and overwhelming and produced over such a long period of time that it's no longer debatable."[429]

Why weren't these statements all over the media? In the same year, a San Francisco earthquake measuring 7.1 in magnitude made national headlines. While 67 people lost their lives from that catastrophic event, how many *tens of thousands* of lives could have been saved had the media shared the surgeon general's report? If Dr. Koop had announced, "Sixty-seven percent of diseases could be cured if you took vaccine X," *that* would have been all over the news! To answer that question, again . . . follow the money. Look at the commercials airing during your favorite TV shows, and you will see who is paying for them to air. You'll quickly notice the biggest media sponsors are the pharmaceutical companies. The same holds true for most of your favorite magazines. What if a national news magazine published an article showing the scientific validity that blueberries may enhance memory loss and could even reverse Alzheimer's disease?[130] [431] Now imagine in that same magazine issue you saw an ad for blueberries with no side effects listed, and on another page there was an ad for the Alzheimer's drug Aricept, with its list of side effects: "stomach ulcers; fecal incontinence; chest pain; painful urination; fainting; fever; flu-like symptoms; depression; shortness of breath; seizures; severe dizziness or headaches; severe stomach pain; irregular heartbeat; swelling of the hands, ankles, or feet; tremors; unusual bruising; weakness; difficulty sleeping, nightmares, vomit that looks like blood or coffee grounds."[432] Given those choices, everyone would buy blueberries. Bye-bye, drug sponsorship money!

From antacids to aspirin to erectile dysfunction medications, Big Pharma's money is what pays for our favorite sitcoms, talk shows, news programs, and reality TV shows. The farmers of this country simply don't have the money to compete with the trillion-dollar pharmaceutical giants. Even if farmers had the funds to put together a massive advertising campaign promoting the health benefits of the produce they sell, they couldn't compete with the media strong arm of Big Pharma, the wealthiest and most powerful industry in the world. Not to mention farmers rely on Big Pharma (or more appropriately termed, Big Farma). It isn't families that are spending the most money on pharmaceutical products, it's the farmers![433] In the United States, 70 percent of antibiotic use is on farm animals, and this leads to more money in the farmers' pockets, too. If the farmers did share the health benefits of the fruits and vegetables they grow, this would compete with Big Pharma's drugs and be a conflict of interest.

For the record, I am not anti-medicine nor do I support boycotting Big Pharma's medications. . . well, except, maybe for the ones that make you vomit up bloody coffee grounds. My father is a medical doctor, as was my grandfather. Medical doctors and many of the medications they prescribe save lives. We are far better off with medicine than we'd be if we had none available. However, considering there are 2.2 million *adverse drug reactions*, 1 million medicine-related *deaths*, and 7.5 million *unnecessary* medical and surgical procedures conducted annually,[434] putting our health *fully* in the hands of the allopathic medical system isn't the answer either.

Let's examine the side effects and annual deaths from eating fruits and vegetables. Wait! There are none! Do you ever have to ask your pharmacist if it's dangerous to mix spinach with asparagus? How about that fruit addict found dead from an overdose of peaches? When's the last time you saw a TV commercial advertising a law firm stating the following: "Have you eaten mangos and suffered a stroke, aneurism, liver failure, or heart attack? You may be entitled to compensation. Call today!"

The *American Journal of Hypertension* presented evidence that a compound in broccoli, glucosinolate, produces a metabolite called sulforaphane, which can significantly improve blood pressure.[435] Sulforaphane is a natural compound that has no side effects nor does it have any negative drug interactions. I challenge you to find a blood pressure medication that can offer that. The health benefits of fruits and vegetables come to us with no side effects or negative interactions. Also, unlike eating animal products, there is no religion, animal rights advocates, culture, or country that encourages people NOT to eat fruits, vegetables, legumes, nuts, or seeds.

Throughout this chapter, you will read statements made by myself and other experts in the fields of medicine and nutrition that espouse a plant-based diet, containing an array of colorful fruits and vegetables. And you will read that, in many cases, to prevent, reverse, and cure disease, it doesn't require taking pharmaceuticals. Nature has provided us, from the beginning of recorded time, all we need for optimum living in the food available on Earth. But why is eating primarily a plant-based diet the most effective and efficient diet for the human body? The answer lies in the plant/human connection.

Nature's Coincidence

The biology of plants is remarkably similar to humans. Much like a fetus is supplied nutrients through an umbilical cord attached to his mother, plant life is fed through a root system from Mother Nature. This portal feeds the plant, which ultimately grows fruits and vegetables. After conception, the fetus shares many parallels with a plant. Human cells and plant cells contain six identical organelles, or active components, which include cell membranes, mitochondria, and a nucleus. The presence of a mitochondria in both plants and humans means we both share a "powerhouse" within us that produces energy for the cells (cellular respiration).

The way humans and plants absorb food is also similar. Our intestines and fertile soil both contain bacteria and fungi that help humans and plants kill off harmful bacteria and break down substances that become food. Bacteria help plants absorb minerals just as the "friendly" bacteria in the human gut do. Human and plant cells are dependent on the same amino acids, nucleic acids, and sugars. Also plants, just like humans, are not able to synthesize minerals, so we both require third-party sources. Plants get their minerals from the soil, while humans get minerals from the plants. Plants require carbon dioxide (the air humans breathe out), water, and sunshine. Humans need oxygen (the air plants breathe out), water, and sunshine.

Plants rely on sunshine exposure to convert carbon dioxide into organic compounds, especially sugars. This is called photosynthesis. Humans rely on sunshine exposure to convert cholesterol to vitamin D3. This is called vitamin D biosynthesis. Ironically, the sun helps plants produce all the vitamins that humans need, except for vitamin D, which humans must get directly from the sun.

Plants are remarkably similar to humans in that each plant will absorb only the nutrients it requires. What each plant pulls from the soil is very specific to protecting it from elements like wind, temperature changes, and diseases that could potentially destroy the plant. The soil, in its most natural state, contains around eighty minerals, but most plants don't need that many. For example, a tomato will only absorb fifty-six trace minerals. Grass requires seventy trace minerals to complete its cycle, so it will innately absorb more than a tomato plant. The more nutrients a plant pulls into its roots, the healthier benefits it offers to humans. Sweet potatoes, for example, absorb more minerals from the ground than white potatoes, which explains why they are the more nutritious of the two. A plant, and the fruits and vegetables it produces, are only as healthy as the foundation in which they are grown. If the soil doesn't have available all the minerals the fruit or vegetable needs, they will grow to look attractive on the outside but remain nutritionally empty on the inside. Thanks to the extended use of fertilizers and mass-farming methods, the soil in the North American continent has had an average of 85 percent mineral depletion over the past one hundred years—the worst of any other country in the world.[436]

Can You DIG This?

Chlorophyll gives plants their green pigment and is what makes life on earth possible. Literally. If there were no chlorophyll, there would be no human life. The oxygen we breathe comes from the chlorophyll. Chlorophyll is very similar in chemical structure to heme, a component of hemoglobin, which is a protein in the blood that has the important job of carrying oxygen to the body's tissues. The main difference between the two ring-shaped compounds is that the center element in the chlorophyll molecule is magnesium, whereas the center element in heme is iron. Research has shown that chlorophyll has the ability to release its magnesium and absorb iron, which aids in the synthesis of human hemoglobin.[437] That means chlorophyll, the blood of a plant, is similar to the blood of a human. Chlorophyll has natural antiseptic and blood cleansing properties.[438] [439]

Chlorophyll helps reverse an acidic environment, meaning it offers great benefits for the digestive tract. People suffering from acid reflux (heartburn), diverticulitis, gastroesophageal reflux (GERD), and irritable bowel syndrome (IBS), have seen a profound improvement by simply increasing their consumption of green leafy plants.[440]

Recommended Daily Servings

So how much of these perfect foods should we be consuming to reap the rewards? The recommended allowance of fruit and vegetables used to be three to five servings per day; however, that number has increased to five to nine. Personally, I'm leery about putting a "number" on fruits and veggies. Do you think people counted how many servings they ate 150 years ago? Is it even possible to place a number on how many fruit and vegetables are needed when each offers a completely different amount of nutrients? Even if you eat the required servings, you might not necessarily be eating the right *variations* to get all the nutrition required.

For example, five servings of apricots each day would not give you the potassium level of five servings of bananas. Additionally, how can a specific daily dosage be the same for all people when we are all different heights, weights, and ages? Would a thirty-year-old, 110-pound female need as many servings of fruit and veggies per day as a thirty-year-old man weighing 295 pounds? What about teenagers? Would a 90-pound thirteen-year-old boy have the same nutritional needs of a girl of the same weight and age? What if the teenage boy got an hour of physical activity every day while the teenage girl stayed inside playing video games and surfing the Internet? Obviously, we all have different requirements, and although a daily fruit and vegetable regimen is vital, there's no definitive way of quantifying exactly how much is needed. Regardless of what the magic number of servings per day is, there is no denying that Americans don't eat enough fruits and vegetables. Nationwide, just 32.7 percent eat five or more fruits and vegetables, two to four days per week, and only 19.4 percent do so just one day per week.[441] That means nine out of ten people don't eat five servings of fruits and vegetables a day, which is the *minimum* most experts say is needed by the body for optimal health.

Eating a Rainbow for Better Health

The saying goes "variety is the spice of life." That's also the #1 rule when it comes to eating fruits and vegetables. As I mentioned above, the servings are important, but they are not as critical as the variety of fruits and vegetables to choose. The best guide to ensuring your choices are providing a healthful range of vitamins and minerals is to think of your fruits and vegetables as a rainbow. Each color of a fruit or vegetable contains unique components that are essential to health.

RED: Tomatoes, red apples (unpeeled), strawberries, rhubarb, cherries, red peppers, raspberries, and watermelon. Red fruits and vegetables are colored by natural plant pigments called lycopene and anthocyanins. Lycopene has been shown to help reduce risk of heart disease and several types of cancer, especially prostate cancer.[442] [443] Anthocyanins act as powerful anti-inflammatories and have antioxidant properties.[444]

ORANGE/YELLOW: Yellow apples (unpeeled), butternut and other winter squash, carrots, lemons, mangoes, oranges, peaches, yellow peppers, pineapples, and sweet potatoes. Orange/yellow fruits and vegetables are colored by a natural plant pigment called carotenoids. Beta-carotene converts to vitamin A, which helps maintain healthy mucous membranes and eyes. Scientists have also reported that carotenoid-rich foods can improve immune system function.

GREEN: Green apples, asparagus, green beans, broccoli, Brussels sprouts, avocados, cucumbers, green grapes, kiwi, lettuce, green peppers, honeydew melon, peas, spinach, and other leafy greens (e.g., kale, chard, collards). Green fruits and vegetables are colored by a natural plant pigment called chlorophyll. As discussed above, chlorophyll has a chemical structure that is very similar to that found within human red blood cells. Chlorophyll protects the DNA of our blood from being damaged.

BLUE/PURPLE: Blueberries, blackberries, figs, Juneberries, purple grapes, plums, eggplant (unpeeled), prunes, and raisins. Blue/purple fruits and vegetables are colored by a natural plant pigment called anthocyanins. These natural chemicals are anti-inflammatory throughout the body, gut, and brain. Anthocyanins (especially blueberries) may help with memory function and reduce or delay the development of age-related neurodegenerative diseases.[445]

WHITE: Cauliflower, garlic, turnips, mushrooms, parsnips, onions, potatoes, and bananas. White fruits and vegetables are colored by a pigment called anthoxanthins and allicin, which may help lower cholesterol and blood pressure and reduce the risk of stomach cancer and heart disease.

Can You DIG This?

There are a plethora of prescription drugs available to help us do everything from sleep at night, wake up in the mornings, have better sex, increase our focus, eat less, and poop more. But many of today's ailments can be successfully treated by eating a whole-food, plant-based diet. The word *drug* comes from the Dutch word *droog*, which means "dried plant."

Almost half of all pharmaceuticals being sold today were derived from research on plants. Most of the plant-based drugs are chemically copied/synthesized by laboratories, and no plant materials are used in their manufacturing. The reason? Pharmaceutical companies can't patent a plant, but if they add "proprietary" chemicals to it, they change its composition, own it, and charge big dollars for it. Chemicals create possible side effects to the prescription drug, which requires a doctor's supervision. So now Big Pharma's drug requires a prescription, filled by a licensed pharmacist, which the insurance company covers . . . and so begins the circle of profits!

Nature's Pharmacy

One of the world's largest organizations devoted to researching the medicinal benefits of fruits and vegetables is the North Carolina Research Campus (NCRC), representing a historic partnership with leading universities to advance knowledge about nutrition and disease prevention. Eight major universities have joined together for fruit and vegetable research, including North Carolina State University, University of North Carolina Charlotte, North Carolina Central University, Duke University, University of North Carolina Chapel Hill, North Carolina A&T State University, University of North Carolina Greensboro, and Appalachian State University. Their leading scientists have used the most state-of-the-art equipment to analyze both plant and human cells at the most sophisticated levels available.[446]

The NCRC is led by a ninety-four-year-old visionary named David H. Murdock. In 2011, his feature on *Oprah* left audience members speechless, as he explained that he does fifty pushups every day and doesn't take *any* medications, not even an aspirin. His doctor told him he has the blood pressure of a teenager. When you ask Murdock if *all his body parts* are working like a teenager, he'll let you in on a little secret . . . he doesn't even need to take Viagra! Where does he get his vigor, stamina, and robust health? Not from any vitamin pills, which Murdock adamantly opposes, but, rather, from a diet rich in fruits and vegetables. Oprah called Murdock's NCRC a "gift to humanity."[447] Based on ongoing research, NCRC has put together its list of the healthiest fruits and vegetables on the planet (see Table 7.1).

Table 7.1: The Healthiest Foods on Earth:[448]

The Healthiest Foods on Earth	
Apple	Supports immunity, fights lung and prostate cancer, and lowers the risk of Alzheimer's disease.
Artichoke	Helps blood clotting, supplies antioxidants, and lowers "bad" cholesterol.
Arugula	Lowers birth defect risk, reduces fracture risk, and supports the health of the eyes.
Asparagus	Nourishes good gut bacteria, protects against birth defects, and promotes heart health.
Avocado	Reduces liver damage, lowers the risk of oral cancer, and balances cholesterol levels.
Banana	Increases fat burning, lowers risk of colorectal, kidney cancer, and leukemia. Also reduces asthma symptoms in children.
Blackberries	Builds bone density, suppresses appetite, and enhances fat burning.
Blueberries	Restores antioxidant levels, reverses age-related brain decline, and prevents urinary tract infections.
Broccoli	Reduces diabetic damage, lowers risk of prostate, bladder, colon, pancreatic, gastric, and breast cancer. Also protects the brain in the event of injury.
Butternut Squash	Supports night vision, combats wrinkles, and promotes heart health.
Cantaloupe	Boosts immunity, protects skin against sunburn, and reduces inflammation.
Carrot	Antioxidants protect the DNA, fights against cataracts, and protects against some cancers.
Cauliflower	Stimulates detoxification, suppresses breast cancer cell growth, and protects against prostate cancer.
Cherries	Alleviates arthritic pain and gout, lowers "bad" cholesterol, and reduces inflammation.

The Healthiest Foods on Earth	
Cranberries	Alleviates prostate and bladder pain, fights lung, colon, and leukemia cancer cells. Also prevents urinary tract infection.
Green Cabbage	Promotes healthy blood clotting, reduces risk of prostate, colon, breast, and ovarian cancers. Also helps with detoxification.
Kale	Counters harmful estrogens that can feed cancer, protects eyes against sun damage and cataracts. Also increases bone density.
Kiwi	Combats wrinkles, lowers blood clot risk, and reduces blood lipids. Also counters constipation.
Mango	Supports immunity, lowers "bad" cholesterol, regulates homocysteine to protect arteries.
Mushrooms	Promotes natural detoxification, reduces the risk of colon and prostate cancer. Also lowers blood pressure.
Orange	Reduces levels of "bad" cholesterol, lowers risk of cancers of the mouth, throat, breast, and stomach, and childhood leukemia. Also helps suppress the appetite.
Papaya	Enzymes aid digestion, reduce the risk of lung cancer, and enhance fat burning.
Pineapple	Speeds post-surgery recovery, promotes joint health, relieves asthma, and reduces inflammation.
Plums and Prunes	Counters constipation, contains antioxidants that protect the DNA from damage. Also protects against post menopausal bone loss.
Pomegranate	Enhances sunscreen protection, lowers "bad "cholesterol, and fights prostate cancer.
Pumpkin	Protects joints against polyarthritis, lowers lung and prostate cancer risk, and reduces inflammation.
Raspberries	Inhibits growth of oral, breast, colon, and prostate cancers. Antioxidant DNA defense and lowers "bad" cholesterol levels.
Red Bell Pepper	Reduces risk of lung, prostate, ovarian, and cervical cancer, protects against sunburn, and promotes heart health.
Spinach	Helps maintain mental sharpness. Reduces the risk of cancers of the liver, ovaries, colon, and prostate.
Strawberries	Protects against Alzheimer's disease, reduces "bad" cholesterol, suppresses growth of colon, prostate, and oral cancer.
Sweet Potato	Reduces stroke and cancer risk and protects against blindness.
Tomato	Reduces inflammation, lowers the risk of developing esophageal, stomach, colorectal, lung, and pancreatic cancer. Also reduces cardiovascular disease risk.

The Healthiest Foods on Earth	
Watermelon	Supports male fertility, reduces risk of several cancers: prostate, ovarian, cervical, oral, and pharyngeal. Also, protects skin from sunburn.

The Fit for Life Challenge!

One of the best-selling health books of all time is *Fit for Life* by Harvey Diamond. This #1 *New York Times* best-selling book achieved a coveted position on the *Publisher's Weekly* Top 25 Best-selling Books in history, alongside *Gone with the Wind* and the Bible! While in Vietnam, Harvey was exposed to the poison Agent Orange (created by those wonderful folks at Monsanto). As a result, he developed a debilitating condition called peripheral neuropathy, which he was able to overcome by changing his diet. Although he still lives with challenges, he is in the record books at Veterans Affairs for being one of the longest known survivors of the condition to be able to get around without a wheelchair.

I've had the privilege of interviewing Harvey several times on my radio show and listening to him share his insights. I asked him what he considers the ONE thing people can do that would create the biggest impact on their health, and he said unequivocally, "Eat more fruit!" He went on to say, "Fruit doesn't digest in the stomach but, instead, goes right into the intestines, so you should never mix fruit with any other food group. Doing so forces the fruit to comingle with other foods and remain in the stomach, where it doesn't belong. This creates a fermentation process which putrefies other proteins. Fruit should be be eaten alone on an empty stomach. When you eat anything else, you need to wait at least three hours before eating fruit. So the best time to eat fruit is when your stomach is absolutely empty, in the morning."[449]

We've all heard that breakfast is the most important meal of the day. Why do people choose this important meal to load up on carbs and fats, including breads, butter, cream cheese, and other such foods? This puts a strain on the digestive system, and when your body has to work hard during that first meal, it makes you tired. Have no fear—coffee to the rescue! It's an endless cycle.

Harvey gave my listeners a ten-day challenge. "From the time you wake up until noon, don't eat anything except fruit." He went on to recommend, "Eat as much as you want but nothing else. Eat them whole, in a fruit salad, or in a smoothie [mixed with cloudy apple juice or water]. And watch what happens."

I have always eaten fruit throughout the day, but until Harvey's recommendation, I've never just eaten fruit until noon. But I decided to give Harvey's advice a try. For two weeks, I didn't put anything into my body except fresh fruits from waking up until lunchtime. Here's what happened: my energy and overall early-morning mood improved *immediately*. After the tenth day, I noticed the puffiness under my eyes starting to disappear, and my skin even looked better. I actually had a patient ask me if I had gotten a facial peel because my skin was "glowing." I felt stronger during my workouts, and my sleep improved! What a profound difference it made taking the fruits I normally eat throughout the day and consolidating them into my morning routine. While I never fully adopted this daily routine (I love organic eggs and steel cut oatmeal in the morning), I do eat only fruit til noon, two to three times a week.

The word *fruition* means "achievement." This word begins with the prefix *fruit*. Try starting your day with some *fruit*, and you'll achieve more, feel better, and live longer. Because fruits have natural sugar (fructose), you may want to curtail eating some varieties and enjoy some in moderation, especially if you have diabetes. We'll cover more on this topic in chapter 10.

Proof for the Plant-Based Diet

Dr. T. Colin Campbell, a biochemist who specializes in the effects of diet on long-term health, has been at the forefront of plant-based nutrition research for more than forty years. His landmark book, *The China Study*, which he co-wrote with his son Thomas M. Campbell II, M.D, was a culmination of more than a decade of research. The *New York Times* summed up the historical impact of this book by stating: "*The China Study* is the most comprehensive large study ever taken on the relationship between diet and the risk of developing disease."

The Campbells examined mortality rates, diets, and lifestyles of 6,500 people in sixty-five rural counties in China and found that people with a high consumption of animal-based foods were more likely to suffer from chronic diseases like cancer, heart disease, and diabetes, while those who ate a plant-based diet were the least likely.[450] The study was conducted in China because this country has a genetically homogeneous population that tends to live in the same way in the same place and eat the same foods for their entire lives.

The Campbells discovered that after individuals adopted a Westernized diet (processed foods, sugar, dairy, and meat), their health proportionality declined. Those who lived healthier and disease-free consumed fewer animals and far less sugar than many other Americans. When I interviewed Dr. Campbell on my show, he shared how cancer cells are triggered:

"Cancer is initiated at the gene level," he said. "These cells are attacked and mutated by various things like chemicals or viruses. That's the starting point. There they lie dormant unless we fertilize them with the wrong nutrient mixture and wake them up. Everyone has these potential cancer cells in most of their tissues, but for the majority of people, they don't cause any mischief. But when they are exposed to the wrong diet, this can cause them to grow, emerge, divide, and spread. When someone eats animal protein in excess, it turns on cancer cells within the body. When you take away animal-based protein, it turns off the cancer cells. When someone eats plant-based protein, it does not turn on these cancer cells."[451]

It doesn't get simpler than that. Dr. Campbell has laboratory analysis that shows dormant sleeping cancer cells "waking up" after a person eats animal protein.[452] Let me ask you two questions. If you walked outside your house and saw a giant pit bull sleeping in the middle of the yard, would you:

A. tiptoe *very* quietly past the dog, trying not to wake him?
B. jump up and down and scream at the top of your lungs?

If you picked B, welcome to a diet of T-bone steaks, hotdogs, hamburgers, and dairy products. When you eat these things, you are waking up the sleeping carcinogenic pit bulls inside of your body. Before ending my interview with Dr. Campbell, he shared a profound statement: "Eighty percent of health-care costs would be eliminated if people ate a whole-food plant-based diet." Again, if the AMA announced vaccine X would eliminate 80 percent of our health-care costs, long lines would form at every doctor's office in America. Why isn't there a long line at the produce section? Follow the money! If everyone listened to Dr. Campbell, hospitals, the health insurance industry, Big Pharma, and the medical profession would lose 80 percent of their income.

Dr. Campbell's close friend and fellow whole-food, plant-based diet advocate is Dr. Caldwell Esselstyn, author of *Prevent and Reverse Heart Disease*. In this book. Dr. Esselstyn discusses his patients' reversals of atherosclerosis (hardening of the arteries) after following a plant-based diet. Dr. Esselstyn believes cardiovascular conditions are not a death sentence and can be reversed by changing one's diet. Many cardiologists are following in the *foodsteps* of Dr. Esselstyn's work. Even Dr. Oz, heart surgeon and prominent television show host, refers many of his patients to Esselstyn for guidance on adopting a whole-food, plant-based diet.[453] After patients with heart disease go on a plant-based diet, angiograms have demonstrated a remarkable *reversal* of their condition.

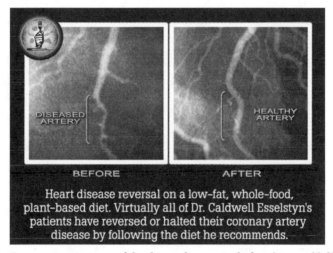

Heart disease reversal on a low-fat, whole-food, plant-based diet. Virtually all of Dr. Caldwell Esselstyn's patients have reversed or halted their coronary artery disease by following the diet he recommends.

Figure 7.1: Coronary angiograms of the descending artery before (pictured left) and after (pictured right) thirty-two months of a plant-based diet without cholesterol-lowering medication.[454]

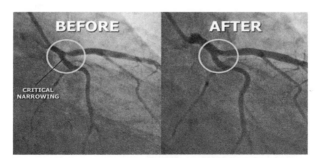

Figure 7.2: Coronary arteries before and after five months on a whole-food, plant-based diet.[455]

People from all walks of life are adopting a plant-based diet and seeing a profound improvement in their blood pressure and cholesterol level, and even a complete clearing of their coronary arteries. Former president Bill Clinton is a vocal supporter of Campbell and Esselstyn's eating plan. In 2010, after years of life-threatening heart issues, Clinton followed a plant-based diet, eating only legumes, other vegetables, and fruit. Within a short period, Clinton dropped 24 pounds, returning him to his college weight, and his blood tests and blood pressure were back to normal.[456]

A large-scale example of how diet plays a profound role in cardio-vascular disease occurred in the 1940s when the Germans invaded and occupied Norway and confiscated all of the livestock and other farm animals to feed their own troops. The people of Norway were forced to eat a plant-based diet. After the Germans arrived, the Norwegian death rate, due to heart attack and stroke, began to decline drastically. Once the hostility ended in 1945 and through the next decade, when meat and dairy were again available, the rate surged to what it had been prior to the war. This analysis proves that eating a plant-based diet prevents heart disease and stroke, and the more farm animals you eat, the more increased risk you have of getting these diseases.[457]

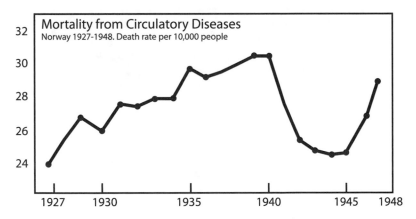

Figure 7.3: Declining death rate in the 1940s after the Germans invaded Norway and confiscated all of the livestock and other farm animals.

A similar phenomenon took place in Finland. After World War II, Finland returned to a diet high in meat and dairy. By the 1970s, the mortality rate from heart disease of Finnish men was considered one of the highest in the world, and so they initiated a countrywide program to decrease their saturated fat intake. A campaign called "dairies to berries" had towns partaking in friendly cholesterol-lowering competitions. Their efforts resulted in an 80 percent drop in cardiac mortality across the entire country when they adopted a whole-food, plant-based diet.[458]

The following bar graph shows the global scale correlation between a diet high in plant foods and a lower incidence of heart disease and cancer. These numbers state that the more unrefined plant foods that are consumed, the lower the percentage of deaths from cardiovascular disease and cancer.

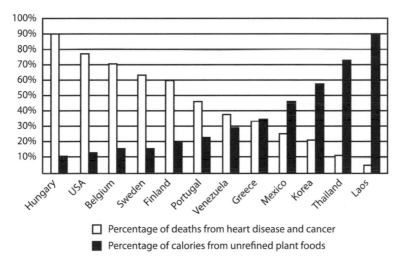

☐ Percentage of deaths from heart disease and cancer
■ Percentage of calories from unrefined plant foods

Statistical database food balance sheets, 1961–1999 Food and Agricultural Organization of the United States.

Living to Your Full Potential

The human body is genetically designed to live 120 years or longer.[459] Following the blueprints for your life span is entirely up to you. John Robbins, Pulitzer Prize-nominated author of *Diet for a New America*, is considered by many to be the poster child for a plant-based diet. After my health issues from eating red meat in college, his book inspired me to completely remove red meat from my own diet. Although I never quite made the complete jump over to being a full vegetarian, 80 percent of my diet consists of fruits, vegetables, whole grains, legumes, and nuts. As we discussed in chapter 1, I choose to follow the *real diet* of our ancestors. I will forever be indebted to John for changing my life and creating a ripple effect that would eventually lead to a career as a nutritionist, formulator of whole-food nutritional products, and syndicated radio and television personality through which I continue to share my passion. I was honored to be able to thank John personally during my radio interview with him, which showcased the benefits of a plant-based lifestyle.

One of John's books is called *Healthy at 100*, which shows that aging gracefully doesn't only mean increasing our life span but also our health span. I highly recommend this book. John explores four very different cultures that have something in common: they have some of the world's healthiest and longest-living people. If you wanted to become the best martial artist, who better to learn from than a Shaolin grandmaster tenth-degree black belt? If you want to live a long, healthy life that is free of disease, learn from those featured in *Healthy at 100*.

One of the men featured in John Robbins's book is Shirali Muslimov, said to be 161 years old.[460] In 1966, *Life* magazine did a feature story on Shirali, who was then married to his third wife, who was 110 years old! His parents had both lived to be over 100, and his brother died at the age of 134.

In the 1970s, *National Geographic* magazine chose world-renowned physician Alexander Leaf to visit, research, and conduct a follow-up on the *Life* magazine article on the world's healthiest and longest-living people. Leaf traveled to remote areas, analyzed lifestyles, diets, vitals, and blood tests.[461] During his journey, he met a woman named Khfaf Lasuria, who was also featured in the original *Life* magazine article. Her memory was excellent, and she was able to speak in great detail about events from her past. After a thorough investigation, Leaf concluded her to be 130 years old. From the age of seventy-five to eighty, she was a midwife who assisted more than one hundred births. Through Leaf's travels, he met many people older than one hundred who were in great health, with blood pressure and pulse rates measuring in at what you'd expect to see in someone in their twenties! These "elderly" people weren't sitting around in rocking chairs knitting either; they were active! Most swam regularly and took vigorous walks down rugged terrain. Only 10 percent had poor hearing, and fewer than 4 percent had poor eyesight.[462] An old man having a healthy sex life in American today would require a lot of prayer and plenty of little blue pills. But for the world's healthiest and longest-living men featured in Robbins's book, continuation of an active sex life into old age is considered to be as natural as maintaining a healthy appetite or sound sleep.

There was one common connection between most of the oldest and healthiest living cultures—the vast majority had no exposure to the processed food, artificial preservatives, and chemical additives that are commonly found in so many modern foods. Their diet primarily contained whole grains, fruits, vegetables, seeds, beans, and nuts. Vegetables were picked fresh from nutrient-rich soils, which had not been destroyed by modern farming techniques so common in the United States. These people usually ate their veggies raw, and when they were cooked, only a very small amount of water was used. Leftovers were rarely eaten because it's believed, in many of these cultures, that food not eaten totally fresh is harmful. The fruits weren't sprayed with preservatives and were eaten fresh off the plant. Very little meat, if any, was consumed, and on the rare occasion when it was, the animals were healthy and freshly slaughtered, never processed. The fat from all meat or poultry was always discarded. Very little salt, butter, or sugar was consumed. This could explain why so many had a perfect cholesterol level of 98.[463] Their protein source was derived from vegetables, whole grains, and a variety of beans. Their carbohydrates came from whole-grain cereals, such as corn, quinoa, wheat, and barley. Their fat mostly came from avocados, seeds, and nuts.

Can You DIG This?

We've come to associate the word *raw* (meaning "uncooked") as something to stay away from when it comes to fish, meat, and poultry. But that's not the case when it comes to vegetables and fruits. Many vitamins are water soluble, and a significant amount of them can be lost when cooking, especially over-cooking. When fruits and vegetables are heated above 107 degrees, natural plant-based nutrients are destroyed. At 130 degrees, vitamin C is destroyed. At 161 degrees, most of the calcium becomes insoluable.[464] [465] If you boil vegetables in water, a lot of the healthy nutrients that were inside them end up going down the kitchen sink. Steaming is one of the best cooking methods for preserving nutrients, including water-soluble vitamins that are sensitive to heat and water.[466]

Cooking also denatures essential enzymes, which are necessary for several bodily functions, including digestion. Broccoli contains an enzyme called myrosinase, which breaks down into sulforaphane—a compound that has cancer-fighting properties. However, when broccoli is cooked, this cancer-preventing compound is lost. Raw carrots supply polyphenols, a group of chemicals with antioxidant properties that have been shown to reduce the risk of heart disease and cancer. Boiling carrots destroys their health-enhancing polyphenols. Raw nuts are another great example. They're an excellent source of protein; however, baking or roasting them reduces the availability and absorbability of the protein they contain by 50 percent.

If you prefer cooked vegetables over raw, steam them. Lightly steaming your veggies is the least nutrient depleting way of cooking them compared to baking, broiling, or boiling. While cooking does destroy some of the healthy phytochemicals (*phyto* means "plant"), it can actually help enhance others. For example, tomatoes contain a powerful antioxidant called lycopene, which has been linked to the prevention of cancer and cardiovascular disease. Cooked tomatoes contain four times more lycopene than uncooked tomatoes. Ohio State University researchers have found that lycopene molecules in tomatoes change their shape, which makes them more usable by the body after being subjected to intense heat during processing. Cooked tomatoes are also better absorbed by the body rather than eaten raw.[467]

In the legume family, there are several that aren't edible unless they are soaked and cooked. Some beans can cause illness and even death if not cooked properly. Black beans, fava beans, kidney beans, lima beans, navy beans, pinto beans, and soybeans are unpalatable raw and may contain toxic compounds only removable by cooking.

Ten-Day Turnaround

If you ask health advocates who inspired them, many put the name Dr. John McDougall at the very top of their list. He's a board-certified internist, author of a dozen nationally best-selling books, and medical director of the ten-day, live-in McDougall Program that has helped thousands of people get off their medications for hypertension, type 2 diabetes, arthritis, indigestion, and constipation. His secret is rather simple—get everyone on a whole-food, plant-based diet. During my radio spotlight on the healing powers of a plant-based diet, Dr. McDougall was part of the panel of experts I interviewed. He shared with my listeners the following:

> If you look at history you'll find those that have lived on a plant-based diet are the healthiest. When people move to the United States, they give up their rice, beans, corn, and potatoes, and they get fat and sick . . . Some try to say it's our modern rich foods, and because our meat is processed and our dairy is contaminated. That is not true. CAT scans have examined pharaohs, priests, and priestesses from three thousand to five thousand years ago and found extensive atherosclerosis, gallstones, and obesity within this group, which accepted the offerings of meat from the temple.[468]

Dr. McDougall brings up a great point. During this era, meat was considered a luxury that only the wealthy ate. Poorer Egyptians never ate meat. Scientists have studied mummies kept in the Egyptian National Museum of Antiquities in Cairo and determined that people of high social status also showed advanced signs of heart disease. Dr. Samuel Wann, one of the researchers, commented, "With today's modern diet, we all sort of live in the pharaoh's court."[469]

Dr. McDougall has treated thousands of patients at his ten-day live-in clinic in California. They spend this time away from their Standard American Diet (SAD) and are allowed to eat only from a 100 percent whole-food, plant-based menu. Dr. McDougall states that in most cases, after the ten days, people with high blood pressure are able to get off their medication. In fact, this is true for many within just twenty-four hours! He is also helping people reverse type 2 diabetes by simply changing their diet.

In my twenty-eight years in practice, I have yet to see any type 2 diabetic cured from the disease by taking diabetic medications. I have never seen anyone cured of hypertension after taking high-blood-pressure medications. However people can be cured of these diseases by simply eating more whole-food, plant-based foods and zero processed foods and cutting back on animal foods. Adult-onset diabetes was very rare fifty years ago, affecting less than 1 percent of the adult population in the United States. Today 29.1 million people over the age of twenty in the United States have type 2 diabetes, but 8.1 million may be undiagnosed and unaware of their condition.[470] Sadly "adult onset" had to be renamed type 2 diabetes because a quarter of a million *children* have it.[471] It is one of the major causes of obesity! The reason? Putting the wrong things into your mouth!

When children and adults weigh more than they should, they are more prone to diabetes. One of the biggest misconceptions people have about type 2 diabetes is that it's caused by having too much sugar in the blood. Although high blood sugar does result from having type 2 diabetes, the real culprit is what's called insulin resistance, a condition in which the body's cells become resistant to the effects of insulin. This makes it difficult for the cells to absorb glucose, which causes a build-up of sugar in the blood. In our body, we have tiny receptors that allow glucose into the cell so it can be used to produce energy. Think of these receptors like doormen who have fallen asleep on the job and are not allowing sugar into the cells, which causes a sugar build-up in the blood. When your diet consists of unhealthful, fattening, and processed foods, it can make the doormen lazy and unable to do their job. Fortunately many people with type 2 diabetes are seeing a complete reversal of their disease after turning to a whole-food, plant-based diet.[472] [473] [474]

SAD, but True

Our Standard American Diet (SAD) is the primary cause of disease. But, no matter how much proof exists on the health benefits of eating a plant-based diet, the fact remains: the majority of people will never totally boycott their SAD lifestyle. But that's okay. If you can at least make an effort to eat more plant-based foods than processed and animal-based foods, the healthier and longer you will live.

A patient, a fifty-three-year-old woman named Susan, came to me with symptoms of fatigue, constant headaches, and difficulty sleeping. An examination showed the following: Susan weighed 182 pounds, her blood pressure was 170/112 (ideal is 120/80), and her fasting triglyceride level was 487 (normal is less than 150 milligrams/dL). Her C-reactive protein (CRP), which measures inflammation in the body, was 5.2 milligrams/L (high risk is anything above 3.0). Susan was a heart attack in the making! She was the typical American and loved her SAD regimen of hamburgers, steaks, processed TV dinners, and fast-food lunches, which she washed down with her favorite beverage, Coke. I explained to her how adopting a diet that was primarily whole-food and plant-based could be the remedy for all her health issues. But old habits die hard, so I struck a deal with her.

Susan agreed to follow a plant-based diet *during the week* as long as she could eat whatever she wanted on the weekends. Considering that meant twenty days a month eating a whole-food, plant-based diet and only eight days a month eating hamburgers, processed foods, and drinking soda, this was a good compromise. Ten weeks later, she came back in for her follow-up visit. Susan was a totally different person! No more headaches, her fatigue was gone, and she was sleeping great. She now weighed 152 pounds, her blood pressure measured normal at 122/78, and her triglycerides were a perfect 148 milligrams/dL. Her CRP had dropped to a healthy 2.8 milligrams/L, and she was no longer in the danger zone of having a heart attack.

Not everyone can walk away from the Standard American Diet and embrace a whole-food, plant-based lifestyle; however, improving one's diet doesn't have to mean "all or nothing." Baby steps are better than taking no steps in the right direction. As John Robbins told me, "An *occasional* scoop of ice-cream isn't going to kill you, but that pint of ice-cream every night before bed most certainly can." So give this "weekend warrior" method a try; see how you feel Monday through Friday, and compare that to how you feel on your weekends. Your body will tell you what days you feel your best. Who knows? You may completely turn over a new leaf (pun intended).

 Discoveries: The nonbiased research showing the healing benefits of eating a whole-food, plant-based diet is undeniable. There is not ONE study showing the opposite. All the vitamins, minerals, amino acids, fiber, enzymes, proteins, and complex carbohydrates needed for human survival exists in fruits and vegetables.

Instincts: If you were trapped in the middle of a forest without a fork, knife, weapon, or other tool—just your bare hands—you could live a healthy life just eating plant-based foods.

God: Our blueprint design (teeth, colon, blood, and pH) is more conducive to eating plant-based foods. There is no religion that disallows eating fruits and vegetables, but many don't allow eating certain animals.

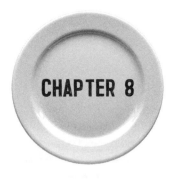

CHAPTER 8

THE WAR ON PLANTS
DESTROYING OUR MOST PRECIOUS
NUTRITIONAL RESOURCE

"The earth is what we all have in common."
—Wendell Berry

We've explored the pros (where they exist) and cons of all the basic food groups. While no one can deny that plant-based foods are good for us, unfortunately, there is also a down side to eating them. Thanks to agriculture, industrialized manufacturing, and Big Pharma, our plant-based foods aren't always what they seem. It all depends on whether they are naturally or chemically grown.

Before World War II, most farming in the United States took place on family farms, without modern herbicides or pesticides, genetically modified seeds, chemical fertilizers, crude irrigation, and gas-guzzling farm equipment. Fast forward to today, and you find mega factory-farms are more like giant-scale industrial operations than great-grandpa's family farm. Sadly, the nutritional value of the crop is the farthest thing from the minds for these modern-day agri-business farmers. The one thing that is most important is maximizing yield and profits. But in order to do that, it means cutting corners.

Grandpa told us that fruits and vegetables aren't like they used to be, and science agrees with him. Soil depletion has caused a significant decrease in the minerals and vitamin content of our fruits and vegetables. The below table shows an analytical comparison of the aggregate mineral content of twenty-seven vegetables and seventeen fruits, between 1940 and 1991.[475]

Table 8.1: Loss of Minerals in Fruit and Vegetables from 1940 to 1991

MINERALS	VEGETABLES	FRUITS
Sodium	-49%	-29%
Potassium	-16%	-19%
Magnesium	-24%	-16%
Calcium	-46%	-16%
Iron	-27%	-24%
Copper	-76%	-20%
Zinc	-59%	-27%

In 1914, an apple was an excellent source of iron (4.6 milligrams). An apple today has only 0.18 milligrams (a disturbing 96.09 percent decline)! That means you would have to eat twenty-five apples today to get the iron content that one apple would give you in 1914![476] I guess the famous saying should be changed to *"twenty-five apples* a day helps keep the doctor away." In 2001, *Life Extension* magazine published an analysis comparing the nutritional content of several fruits and vegetables from 1963 to 2000. The vitamin C content in sweet peppers dropped by 31 percent, vitamin A in apples dropped by 41 percent, and broccoli saw a 50 percent drop in calcium and vitamin A. Watercress lost 88 percent of its iron, and cauliflower lost 40 percent of its vitamin C. One of my favorite veggies is collard greens, but I would have to eat six-and-a-half cups of collard greens today to equal the nutritional content of one cup of collards from 1963. (I don't love them *that* much!) The vitamin A in collard greens has dropped from 6,500 IUs to 3,800 IUs. The potassium content in collards plummeted from 400 milligrams to 170 milligrams, and magnesium fell sharply from 57 milligrams to a measly 9 milligrams.[477] And the list goes on and on and on.

Our vegetation has become so void in nutrients that if we're not careful, the cardboard boxes they're shipped in may end up being more healthful for us to eat. Aside from mineral depletion, our fruits and vege-tables have lost their superfood value for many other reasons, beginning with the deforestation of the planet.

Fertilizer: Friend or Foe?

Our ancestors didn't use fertilizer to grow their gardens; why do plants need it today? To answer that, it's important to note that the minerals plants need are received from the soil. They do not produce any themselves. There's a big difference between plants that grow in the wild compared to those harvested at commercial farms. After a plant matures, nature creates a replenishment of minerals through dry leaves, grass clippings, dried ani-mal manure, rain, and wind. All of these help recycle the soil and deposit minerals and nutrients back into the land. But these natural processes take time, and in the farming business, time costs money. The quicker the turn-around, the more profits to be made. Have no fear—fertilizer to the rescue!

In the early 1900s scientists discovered that crops would grow on a mixture of just three minerals: nitrogen (N), phosphorus (P), and potas-sium (K). That would allow the fruits and vegetables to look healthy enough to sell even though they didn't contain close to the amount of minerals required. When news broke that just three inexpensive minerals would be all it takes to grow plants, chemical manufactures began selling synthetic NPK mixtures to farmers.

In 1908 Fritz Haber was credited for inventing an inexpensive nitro-gen fertilizer after he discovered how to make ammonia, a molecule made of hydrogen and nitrogen atoms, from inert nitrogen gas in the air. Haber received the 1918 Nobel Prize in chemistry for his work and became a hero among farmers. By the 1960s, in order to compete in the global mar-ket, almost all farmers had become totally dependent on fertilizers. NPK gave the farmers the three main elements essential for plant growth with a very quick rate of return. But plants need more than a measly three min-erals and so do the humans that consume them. We need calcium, magne-sium, selenium, chromium, iron, copper, cobalt, molybdenum, vanadium, boron, zinc, and many more. Chemical fertilizer sales have increased every decade, with 100 million tons of nitrogen produced per year![478]

Unfortunately Haber didn't research the long-term repercussions of adding large amounts of artificially made nitrogen into the soil. Artificial nitrogen fertilizers increase the level of potentially toxic nitrates, and they also decrease the fiber content in plants.[479] Artificial nitrogen can also destroy the calcium, magnesium, and potassium normally found in the soil.[480] It kills microbes that are naturally occurring in the dirt and essential for plant health. But it's not just the plants that are suffering. When humans eat fruits and vegetables grown in synthetic nitrogen fertilizers, it increases the amounts of toxic nitrates in their blood stream.

According to the National Research Council, nine of the top fifteen foods with cancer-causing risk are produce items that contain a high nitrate content from nitrogen fertilizers and pesticides. A twelve-year study that compared naturally grown versus chemically grown fruit and vegetables showed that those that are chemically grown have sixteen times more nitrates.[481] Synthetic nitrogen fertilizers can also reduce carbohydrate synthesis,[482] which results in lower glucose content and affects the taste of fruit and vegetables. Grandpa was right! His generation did have more flavorful fruits and vegetables.

Ammonium nitrate is used as an oxidizing agent in explosives and terrorist weapons. In fact ammonium nitrate–based explosives were used in the Oklahoma City bombing and in the 2011 Delhi bombing! And this is also the ingredient placed at the roots of the plants we eat? But here's the really scary part: the warning label on ammonium nitrate states, "Avoid contamination with inorganic material, including chlorides and metals such as aluminum, antimony, bismuth, cadmium, chromium, cobalt, copper, iron, lead, magnesium, manganese, nickel, tin, and zinc, as it may react violently or explosively."[483] [484]

Say what? These metallic minerals naturally found in the soil shouldn't come in contact with an ingredient in the fertilizer? Maybe it's a good thing our soil is depleted of these vital minerals. Sure beats having carrots end up as dynamite sticks! Okay, I'm being dramatic here. I know there are more moving parts to creating an explosive out of fertilizer, but do you really think our ancestors grew their fruits and vegetables with a synthetic ingredient that was also used to blow up buildings?

Another problem with these artificial fertilizers is that they contain excessive sodium. This salt content reduces the soil's ability to hold moisture, making it more difficult for the plant to attain the right amount of water it needs. This constant salt exposure also harms the delicate roots and disables their ability to absorb water, even when the ground is saturated. This added salt kills the beneficial microorganisms and earthworms living in the soil. They also create a thatch that ends up becoming a fertile breeding ground for diseases and destructive insects. Have no fear! It's toxic pesticides to the rescue! The irony of this is that vegetables grown in organic fertilizers (mulch and compost) attract significantly fewer pests than those grown in artificially fertilized soil.[485]

GMO—OMG!

Four years ago, a Trader Joe's healthy grocery store opened up in my town. The line of shoppers literally wrapped around the building. A man in front of me at the cash register asked the lady, "I don't get it. What's all the excitement about?" She replied, "Well, for starters, we don't sell GMOs here." He looked at her very puzzled and said, "Why on Earth would anyone purchase a car from a grocery store?" For anyone perhaps still living under a rock, a GMO is not a car. It's a genetically modified organism (GMO), which has been altered in a lab through genetic modification, whether by high-tech modern genetic engineering, or long-time traditional plant-breeding methods.

This genetic altering technology uses DNA molecules from different sources, which are combined into one molecule to create a new set of genes. Molecular engineers working in laboratories are gene-splicing vegetable seedlings with poisonous pesticides and herbicides so the plants are inherently protected from the worms and insects that damage them. Who is the company playing God and creating these Frankenstein seeds? None other than Monsanto, the biotech giant and creator of the most popular herbicide/pesticide in the world: Roundup. In fact these gene-spliced seeds produce what is referred to as "Roundup Ready" crops.

The dangers of eating pesticides and herbicides are well documented. The primary poison in these products is a toxin called glyphosate. This chemical was first introduced as a weed killer in 1974, prior to the introduction of genetically modified crops. This chemical is strikingly similar to dichlorodiphenyltrichloroethane, better known as DDT, another poisonous pesticide Monsanto manufactured in the 1940s. DDT was banned in 1972 after it was linked to serious health hazards to humans and several environmental issues. Glyphosate and DDT are very difficult compounds to degrade, and both promote the proliferation of disease-causing pathogens; however, many experts consider glyphosate to be an even greater health risk than DDT.[486] Dr. Don Huber, a professor at Purdue University, is considered one of the leading experts on the toxicity of genetically engineered (GE) foods. He's taught plant pathology and soil microbiology for more than thirty-five years. When asked which toxin he would prefer to use if he had to make a choice between two evils, DDT or glyphosate, Dr. Huber said he'd take DDT any day.[487]

Statistics from the California Environmental Protection Agency's Pesticide Illness Surveillance Program shows that glyphosate-related health incidents are reported with more frequency than incidents related to any other pesticides.[488] Glyphosate herbicides damage DNA in human cells, causing birth defects, endocrine diseases, and cancer. Scientists hired by Monsanto have been accused of deliberately trying to conceal the dangers of glyphosate by falsifying tests.[489] In 1983 the EPA found "routine falsification of data" when investigating Industrial Biotest Laboratories.[490] [491] In 1991 Craven laboratories also conducted studies for Monsanto. The owner and three employees of this lab falsified lab results and were indicted on twenty felony counts. The owner was sentenced to five years in prison and fined $50,000; the lab was fined $15.5 million and ordered to pay $3.7 million in restitution.[492] Yes, folks, it's another monumental Monsanto monstrosity!

I'm a big advocate of a product called Veggie Wash. This is an all-natural spray that helps remove wax, soil, and agricultural chemicals from produce before eating them (veggie-wash.com). Unfortunately, washing produce cannot remove any of the dangerous glyphosate residue *inside* it. This is because the chemical starts from the seed, and as the plant grows, it becomes systemic inside of the plant. The EPA considers glyphosate a Class III toxic substance, fatal to an adult at 30 grams.[493] Scientific peer-reviewed, biomedical literature links it to two dozen adverse health effects. This toxic chemical also causes groundwater contamination! The *Journal of Environmental Toxicology and Chemistry* showed the chemical is present in 60 to 100 percent of all air and rain samples tested, indicating that glyphosate pollution and exposure is now nearly omnipresent in the United States.[494]

The amount of glyphosate humans ingest after eating genetically engineered Roundup-ready crops is appalling! In fact, there was so much glyphosate measured in genetically modified soybeans when they were first introduced, Europe had to increase their legally allowable levels by 200 percent! There's no denying the facts: If you are eating genetically modified plants, fruits, or vegetables, you are eating this chemical. And when you eat glyphosate, it ends up in your colon where it potentially destroys some of the good bacteria of your gut. This can compromise your immune system, making you more prone to many diseases. Serious health risks associated with GMO consumption include infertility, accelerated aging, insulin dysregulation, and dysfunctional changes in the liver, kidney, spleen, and gastrointestinal system.[495]

Okay, then just stay away from the big, bad GMO products, right? Unfortunately it's becoming very difficult to find anything that *doesn't* contain GMOs. Eighty-five percent of U.S. corn is genetically modified; 91 percent of soybeans, 88 percent of cotton (cottonseed oil is often used in food products), and 70 percent of all processed foods on supermarket shelves—from soda to soup, crackers to condiments—contain genetically modified ingredients.[496] [497] Thanks to a nonprofit organization called Non-GMO Project, we are seeing more transparency with food products. The project is educating consumers and providing verified non-GMO choices. Because more consumers are becoming aware and demanding GMO-free foods, manufacturers are starting to offer more GMO-free options. To find Non-GMO Project Verified products and restaurants visit nongmoproject.org.

Can You DIG This?

Genetically modified foods were introduced into the marketplace in 1996, and the incidence of people in the United States with several chronic diseases almost doubled, going from 7 percent to 13 percent. Allergies and food-related illnesses increased 200 percent within five years of modified foods becoming mainstream.[498] The Lyme Induced Autism Foundation, a patient advocacy group, found a plethora of evidence showing harm for individuals eating GMOs, especially those with autism, Lyme disease, and associated conditions.[499]

Eat Organic

When eating processed and plant-based foods, avoid anything that is genetically modified or grown in artificial fertilizers. Look for the "Non-GMO Project" seal. Another proactive step you can take is to shop at local farmers' markets and health food grocery stores. Buying fruits and vegetables from *local* farmers' markets not only supports local agriculture, it also saves countless pounds of carbon emissions, since your food has not been shipped from afar to your supermarket.

In 2014, the Center for Urban Education about Sustainable Agriculture shared findings showing how long produce takes to travel from the farm where it is grown to your refrigerator. Apples travel the shortest distance (766 miles); grapes travel the longest distance (2,143 miles).[500] In the United States, 50 percent of our fruits and 20 percent of our vegetables are imported from overseas.[501] The farther produce travels, the less nutritious it is, and the more preservatives it is likely to contain. There is no such thing as fresh fruit from California if you are eating it in Georgia. Support your local farmers' markets and roadside produce stands. Also look for "USDA-Certified Organic." USDA's National Organic Program regulates the standards for farms, wild-crop harvesting, or handling operations that want to sell an agricultural product as organically produced. Organic foods are free from artificial fertilizers, herbicides, pesticides, and GMOs and are nutritionally superior to conventionally produced food. In fact, organic fruits and vegetables give us between 20 and 40 percent higher antioxidants than non-organic varieties.[502]

I can't tell you how many times I've heard people use the excuse, "I'm on a budget and can't afford to buy organic foods." The fact is, you can pay a little more now or pay a lot more later. It's a whole lot cheaper to buy organic foods to enhance your health than pay later for the Clarinex you'll need to treat your allergies, corticosteroids to treat your arthritis pain, Ciprofloxacin to treat your gastrointestinal disorder, Avanafil for your impotency, Fosrenol for your kidney dysfunction, or the tens of thousands of dollars it will cost for chemotherapy to treat your cancer. To find farmers' markets, family farms, and other sources of sustainable, organically grown food in your area, where you can buy USDA organic, GMO-free produce, visit Local Harvest (localharvest.org). For a list of foods and common brand names containing GMOs that you should avoid, visit TrueFoodNow.org/shoppers-guide.

10 TIPS FOR AVOIDING GMOs

1. Avoid ALL processed foods that contain corn or soy that is not labeled 100 percent "USDA-Certified Organic."

2. Avoid vegetable oil, vegetable fat, and margarines (made with soy, corn, cottonseed, and/or canola). Instead use organic sources of grape-seed oil, virgin coconut oil, hempseed oil, and olive oil, which are available at organic and whole-foods markets.

3. Avoid ingredients derived from soybeans: soy flour, soy protein, soy isolates, soy isoflavones, soy lecithin, vegetable proteins, textured vegetable protein (TVP), tofu, tamari, tempeh, and soy-protein supplements.

4. Avoid ingredients derived from corn: corn flour, corn starch, corn syrup, cornmeal, corn gluten, corn masa, and high-fructose corn syrup (HFCS).

5. Avoid popcorn that is not labeled 100 percent USDA-Certified Organic.

6. Avoid non-organic products made in North America that list "sugar" as an ingredient (and NOT pure cane sugar). It is almost always a combination of sugar from both sugar cane and GM sugar beets.

7. Avoid sweeteners that use aspartame. This artificial sweetener is derived from genetically modified microorganisms and is the sweetener used in products such as NutraSweet and Equal. Artificial sweeteners in general are worse for your health than sugar and should always be avoided.

8. Buy fruit juices that are 100 percent juice. Most fruit juices, apart from papaya, are not from GM foods, but the sweetener used in many fruit juices (and sodas) is high fructose corn syrup, which is almost always derived from genetically modified corn.

9. Avoid any grains derived from corn. Instead, eat 100 percent whole wheat (including whole-wheat couscous), rice, quinoa, oats, barley, or sorghum.

10. Avoid eating produce with PLU labels that don't begin with a 9. The numbers on the stickers you find on produce indicate how the product was grown:

- A four-digit number indicates the food was conventionally grown.
- A five-digit number beginning with an 8 is a genetically modified food. However, not all GM foods can be identified because PLU labeling is optional. An easy way to remember this: "The eight isn't great."
- A five-digit number beginning with a 9 indicates it is organic.

The Soy Scam

The soybean industry wants us to believe that soy is the healthiest food we can put into our bodies. What they neglect to share is evidence that it can cause life-threatening allergic reactions—such as food anaphylaxis—hormonal imbalances, and immune disorders that can lead to all types of conditions, including cancer.[503]

How can something "natural" cause such health issues? Soy was originally used by modern Western populations as an industrial product to manufacture paints and shock absorber fluid. In fact, it was Henry Ford in 1940 who used two bushes (120 pounds) of soybeans in each Ford car.[504] Ford also developed soy-based plastics, which he used to make a vehicle that he colloquially titled, the "Soybean Car."[505] Soy farming started around 1100 BC in China, where it was used to build soil fertility and feed animals. Soybeans were not considered fit for humans until the Chinese learned to ferment them, which makes them digestible. Asian diets now include fermented soybeans in the form of natto, miso, tamari, and tempeh. Unfermented soybean products such as tofu (bean curd), soy milk, and soy protein powder contain large quantities of natural toxins. Asian cultures utilize time-consuming fermentation processes to remove most of the toxins from soy, making it safer to consume. Doing this in America would take too much time and create lost revenues. Today, the United States high-tech processing methods not only fail to remove the anti-nutrients and toxins that are naturally present in soybeans but leave toxic and carcinogenic residues created by the high temperatures, high pressure, alkali and acid baths, and petroleum solvents.[506] Also in Asia, soy is primarily used as a condiment or side dish and not eaten as a meal like it is in the United States.

Several chemicals found in soy are considered to be dangerous for human consumption.

Phytoestrogens. A plant estrogen found in abundance in soy that may damage the endocrine system and the thyroid gland, possibly contributing to autoimmune disease. Parents, would you give your child birth control pills? If you are feeding them a soy-based formula, you are feeding them a substance that contains estrogen compounds, the thing used in many oral contraceptives. Infants who are fed soy-based formula have up to 22,000 times more estrogen compounds in their blood than babies fed milk-based formula. This is the estrogenic equivalent of five birth control pills per day.[507] This may be linked to premature development of girls and small testes and underdevelopment in boys.[508] Looking at worldwide trends, Puerto Rico has the highest known incidence of premature breast development. Girls as young as two were developing breasts. Analysis revealed that most of these children were fed soy-based infant formulas.[509] Soy has also been correlated with childhood leukemia.[510] In adults, soy has been linked to an increased risk of thyroid disease, breast cancer in females, and infertility in males.[511 512 513]

Phytic acid. Found in high levels in soy products like soy milk, phytic acid binds with, and reduces, the absorption of vital minerals such as niacin, calcium, iron, magnesium, and zinc. When soy is soaked and/or boiled (a common practice in the United States), this does not lower the amount of phytic acid.[514] However, when soy is fermented, it removes over half of the phytic acid, and when it is fermented and fried (common preparation in Asian cuisines), all the dangerous properties of phytic acid is removed. Scientists are in general agreement that phytic acid contributes to widespread mineral deficiencies among people who eat large amounts of soy beans.[515] Because phytic acid can cause zinc deficiency, consuming it can lead to a wide variety of health issues, including skin problems, impaired appetite, fatigue, altered gene expression, and weakened immune system.[516 517] The phytic acid in soy is a trypsin inhibitor, which means it blocks the enzyme trypsin, which is needed to digest protein. When blocking happens, the pancreas has to work harder to produce more enzymes, which can lead to hypertrophy and cancer of the pancreas in humans.[518] [519]

Lysinoalanine. An unusual amino acid that is found in the proteins of cooked foods, lysinoalanine is formed when soy is heated. Lysinoalanine has been linked to kidney damage and is eliminated when soy is fermented, but not when it is heated.[520]

Nitrosamines. Nitrosamines are strongly suspected of being human carcinogens. For example, tobacco-specific nitrosamines are one of the major groups of chemical carcinogens in tobacco products, and no doubt remain the causal link between tobacco use and cancer.[521] Nitrosamines promote the formation of liver and gastric cancer.[522]

Hemagglutinin. This is a clot-promoting substance in soy that causes red blood cells to clump together. When red blood cells cluster together, they can cause dangerous blood clots in the legs, lungs, and heart. Hemagglutinin is a growth depressant, and animals that are fed soy must be given lysine supplements to combat stifled growth. Fermenting soybeans, as is common practice in Asia, neutralizes hemagglutinin.

Goitrogens. Goitrogens are substances that suppress or reduce the production of hormones by the thyroid by blocking the gland's ability to absorb iodine. Goitrogens can also trigger thyroid disease. Concerns that soy is a goitrogen have been studied for years, but were raised specifically by FDA researchers Daniel Doerge and Daniel Sheehan, key experts on soy. In 2000, they wrote a report protesting the positive health claims of soy, which the FDA was approving at the time. They showed a significant body of data demonstrates that soy contributes to goitrogenic and carcinogenic effects.[523]

Aluminum. Due to industrial washing, soy often contains high levels of aluminum. This occurs when producers soak the beans in harsh alkaline solutions that leach aluminum from the processing equipment. The soaking solutions are used mainly in the production of modern soy foods such as soy protein isolates, soy protein concentrates, soy supplements, soy protein shakes, and textured soy protein.[524]

Soy Causes Memory Loss

Consuming soy foods and soy milk has been linked to memory loss and even Alzheimer's disease. Experts at Oxford University researched the impact of soy consumption of 719 senior citizens and determined that people who regularly consumed soy had 20 percent less memory function than those who didn't.[525]

In April of 2000, a study from Hawaii showed that eating tofu on a regular basis might actually shrink the brain. This research showed a positive correlation between tofu consumption and brain atrophy in a large sample of men over several decades. Men who eat tofu, often during midlife, are two-and-a-half times more likely to develop Alzheimer's disease. The researchers with the Hawaii study concluded that soy should be considered a dangerous drug and not a food.[526 527 528]

For those of you who are reading this while enjoying your glass of soy milk, you may not remember reading this tomorrow. Please take a minute now and type the following reminder into your smart phone, "Stop drinking soy milk; it causes memory loss." Go ahead. Do it now before you forget.

FDA Looking the Other Way

The FDA lists soy on its Poisonous Plant Database.[529] Some of the published studies have shown possible side effects ranging from skin conditions to pancreatic disease. Yes, our government clearly knows the dangers of soy but chooses to look the other way, just as it does with the dangers of hormones and antibiotics used in cow's milk. After all, soy is a multi-billion-dollar industry! Lawmakers whose campaigns are underwritten by agribusinesses use these billions of taxpayer dollars to subsidize the commodities that are the key ingredients of the soybean industry, including the hundreds of items made from them.

An extensive review of two hundred different studies on soy has shown very limited evidence of any health benefits. Soy may cause a small reduction in "bad" LDL cholesterol, and a small percentage of women have reported a minor reduction in hot flashes when using soy during menopause. The American Heart Association backtracked on its earlier support of soy and now says there is no evidence that soy has specific benefits for heart health or for lowering cholesterol.[530]

Sea Vegetables: Nature's Perfect Food

Far away from the Monsanto mafia, with their GMO seeds grown in nutrient-deficient soil, loaded with toxic pesticides and chemical fertilizers tilled with gasoline-guzzling tractors, there still exists the perfect place on Earth for our nutritional needs—the sea! You don't have to DIG through any soil to discover that sea vegetables offer the most nutrients on the planet. In fact, unlike land vegetables that get their minerals from the land below them, sea vegetables get theirs from the water that surrounds them. Sea vegetables are often referred to as sea "weed," but they are nothing like the scavenger weeds that grow on land. They are actually marine algae that grow in the coastal waters.

Humans have deforested our planet to build houses, malls, skyscrapers, roads, airports, and factories. Much of the remaining land that surrounds us is used for landfills contaminated with chemicals, artificial fertilizers, pesticides, and petroleum. But we have not destroyed our ocean waters . . . yet. Every naturally occurring nutrient exists in the sea. This mineral-rich, abundant sanctuary of nourishing water produces plant life containing every nutrient known to man. I emphasized "known to man" because there are elements of the ocean that man has yet to discover. The story of how the B vitamins were detected provides a great example of how scientific discoveries can unfold gradually. In 1925 only one B vitamin was known. By 1975 ten other B family members had been discovered, bringing the total number of B factors to eleven. All of the B vitamins existed before 1925; humans just hadn't discovered them. There's no telling how many more vitamins in the B family scientists will discover in the decades to come.

Sea vegetables are very popular in Asian cultures. Archaeological evidence suggests that Japanese cultures have been consuming sea vegetables for more than ten thousand years. The consumption of health-enhancing sea vegetables has been attributed to Asians' overall health and lower mortality rate. In the eighteenth century, kelp was introduced as a vital source of iodine and was used to succesfully treat goiter (a enlarged thyroid gland). Iodine was later added to table salt to prevent iodine deficiency in the United States, and the rate of goiter drastically declined. Sea vegetables are virtually fat-free, low in calories, and offer the richest sources of minerals in the entire vegetable kingdom. Unlike land vegetables that have declined in their nutritional content because of mineral deficient soil, seawater contains almost the same mineral composition today as it did a billion years ago.[531] The average land plant today contains less than twenty minerals and vitamins, while sea vegetables contain up to ninety-two (460 percent more than land vegetation). Sea vegetables also provide vital fiber, enzymes, proteins, and complex carbohydrates. They contain sodium alginate, which actively helps remove radioactive elements and heavy metals from the body. Sea vegetables offer sterols, which are reported to help lower cholesterol in humans, and they have the only natural source of vitamins D and B12 in the entire vegetable kingdom.[532] [533]

About 70 percent of Earth's surface is covered in water. An average adult's body is 60 percent to 70 percent water; for children that figure is closer to 75 percent.[534] But the similarities don't stop there. Seawater and human blood contain many of the same minerals in similar concentrations. The pH range for blood and seawater are also similar, normally around 7.4. The pioneer researcher who first studied the composition of ocean water compared to human blood was a French doctor, biologist, and biochemist named René Quinton. In 1897 he was credited as the first doctor to study the amazing healing properties of phytoplankton (sea vegetables) and seawater. After successfully treating thousands of patients for many degenerative diseases, the pharmaceutical industry (who wants profits not cures) stepped in and forced him to stop. Sea veggies also contain fucoidans, a natural compound that has been shown to have antibacterial, antifungal, antioxidant, anti-cancer, and blood-thinning properties.[535]

Sea Vegetables, Radiation, and Environmental Pollutants

One of seaweed's most prominent health benefits is its ability to remove radioactive strontium and other heavy metals from our bodies. Brown seaweeds such as kelp contain alginic acid, which binds with the toxins in the intestines, rendering them indigestible, carrying them out of the system through the feces. This means that regularly eating seaweed (especially the brown variety) can effectively reduce toxic elements in our body. In fact, kelp reduces radioactive strontium absorption in the intestines by 50 to 80 percent.[536]

The U.S. Atomic Energy Commission recommended taking five grams of powdered kelp daily for protection from the radioactive fallout from atmospheric nuclear testing. Radiation exposure originates from many sources, not just the fallout from nuclear weapons or power plants. Other sources of radiation exposure include X-rays, microwave ovens, florescent lights, power lines, cell phones, computer monitors, and even your alarm clock. These electro-magnetic radiation (EMR) waves pass through the body, causing DNA damage and the formation of harmful free radicals. Because sea vegetables are rich in both sodium alginate and iodine, they offer a very effective protection from these dangerous radioactive waves.[537] The iodine in sea veggies also keeps the thyroid from absorbing radioactive iodine-131.[538] [539] If this is allowed to accumulate in the body, it can cause thyroid mutations and cancer. Consuming the natural plant-based iodine in sea vegetables protects the thyroid from this dangerous element.

Can You DIG This?

Since growing your own sea veggies isn't possible, they must be purchased from outside sources. You can find fresh sea vegetables at most Japanese sushi restaurants and some health food stores. Check for online retailers of organic produce if you can't find local organic sea vegetables. One of the healthiest sea veggies is called nori. You can find organic strips of this plant at noridirect.com. For fresh seaweed salad shipped to your front door, I recommend alwaysfreshfish.com. Sea vegetation can be added to cold dishes or hot soups, and in the roasted crumbled flake form, they are easily blended and added to smoothies. Nori strips also make a perfect garnish for anything from rice to noodles, pasta, or salad. Simply sprinkle them on just before serving, as no preparation is required.

Organic Garden Time!

If you truly don't want to be at the mercy of subsidized farmers, Big Pharma, Monsanto, and all the chemicals and pesticides they use to grow our plants, fruits, and veggies, there's a simple solution: grow your own! Growing your own organic garden is a great way to save money and truly enjoy eating healthy produce. This gives you the power to take full control of what you eat!

If you live in the city, you can grow plants in window pots. If you live in the country, you can set up a backyard garden, and if you reside in a small apartment, go with a small container garden. You can adapt your garden to what you have available and meet nearly all your produce needs easily and inexpensively. I grow my own organic tomatoes, lemons, carrots, bell peppers, kale, lettuce, cucumbers, and herbs. This saves me hundreds of dollars I'd be spending at the market. I even grow my own stevia, which I use to sweeten the lemonade I make from my freshly squeezed backyard lemons.

For many of you, it's not about the money; it's about that four-letter word we all don't have enough of: T-I-M-E! You just don't have the time to take care of a garden, right? Do you have children or pets? Do you have a house you clean? Do you do your own laundry? Taking care of a garden is less time consuming than these tasks. And, if you have children, they will learn so much and love tending to a garden. It's a terrific family endeavor. Your garden needs regular water and sunshine. Try it, and you'll quickly see, there's nothing more satisfying than eating fruits, vegetables, or other plants grown at home. For all your needs to growing your own organic garden visit groworganic.com.

 Discovery: The nutritional value of our fruits and vegetables is declining. Cost-cutting practices, nitrogen-laden mineral-deficient fertilizers, chemicals, and pesticides used in the harvesting process are among the culprits. Couple that with insidious GMO plants, and we become hard-pressed to find a suitable food. Looking deeper than the topsoil of our land, we can find nature's remaining miracle food—sea vegetables. Or learn to buy organic land plants or, better yet, grow your own.

Instincts: Grandpa said it best, "The fruits and veggies were better when I was a kid." Try this quick test. Eat a tomato grown in your own garden or one that's certified "organic" and compare the color, taste, and texture of a conventionally grown tomato you purchase at the grocery store. Trust your conclusion.

God: When scientists tamper (play Dr. Frankenstein) with our food supply by creating genetically modified seeds and processed fruits and vegetables, we are no longer eating as nature intended.

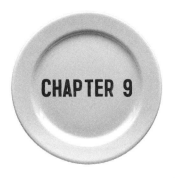

CHAPTER 9

THE GREAT VITAMIN CONTROVERSY
A BILLION DOLLARS DOWN THE DRAIN

"Earth provides enough to satisfy every man's needs,
but not every man's greed."
—Mahatma Gandhi

I used to be a big believer in dietary supplements. After graduating college, I applied everything I learned about supplementation to my practice. Just like the experts taught me, I sent my patients to the health food store to purchase a bag full of pill bottles. Always one to practice what I preach, I personally took twenty-six supplements a day.

However, my views on nutritional supplements took a drastic turn in 1992, after a patient told me a story about her clogged septic tank. The repairman shared with her the cause of this tank blockage: hundreds of undigested daily multivitamins, some of which still had the brand names readable! A few weeks later, a man named Andy came in for his monthly treatment and told me he had been experiencing abdominal pain. After his doctor ran some tests, he asked Andy if he had been taking a high volume of vitamin pills. When Andy told him he was taking thirty supplements a day, the doctor told him to stop because they weren't being digested and were becoming lodged in his intestines. Who on Earth would recommend that Andy swallow thirty pills every day?

Guilty as charged.

After the septic-tank story and the disheartening news from Andy, I began to question *everything* I thought I knew about nutritional supplementation. If these pills weren't being absorbed, then how could they help fight and prevent disease as the textbooks had taught me? Had I been lied to all these years? Had I been lying to myself, my patients, friends, and my family? Sadly, the answer was a resounding "Yes!"

I took my blinders off and investigated the absorption of vitamin and mineral pills. I learned that city disposal plants filter out thousands of pounds of vitamins every year. In the mid-'90s, I discovered in the *Physicians' Desk Reference* (PDR), often referred to as "the Medical Bible," that just 10 percent of a vitamin or mineral pill is absorbed![540] That means for every $100 spent on vitamins, $90 is flushed down the toilet. After conducting tests on seventeen brand-name vitamins for dissolvability, Integrated Biomolecule Corporation, a research institute in Arizona, concluded that none of the supplements tested were considered fully dissolved in two hours. In fact, some of the pills were not completely dissolved even after twelve hours.[541] After you eat food, within an hour it leaves the stomach and begins to travel through the intestines. Since most pills take between two and twelve hours to digest, intact pills are traveling through the intestines. It is not uncommon for radiologists to find undigested vitamin supplements in X-rays of patients' lower intestines.[542] Nurses and hospital orderlies find so many undigested vitamin pills in bedpans, they've nicknamed them "bedpan bullets."

A Tough Pill to Swallow

The human body doesn't fully absorb vitamins and minerals in pill form for several reasons. Rocks and shells (oyster shells, carbonates, oxides, and dolomites) are used to create mineral supplements like calcium, copper, zinc, and iron. But the human body isn't designed to digest rocks and shells, so they pass right through. Nor was the body made to swallow anything whole. Digestion begins in the mouth, not in the stomach. Our teeth crush what we eat into small particles, enabling three digestive enzymes found in saliva to break down and begin assmillating the nutrients, carbohydrates, fats, and proteins before they ever make their way to the stomach. Swallowing a vitamin pill bypasses this critical part of the digestion process.

Add to the mix the binders, fillers, coloring, flow agents, and added coating (glue) that holds the pills together, and it's obvious that pills don't come close in absorbability compared to the nutrients in whole foods. Vitamins from whole foods contain proteins that act as a "chaperone," as Nobel Prize winner Dr. Günter Blobel put it. In 1999, Blobel said that this chaperone protein is the key to getting a vitamin into the bloodstream.[543] Studies have demonstrated that while the body only absorbs 10 percent of synthetic vitamins, whole-food vitamin sources absorb 77 to 93 percent.[544] Almost every vitamin supplement on the market is synthetic and contains no whole-food vitamins. I used to rationalize that absorbing 10 percent of synthetic vitamins was better than nothing, until I learned that some of these vitamins and minerals can lead to severe health issues, hormonal imbalances, lowered immune system, and increased risk of death.

The word *synthetic* means "unnatural or fake." Think of this as being a counterfeit. Chemists in lab coats have tried their best to recreate nutrients from nature, but just like a good counterfeit fifty-dollar bill, it's still a fake! The naked eye may have a hard time detecting counterfeit money, but try putting that counterfeit money into a bill changer. That machine is designed to analyze everything from the weight, composition, and tiny details of its design. When it detects a fake fifty-dollar bill, it spits it right back out. The same holds true with counterfeit nutrients. The cellular receptors in our bloodstream are designed to be just as picky when allowing nutrients access. Because our cells are selective and accept only whole-food (non-counterfeit) sources, most synthetic vitamins are never utilized by our organs, muscles, or bones.[545] Chemists may be smart but, as the saying goes, they can't fool Mother Nature!

Unfortunately, this doesn't stop Big Pharma, who manufactures today's most popular synthetic vitamins, from trying to fool us by labeling their supplements as containing "natural" ingredients. In fact, Big Pharma owns all of the major-brand vitamins. Bayer HealthCare (of aspirin fame) makes One A Day and Flintstones Chewables. Theragran-M is manufactured by Bristol-Myers Squibb. Centrum, the giant in the vitamin industry, is owned by the largest pharmaceutical company, Pfizer. What's worse is the U.S. government doesn't have a definition of *natural*, which means most manufacturers misuse the term. If a product states, "Contains 100 percent natural ingredients," it could be derived from 90 percent synthetic chemicals with only 10 percent from natural sources. Deception? You bet! If you purchase a supplement that says, "Contains whole-food, all-natural ingredients," that could mean that only two whole-food, natural ingredients are mixed with thirty synthetic ones, making the statement true in the eyes of the legal system.

Many people choose supplements in lieu of taking drugs. Some individuals take them to boycott giving their money to Big Pharma. But with Big Pharma in the vitamin business, every time you swallow your vitamin pill, you pass the buck to a pharmaceutical company. Isn't this a conflict of interest? These same companies make billions of dollars in revenue each year on prescription drugs, cancer medications, vaccines, pain meds, and cardiovascular and diabetic treatments. Do they really have an interest in seeing preventative vitamins help us stay healthy and away from doctors? Big Pharma has bought out all of the major vitamin companies on the market so they can get a big piece of the multibillion-dollar pie. Many of the chemicals pharmaceutical companies use to make drugs are also used to make vitamins.

Table 9.1: Composition of Food and Non-Food Vitamins[546]

Vitamin	Examples Of Good Food Sources	Chemicals Used To Make The Synthetic Version
Vitamin A/ Beta-carotene	Carrots	Methanol, benzene; refined oils; acetylene; petroleum esters (also used to make antibiotics)
Vitamin B1	Yeast, rice bran	Coal tar derivatives, hydrochloric acid; acetonitrile with ammonia (also used to make immuno-suppressant drugs)
Vitamin B2	Yeast, rice bran	Synthetically produced with 2N acetic acid (also used to make antimicrobial and antifungal medications)
Vitamin B3	Yeast, rice bran	Coal tar derivatives, ammonia; 3-cyanopyridine (also used to make anticonvulsion and sedation drugs)
Vitamin B5	Yeast, rice bran	Condensing isobutyraldehyde with formaldehyde (also used in cardiovascular medications)

Vitamin	Examples Of Good Food Sources	Chemicals Used To Make The Synthetic Version
Vitamin B6	Yeast, rice bran	Petroleum ester and hydrochloric acid with formaldehyde (also used to make vaccinations)
Vitamin B8 (Inositol)	Rice	Phytin hydrolyzed with calcium hydroxide and sulfuric acid (also used to make antibacterial/microbial medications)
Vitamin B9 (Folate)	Broccoli, rice bran	Processed with petroleum derivatives and acids; acetylene (also used to make sedatives)
Vitamin B12	Yeast	Cobalamins reacted with cyanide (also used to make ulcer medications)
Vitamin "BX" (PABA)	PABA yeast	Coal tar oxidized with nitric acid from ammonia (also used to make psoriasis medications)
Choline	Yeast, rice bran	Tartaric acid, ethylene and ammonia with HCl (also used to make cough medicines)
Vitamin C	Acerola cherries, citrus fruits	Hydrogenated sugar processed with acetone (also used to make nail-polish remover)
Vitamin D	Yeast	Irradiated animal fat/cattle brains or solvently extracted
Vitamin E	Rice, vegetable oils	Trimethylhydroquinone with isophytol (also used to make acne and skin medications)
Vitamin K	Cabbage	Coal tar derivative; produced with p-allelic-nickel (also used to make eczema medications)

Can You DIG This?

Try this simple experiment at home. Take your multivitamin and place it on the countertop next to a sliced banana or apple. Come back in a few hours, and you will notice that the fruit has turned brown and withered. Why? Because at a cellular level it's ALIVE, and after being exposed to the free radicals in the air, it begins to oxidize and die. Now look at your multivitamin sitting next to these pieces of exposed fruit. Whether it's a One A Day, Centrum, Theragran-M, or a Flintstone's Chewable, you will see no change in color. No browning or withering away because nothing can die that is never alive to begin with. Come back the next day, and you will still see no change. Next week, next month, the dead vitamins will still be dead. These multivitamins contain no fruits, vegetables, herbs, or whole grains—not a single natural vitamin, phytochemical, macro mineral, enzyme, or amino acid exists. When you swallow your multivitamin pill, you are ingesting chemicals that used to be inside of a test tube.

"And Other Ingredients . . ."

Many potentially dangerous chemicals are used to make nutritional supplements, but you'll never know about them because they're usually generically listed on the ingredients label as "other ingredients." These "other ingredients" include binders that hold the substances together; synthetic dyes, which give them their color; and coatings of plastic derivatives or shellac (made from ground insects) to make pills easier to swallow, prevent them from dissolving too soon in your mouth, and cover up their smelly active and chemical ingredients. Further, "active ingredients" include carnauba wax—similar to what is used to coat wood floors and boats—to give the pill that shiny appearance. The wax coat also keeps the pills intact during the phases of cleaning, inspecting, counting, and bottling them at the manufacturer's plant. Vitamin pills also have to stand up to being shaken by the consumer every day when pouring the pills into his or her hand. To solve that problem, many vitamins contain flow agents to keep the supplement from sticking during production and bottling. This allows the machinery to run at maximum speeds, requiring minimal cleaning, and thereby maximizing profits. The Organic Consumer's Association estimates that at least 95 percent of off-the-shelf multivitamins are synthetic and contain unnatural additives, fillers, and dyes. Even supplements labeled "natural" contain traces of artificial chemicals.[547]

Unfortunately, many manufacturers fail to list these "other ingredients," and even when they do, some are disguised using vague terms such as gum, gelatin, emulsifiers, stabilizers, anti-caking agents, or sometimes as "other unnatural ingredients." The additives used to make vitamins are also used to manufacture items like shaving gel, cement, sheetrock, paint, laundry detergent, nail polish, and tires.

Humans weren't born in a pharmaceutical lab, and our nutritional products shouldn't be created in one. Consumers have been brainwashed into believing their supplements are "natural" and "prevent disease," when in fact they contain the same chemicals used to make inedible items that you would never fathom putting into your mouth. Even if a supplement contains healthful whole-food nutrients, the "other ingredients" may reduce their good benefits, creating an unhealthful balance within the body. Sadly, even informed consumers find it difficult to rely on labels for accuracy. The FDA is not responsible for labels' accuracy, and the law doesn't require any nutritional manufacturer to submit proof of either what's inside or its safety or potency.

The following was extracted from the FDA website:

> Under the Dietary Supplement Health and Education Act of 1994 (DSHEA), the dietary supplement or dietary ingredient manufacturer is responsible for ensuring that a dietary supplement or ingredient is safe before it is marketed. FDA is responsible for taking action against any unsafe dietary supplement product after it reaches the market. Generally, manufacturers do not need to register their products with FDA nor get FDA approval before producing or selling dietary supplements. Manufacturers must make sure that product label information is truthful and not misleading.[548]

This means that the FDA is responsible for taking action against any unsafe dietary supplement product *after* it reaches the market and causes a concern. Because manufacturers aren't held accountable, anyone can create their own nutritional product line and sell it on the market. Several years ago, it was discovered that a manufacturer in Florida was selling bottles of the herb echinacea, but the capsules actually contained only grass and hay! Okay, that's not harmful to the body, just the wallet, but sometimes the opposite takes place and consumers can get more than they bargained for. One example of such a case is a product called Total Body Formula, which stated on the label that it contained the mineral selenium. And indeed it did. The problem is the amount of selenium was in milligrams (mg) instead of micrograms (mcg). Since it takes a thousand micrograms to make one milligram, Total Body Formula contained lethal dosages of selenium! In fact, it caused hair loss, heart dysfunction, and stage 3 kidney failure! The Wright Group, the research and development company for Total Body Formula, was supposed to test the product before it went to market. Instead, the company issued a fake certificate of analysis (COA).

In May 2012, *Dateline NBC* did an investigation on Total Body Formula. Investigative reporter Chris Hansen interviewed Frank Jaksch, co-founder and chief scientific officer of ChromaDex Corp—a third-party lab that analyzes the quantity and quality of nutritional products. Jaksch said many nutritional manufacturers do a "dry lab," which means the samples that come in go straight into the trash and a fake COA is rubber stamped as "tested and approved."[549] Millions are risking their lives by blindly taking products without knowing for sure the ingredients' quality and quantity. Manufacturers of nutritional products are so unregulated that, in one case, to cut corners from purchasing an expensive filtering device, one manufacturer used nylon panty hose to filter out unwanted debris from their formulas. That's right, women's panty hose![550] Now that's what I call a bit of *a stretch*.

Liquid Nutrition

A liquid alternative means not ingesting binders, fillers, or wax coatings, and, therefore, would digest better than pills. Also, a whole-food liquid product would bypass the digestion issues associated with gagging down a bunch of pills. It's also convenient and better absorbed. The challenge with liquid nutritional products is they are often pasteurized, and this heat process destroys many of the whole-food nutrients. They also contain de-foaming agents and unnatural chemical preservatives.

Liquid products contain water, which is the number-one breeding ground for bacteria, so chemical preservatives are used. Sodium benzoate is the most common preservative/antimicrobial agent. This chemical is also used to make fireworks and silver polish! As soon as you open a liquid product, it is exposed to air, which breeds bacteria, yeast, and fungi. Common sense time . . . if sodium benzoate is used to kill living bacteria, wouldn't it also destroy the natural components found in fruits, vegetables, and herbs? You will find wonderful liquid products on the market, containing whole-food, health-enhancing exotic super fruits like acai berry, goji berry, mangosteen, and noni fruit. Leading nutritionists (myself included) consider these the most nutrient-rich fruits in the entire world. But they aren't supposed to be eaten mixed with antimicrobial fluid. Natural alternatives to sodium benzoate do exist, but the cost is significantly higher than that of sodium benzoate, which is why most manufacturers go with the unnatural cheaper chemicals.

Another chemical used in liquid vitamin supplements is a de-foaming agent called polydimethylsiloxane. De-foaming agents allow the bottles to be filled at high speeds. Without de-foaming, your liquid supplement would look like a cappuccino half filled with foam. Unfortunately, de-foaming agents aren't required to be listed on the label because they are not considered part of the actual ingredients. The good news is this chemical has not been shown to have any toxic effects in humans. That is, unless it's heated to temperatures in excess of 150 degrees. When that happens, dimethylsiloxane breaks down into formaldehyde. Yes, that's the same stuff used to embalm dead people! Liquid products are required to go through a pasteurization process, which means they are heated to over 160 degrees, which can cause de-foaming agents to turn into corpse embalming juice!

Fortify Me?

I remember one day asking a patient if she took any vitamins or minerals, and she told me, "I don't need to. I eat something every morning that supplies me with essential vitamin A, thiamin, riboflavin, folic acid, iron, and vitamin B6." When I asked her what gave her this daily nourishment she replied, "Pop-Tarts!"

There's a difference between the vitamins listed on the label of food items and those that are naturally occurring. The former are called "fortified" nutrients, which means they are derived from the same worthless chemical compounds found in the daily multivitamins discussed earlier. Sadly, most people believe the nutrients in their vitamin bottle, their cornflakes, or weight-loss shake are natural. Not so. The fact is that 95 percent of dietary supplements on the market are not derived from any natural sources. The true definitions of the terms *natural* or *whole food* mean the foods are derived from something that is alive and contains a complex family of vitamins and micronutrients (known and unknown), exactly as they are found in nature. These natural nutrients contain a synergistic balance that the body recognizes for proper absorption and optimal utilization. Nutrients from synthetic chemical compounds lack the synergist properties created by nature to help the body properly utilize the nutrients it contains.

Rather than go through the entire alphabet of dietary supplements and the health risks of taking synthetic nutrients, I will provide information on the four most popular—vitamins C, D, and E, and calcium. People buy these four nutrients more than all the others combined.

DNA Destroyer: Vitamin C

Vitamin C is the most popular supplement in the world. When I lecture across the country, I ask people to raise their hands if they are taking, or have taken, a vitamin C supplement; almost every hand goes up. When I ask people to share why, the two most common reasons are "To protect against the common cold" and "To protect against cancer!" Most of those raising their hands have never actually taken vitamin C but rather ascorbic acid, its synthetic chemical counterfeit created in a lab. As with other counterfeits created in a lab, most vitamin C supplements are produced using a concoction of toxic chemicals you would never consider putting in your mouth.

"Vitamin C causes genetic damage!" read the headlines. This *New York Times* article sent shockwaves through millions of vitamin advocates who would learn that ascorbic acid was damaging their DNA. In 1998 British researchers found that 500 milligrams of vitamin C daily produces cellular damage and cancer-inducing free radicals. Vitamin C supplements convert harmless ferric iron found in the body into harmful ferrous iron, which can lead to heart damage and other organ dysfunction.

Dr. Victor Herbert, from the Mount Sinai School of Medicine, told the *New York Times*, "Unlike the vitamin C naturally present in foods like orange juice, vitamin C as a supplement is not an antioxidant." He went on to say, "Vitamin C naturally present in food has no [negative] oxidizing effects." Vitamin C supplements in large doses have been linked to genetic damage as far back as the mid-1970s. In the late '90s, Canadian researchers discovered vitamin C damages genetic material in three systems: bacterial cells, human cells grown in test tubes, and live mice.[551] For years I took

3,000 milligrams of ascorbic acid every day. That was the amount I learned was ideal for optimal health and to keep me from getting cancer. Here I was taking 600 percent above the daily dosage found to cause genetic damage linked to cancer!

My office was located fifteen minutes from Takeda Chemical Industries, Ltd (the U.S. office), Japan's largest pharmaceutical company. Some of Takeda's U.S. products include the cancer drug, Lupron; the ulcer medication, Prevacid; the blood-pressure drug, Blopress; and the popular antibiotic, Cephalosporin. In addition to the drugs Takeda has created, they also manufactured ascorbic acid for vitamin supplements, cereals, and sodas. At the time the aforementioned article was published, I was treating one of Takeda's top chemist PhDs. During his next visit, I handed him the *New York Times* article and asked, "What do you think about this? This says the vitamin C you are making is destroying people's genes!"

His reply? "Oh, it doesn't surprise me. If you knew the toxic chemicals we use to make ascorbic acid, you would understand how it could damage a person's genes. I personally would never put the stuff into my body!"

Exactly how is ascorbic acid made? First they start with sorbitol and add tiny beetles, which are flown in from overseas. Their excrement (that is, bug crap) is treated with acetone, which is the same chemical used in nail-polish remover. Then perchloric acid is added to the mix, the same ingredient used in rocket fuels and explosives. These ingredients are filtered out and then benzene is added (a toxic chemical used in gasoline). It's distilled and centrifuged before caustic bleach and nickel are added to the recipe, along with the chemical toluene, a poisonous solvent used in glues and paints.[552] [553] Then these chemicals are filtered and processed and sold to you as vitamin C (ascorbic acid). Your kids eat them in their toaster pastries; you eat them when you take vitamins and drink sodas or fruit drinks.

Let me reiterate: natural vitamin C doesn't cause genetic damage; only the kind made by chemists in a lab does. I confirmed what the chemist told me was true and wrote an article on the topic for a local publication, *Encore* magazine. After reading this article in my waiting room, one of my patients, who owns a plumbing company, said to me, "Now it all makes sense! I was the plumbing contractor for Takeda, and they had me put in titanium pipes! I never understood why manufacturing vitamin C would require unorthodox extra-strength pipes, but after reading about all the toxic chemicals being used, it makes sense now. Had they used regular piping, those caustic chemicals would have eaten holes in them in less than a month!" Folks, what do you think happens to our delicate colon, blood vessels, organs, and muscles when we ingest this synthetic ascorbic acid? We don't have the option of lining ourselves with titanium.

If you're drinking nutritional products, sodas, juices, or vitamin supplements with "ascorbic acid" on the label—stop! While the benefits of vitamin C from nature have been shown to help the body stay healthy and combat disease, dozens of double-blind studies prove supplementing with ascorbic acid does not help combat, cure, or prevent anything . . . not even the common cold.[554]

Vitamin C: "C" for Corruption

Who created all the vitamin-C hype? That credit goes to a man named Dr. Linus Pauling, chemist, biochemist, peace activist, author, and educator. Pauling received more than two dozen awards and honors during his career. He's considered one of the most influential chemists in history and ranks among the most important scientists of the twentieth century. He's largely responsible for the widespread belief that people needed a minimum of 1,000 milligrams of vitamin C to reduce the incidence of colds (the RDA of vitamin C is 60 milligrams).[555] In 1976 he revised his recommendations and said people needed a minimum of 3,000 milligrams per day of vitamin C to be effective against cancer, heart disease, and other illnesses.[556] Pauling himself reportedly took 12,000 milligrams of vitamin C every day![557] Let's see if those numbers line up with how much vitamin C the human body is designed to take. The highest natural source of vitamin C comes from an orange, which offers approximately 30 milligrams of vitamin C. If the human body requires 3,000 milligrams of vitamin C per day, that would be equivalent to eating one hundred oranges! Do you think the human body was designed to eat that many oranges per day? Dr. Pauling took the vitamin C equivalent of eating four hundred oranges every day!

While Dr. Pauling said he was using mega doses of ascorbic acid to cure cancer, the Mayo Clinic conducted three double-blind studies involving 367 patients with advanced cancer. Patients given 10,000 milligrams of ascorbic acid daily did no better than those given a placebo.[558] Pauling's long-time associate, Arthur Robinson, Ph.D., eventually blew the whistle showing Pauling's suggested mega dosages of vitamin C was deceptive. According to an investigative report published in *Nutrition Forum Newsletter*, Robinson's own research led him to conclude in 1978 that the momentous doses of vitamin C being recommended by Pauling might actually cause cancer in mice.[559] After Robinson shared this with Pauling, he was asked to leave the institute. Pauling had all Robinson's incriminating research destroyed.

Throughout his career, Pauling was opposed to natural vitamin C and attacked the health-food industry for misleading its customers by saying "natural vitamin C is a waste of money" and synthetic vitamin C (ascorbic acid) was identical, cheaper, and just as potent. Why would Pauling be so supportive of fake vitamin C instead of that found in nature? Was there any ulterior motive? For that answer, let's follow the money. The Linus Pauling Institute of Science and Medicine was founded in 1973 and operated under that name for twenty-two years. During that time, Pauling's largest financial supporter was none other than Hoffmann-La Roche, the pharmaceutical giant that produces a huge share of the world's ascorbic acid. That's right; Big Pharma financially supported Pauling's work. Had Tropicana orange juice donated more money to Pauling's institute, perhaps he would have taken a stance that said oranges were a better source of vitamin C. He remained adamant that taking massive amounts of ascorbic acid every day would prevent everything from the common cold to cancer. In August of 1994, Dr. Linus Pauling died . . . from *cancer*.

Natural Whole-Food Sources of Vitamin C

- Citrus fruits, red sweet peppers, kiwi, strawberries, and Brussels sprouts
- When choosing a vitamin C supplement, avoid supplements with ascorbic acid, Ester-C, and ascorbyl palmitate. Look for an all-natural supplement using whole-food sources derived from the acerola cherries, rose hips (fruit from a rose plant), camu camu berries, or other fruits/vegetables that are naturally rich in vitamin C. Two great options I recommend are Complex C by MegaFood Inc. (www.megafood.com) and Pure Radiance C by The Synergy Company (www.synergy-co.com).

Calcium Supplements: Help or Harm?

Osteoporosis (lack of calcium in the bones) is the fourth-leading cause of death among women, following heart disease, cancer, and stroke.[560] Death from osteoporosis is usually a result of complications that may follow bone fractures. Calcium supplements to the rescue? Unfortunately, no. Most calcium supplements on the market today are worthless garbage, doing absolutely nothing but giving people false hope and hype on building strong bones. The only thing being "strengthened" is the bank accounts of the manufacturers who are deceiving people. Most calcium supplements are made from rocks and shells, which we've already determined the human body was not designed to digest. The most popular calcium sold in America is called "oyster shell" calcium. Do you think our ancestors walked along the beach picking up pieces of oyster shells, crushing them up, and swallowing them with a glass of water? Nope. Why would modern man take oyster-shell calcium? Calcium in rock and shell form is less than 5 percent absorbed. So if you are taking 1,000 milligrams of calcium, you are getting 50 milligrams. Of that 50 milligrams that does end up in the bloodstream, none of it is allowed access into the bones. Calcium is an alkaline mineral and requires an acid to absorb it; therefore, scientists have tried to add acids like citric, gluconic, and lactic acid into our supplements. These additions do help the rocks and shells absorb better into your body, but do you really want them there? Rocks and shells circulating around the body could end up sticking to the arteries, form stones and spurs, and become a building block for fibroids and cysts.[561]

Oyster shells have also been shown to contain small amounts of lead, which is a toxin. Reports of lead in dolomite (another rock calcium source) have also shown to contain lead.[562] How does lead end up in calcium tablets? Many calcium products labeled as "natural" come from mineral beds that naturally contain lead. Researchers at the University of Florida at Gainesville reported that eight of the twenty-two calcium products they tested—including popular national brands such as Caltrate 600—contained lead, which can lead to anemia, high blood pressure, and brain and kidney damage in adults, and developmental damage in children.[563]

Rocks and shells are not whole foods and do not contain the balance of other vitamins and minerals needed to absorb calcium into the bones, such as zinc, magnesium, vitamin D, phosphorus, and boron. The body needs whole-food calcium sources in order to get completely absorbed by the body (not the measly 5 percent absorption of most calcium supplements).

Natural Whole-Food Sources of Calcium

- Green leafy vegetables are a perfect example because plants take the inorganic calcium "rocks" in the ground and convert it into living, organic calcium.
- Sea vegetables are another great source of calcium thanks to the rocks, shells, and coral lining the bottom of the sea. Plants convert this calcium into an organic source usable by the body.
- When we eat fish that have eaten other fish or krill and shrimp that has fed off the calcium-rich plankton and seaweed, we are consuming usable whole-food calcium. Scientists have gotten this crazy idea that because rocks, shells, dolomite, and coral have high calcium content, we can go right to these nonliving sources for our calcium needs. How absurd! When humans consume rocks and shells, it can lead to major health issues.
- Chia seeds are flavorless and make great additions to salads, soups, veggies, and smoothies.
- Sesame seeds are an excellent source of calcium. Sesame seed butter, also known as tahini, is another option and a great alternative to peanut butter.
- Dried plums are another good source of calcium. Ironically, plums—and by extension prunes—are one of the few fruits that contain very small amounts of oxalates, a substance that can bind to calcium, thus making it less bioavailable.
- A calcium supplement I recommend is called AlgaeCal (www.algaecal.com). This is a wild-harvested, plant-sourced calcium derived from a South American marine algae called *Algas calcareas*. Researchers from Harvard Medical School and the University of Connecticut collaborated on a landmark study published in the peer-reviewed journal *Molecular and Cellular Biochemistry*. In direct head-to-head tests, the scientists compared the effects of AlgaeCal with the two top sellers, calcium carbonate and calcium citrate. The study results showed that AlgaeCal increased alkaline phosphatase activity 200 percent more effectively than calcium carbonate, and 250 percent better than calcium citrate. In addition, AlgaeCal

outperformed calcium carbonate and calcium citrate by 400 percent! It also increased osteoblasts to produce new bone-building cells.[564] Research shows this plant-based calcium also increased bone density of postmenopausal females in a six- to twelve-month time span.[565]

The Big "D-Lemma": Vitamin D

We have become a "vitamin D-ficient" nation. According to the National Vitamin D Council, 70 percent of Americans are vitamin D deficient and this trend is reaching epidemic proportions.[566] [567] Technically, vitamin D isn't a "vitamin"; it's actually a hormone produced by the body when it's exposed to sunshine. Vitamin D helps ensure adequate serum calcium to aid in mineralization of bone. Without sufficient vitamin D, bones become brittle. In 1918 it was discovered as the agent that prevents rickets, a disease of the skeleton. It was later found to be what regulates calcium absorption from food. Since then, scientists have tried their best to recreate the "sunshine vitamin" in a laboratory.

The first attempt was eradicating fungal sterols into vitamin D1, but this was later found to be ineffective. Then, they recreated vitamin D2 (ergocalciferol), synthesized by plants. Later, scientists would discover vitamin D3 (cholecalciferol), which is the type of vitamin D that is synthesized by the skin in humans when exposed to ultraviolet-B rays from sunlight. Scientists found that vitamin D3 also has antitumor properties and prevents cancer. A growing body of research suggests that vitamin D3 plays a significant role in the prevention and treatment of type 1 and type 2 diabetes, hypertension, glucose intolerance, multiple sclerosis, cancer, and many other medical conditions.[568]

Synthetically made vitamin D3, although better than synthetic D1 and D2, still doesn't offer the same benefits as the vitamin D3 found in nature. In fact, when attained naturally by the body, vitamin D3 is ten times more effective than the man-made counterfeit.[569] Some manufacturers tried adding two times the amount of synthetic vitamin D in each capsule, thinking this would increase its potency; however, neonatal problems and hypercalcemia (dangerous levels of calcium in the blood stream) resulted.[570] More is not always better. Many doctors prescribe 50,000 IUs of vitamin D2 to patients, which is more than 1,700 percent above the recommended daily allowance (RDA). Why are they prescribing so much D2 when science has proven it's not as effective as D3? Because 50,000 IU of D2 is only available through a prescription. Big Pharma wants a piece of D pie! They know seven out of ten people are deficient, and instead of your doctor telling you to get more sunshine or stop by your local health food store, it's modus operandi time—and they tell you to get a prescription!

Causes of Vitamin D Deficiency

To get adequate amounts of vitamin D, the body only requires ten to fifteen minutes of sunshine per day. Just like a plant needs sunshine to thrive, so do humans. When a plant is deprived of sunlight for too long, it will eventually die. Likewise, when we deprive ourselves of vital sunlight, our vitamin D levels decline, causing an increase in mortality.[571]

People are more vitamin D deficient than ever in history because we avoid sunshine like the plague.[572] Society has been brainwashed into believing that the sun is an evil cancer-causing entity that must be avoided at all costs. That is absolutely not true. Sunshine produces vitamin D, which helps us combat cancer. The use of sunscreen with a sun protection factor (SPF) of 8 or higher inhibits more than 95 percent of vitamin D production in the skin.[573] Only *overexposure* to sunshine (when it leads to sunburn) carries any risks. Not getting enough sunshine also causes an increased risk of colorectal and breast cancers.

According to researchers from the Moore's Cancer Center at the University of California, San Diego, if vitamin D levels among populations worldwide were increased, 600,000 cases of breast and colorectal cancers could be prevented each year. Even beyond cancer, the researchers pointed out that increased levels of vitamin D3 could prevent diseases that claim nearly one million lives throughout the world each year.[574] In 1992 Dr. Gordon Ainsleigh published a paper in the journal *Preventive Medicine* in which he reviewed fifty years' worth of medical literature on cancer and the sun. He concluded that the benefits of regular sun exposure (fifteen minutes per day) outweigh the risks of squamous-basal skin cancer, accelerated aging, and melanoma. Regular moderate sunbathing would result in a decrease of breast and colon cancer death rates in the United States by one-third. Even just exposing your face or arms will absorb enough Vitamin D into your system.[575]

It's not sunshine, but the lack of it that is killing us. The cosmetic skin care industry has misled the public into believing that ultraviolet (UV) exposure is harmful and causes aged skin and skin cancer. The truth is there is no research showing that regular, nonburning exposure to UV sunlight poses any risk of skin damage or cancer. But even scarier, there is no evidence that sunscreen protects people from skin cancer at all. Malignant melanoma has been found more frequently in sunscreen users compared to nonusers.[576] Other studies have found that fair-skinned people that used more sunscreen have a higher incidence of skin cancer.[577] [578] A wide range of public health agencies (including the FDA) have found very little evidence that sunscreen prevents most types of skin cancer. The International Agency for Research on Cancer says the best choice for skin cancer prevention is to avoid getting burned by wearing clothing and hats and making use of shade as primary barriers to UV radiation.[579]

It seems as if everything on the market has sunscreen protection added to it to keep us safe from getting skin cancer. From face and body creams, to makeup and shampoos—even some nail polishes have added sun protection. Heaven forbid you absorb a little sunshine through your fingernails! Many retailers, including GAP and L.L. Bean, sell shirts, shorts, and other clothing infused with sun-blocking titanium and zinc oxide. Apparel stores sell shoes with added sun protection. For those of you who don't want to spend money on sun-protecting clothing, you can use your own. Sun Guard, a laundry additive, contains Tinosorb, an ingredient that its manufacturer, Phoenix Brands, says gives everyday clothes UVA and UVB protection (up to twenty washes)!

We live in constant fear of the sun and go to great lengths to make sure we remain hidden from its "dangerous" rays. People spend billions of dollars on sunscreen protection, yet cases of skin cancer continue to rise. Since the 1970s, skin cancer has increased 700 percent. More than thirteen thousand people a year develop malignant melanoma—the most deadly type of skin cancer. The total is expected to surge to twenty thousand a year by 2027. In 1975 that figure was only 1,800.[580] Research published in the *European Journal of Cancer* found regular, moderate sun exposure may actually *reduce* the risk of melanoma, stating that people who spend time in the sun are *less likely* to develop skin cancer.[581]

Why did we have less skin cancer forty years ago, during a time when we didn't use sunblock? For the answer to that question, simply look at some of the ingredients used in sunblock. The items people buy to *protect us* from cancer may actually be *causing us* to get cancer!

What you put on your skin gets absorbed into your bloodstream. The Environmental Working Group (EWG) compiled a review of more than 1,700 market brands of sunscreen products and found that 84 percent of sunscreen products offer inadequate protection from the sun, or contain ingredients of significant safety concerns.[582] One of these ingredients is called octinoxate, which has been shown to increase sun sensitivity and lead to estrogen and thyroid hormonal imbalances. This can lead to a lowered immune system, making you more prone to cancer. Another chemical used in sunblock is oxybenzone, which has been shown to release free radicals that actually contribute to the development of skin cancer. Oxybenzone has been associated with a significant drop in testosterone levels in men during a one-week application period. Low serum testosterone levels are predictive of prostate cancer.[583] Fifty-six percent of beach and sport sunscreens contain oxybenzone.[584]

Another dangerous chemical found in 80 percent of commercial sun block is called octylmethoxycinnamate. This chemical was found to kill mouse cells even at low doses. Recent studies on childhood illnesses linked the chemical to a possible cause of ADHD, asthma, and allergies.[585] Retinyl palmitate is another high-risk ingredient found in many sunscreens. According to a CNN report, "Government-funded studies have found that this *retinyl palmitate* may increase risk of skin cancer when used on sun-exposed skin."[586] According to EWG's chemical database, retinoic acid increases following topical application of retinyl palmitate and is listed as moderately hazardous due to potential toxicity to organ systems.

Professor Julia Newton Bishop, an epidemiologist who led the research on weekend sun exposure, said, "It seems regular exposure helps the skin adapt and protect itself against the harmful effects of sunshine. Increased levels of vitamin D made in the skin while exposed to sunlight are also protective."[587] There is no substantial evidence that sunscreen protects against any of the three forms of skin cancer, and more and more research is showing quite the opposite. While sunscreens do help keep you from burning, the dangerous cancer-causing ingredients of sunscreen along with the fact that they don't allow cancer-protecting vitamin D absorption, are doing more harm than good. When outside for extended periods of time, you are far better off covering up your skin than using sunblock! One of the best ways to prevent burning is to get sunshine exposure after 2 p.m., since that is when the body produces more vitamin D from the sun. We only need ten to fifteen minutes of sunshine each day to get enough vitamin D. Quite interesting, considering the skin begins to burn after twenty minutes in the sun. If you are out in the sunshine longer than this, simply put on protective clothing, use an umbrella, and wear a hat. If you want to apply sun protection, stay away from sunblock products made from harsh chemicals that are linked to cancer.

Natural Source of Vitamin D

- In addition to sunshine, a select number of foods contain the whole-food natural form of vitamin D: shiitake and button mushrooms, mackerel, salmon, herring, sardines, tuna, catfish, cod liver oil, eggs, and sea vegetables.
- For a Vitamin D supplement, I recommend Megafood (www.megafood.com). For skin products, I like Raw Elements (www.rawelementsusa.com). Its maker uses all-natural and certified-organic ingredients, which they claim will nourish and protect the skin from being burned. The EWG has given Raw Elements their #1 rating for safety and efficacy. The product doesn't restrict the body's vitamin D absorption the way other products do.

Vitamin E

Let's look at one more example of the sinister side effects of counterfeit supplements—vitamin E. This vitamin is essential to body metabolism, cell growth, and function. It is also a potent antioxidant crucial in the formation of red blood cells. We've been told this vitamin helps support the brain as well as the cardiovascular, reproductive, and respiratory systems. All this is true. Vitamin E is a very important nutrient; however, that is true only when you get it from *naturally occurring* sources. The liver is picky and accepts vitamin E sources from food more readily than it does from the counterfeit version made by scientists.[588]

Researchers at Oregon State University, Corvallis, found the human body retains natural vitamin E three times better than synthetic forms.[589]

Natural vitamin E in whole-food form is called d-alpha tocopherol. Synthetic (counterfeit) vitamin E is labeled as dl-alpha tocopheryl or dl-tocopheryl acetate. The differences are easy when you know what to look for. When looking for a natural form of Vitamin E, always select one that is "d" (not "dl") and the word tocopherol ends with "ol" (not "yl"). As with the other vitamins we've discussed, when you fractionize pieces of a vitamin complex in a lab, you don't create the intricate synergistic properties needed for the proper absorption and assimilation of vitamin E. Even before birth, a fetus refuses to use synthetic vitamin E compared to natural sources. The *American Journal of Clinical Nutrition* published research that shows, "The placenta and the fetal liver are able to discriminate between natural vitamin E and the synthetic version.[590]

Vitamin E Causes Prostate Cancer

Many men regularly take vitamin E supplements because they have been shown to help decrease hair loss, lower LDL, reduce inflammation, combat arthritis, and increase libido.[591] [592] But a study of 35,000 men was conducted using the synthetic (dl-alpha tocopheryl) rather than the natural, whole-food source (d-alpha tocopherol). The results reported by the *Journal of the American Medical Association (JAMA)*, showed that vitamin E supplements cause an increased risk of prostate cancer among healthy men.[593] The dosage found to put men at risk is 400 international units (IU), which happens to be the amount found in most over-the-counter vitamin supplements. Except for skin cancer, prostate cancer is the most common type of cancer in men in the United States. Eric Klein, M.D., an internationally renowned prostate cancer expert who served as the national study coordinator, stated, "There is no reason for men in the general population to take the dose of vitamin E used in the trial, as the supplements have shown no benefit and some very real risks."

Vitamin E Increases Risk of Untimely Death

Researchers at Johns Hopkins report that high doses of vitamin E supplements, in excess of 400 IU, is associated with a higher overall risk of dying. This study, published in the *Annals of Internal Medicine*, took place between 1993 and 2004 and involved more than 136,000 patients. Risk of death was estimated by comparing the mortality rates of takers of high doses of vitamin E and those taking a placebo (sugar pill). Follow-up periods ranged from 1.4 years to 8.2 years. When the data for these trials was re-evaluated, nine of eleven trials involving 400 IU per day or more of vitamin E showed an increased mortality risk.[594]

Lead author Edgar R. Miller III, M.D., Ph.D. said, "Our study results do not support the use of high-dose vitamin E supplements. If people are taking a multivitamin, they should make sure it contains no more than a low dose of vitamin E. A lot of people take vitamins because they believe it will benefit their health in the long term and prolong life. But our study shows that use of high-dose vitamin E supplements certainly did not prolong life but was associated with a higher risk of death!"[595]

Vitamin E supplements typically contain 400 to 800 IU, which has been shown to be too high and dangerous. What a difference from what I was taught in college! The nutritional experts that I learned from recommended we take *up to* 1,500 IU per day for the health of the heart. Not so, according to a Physicians' Health Study, which assessed the effects of vitamin E supplements (dl-alpha tocopheryl) on the risk of major cardiovascular disease among 14,641 male physicians. Compared with placebo, vitamin E did not have an effect on the prevention of major cardiovascular events. In fact, vitamin E was associated with an *increased risk* of hemorrhagic stroke![596] Both the Johns Hopkins research and the Physicians' Health Study were conducted using the synthetic and not the natural (d-alpha tocopherol) form of vitamin E.

Vitamin E Linked to Osteoporosis

Scientists discovered a link between consumption of vitamin E and osteoporosis. Giving mice increased doses of the vitamin at a level similar to that found in supplements caused the animals' bones to thin. The mice developed osteoporosis after eight weeks on the diet, which had levels of vitamin E significantly higher than those found in a mouse's natural diet, according to the study, published in the March 2012 edition of the journal *Nature Medicine*. This research showed vitamin E stimulates the osteoclasts, which causes the bones' cells to degrade and lose their strength.[597] Again, this test was conducted using the synthetic source of vitamin E and not whole-food vitamin E sources.

Natural, Whole-Food Sources of Vitamin E

When taking natural, whole-food sources of vitamin E, there are no deaths or associated risks of cancer or fear of getting brittle bones! Natural sources of vitamin E (d-alpha tocopherol) include wheat germ, nuts, seeds, olives, spinach, asparagus, and other green leafy vegetables.

The Wonders of Wheatgrass

Wheatgrass is nature's perfect multivitamin. It is the name of tender green shoots of the wheat plant. The grass is composed of the young shoots of wheat before stalks form a head with grain. It contains no wheat gluten and offers phenomenal healing properties. Wheatgrass is a superfood containing an array of nourishing vitamins, minerals, amino acids, enzymes, and fiber.

Wheatgrass contains high amounts of vitamins A, E, and B-complex, as well as many minerals and trace elements including calcium, phosphorus, selenium, sodium, potassium, magnesium, iron, and zinc. Wheatgrass boasts twelve amino acids, including the eight essential amino acids: phenylalanine, valine, threonine, tryptophan, isoleucine, methionine, leucine, and lysine. Essential amino acids are vital to the cells of the body, but they are something the body cannot create and, therefore, must be obtained through diet. A deficiency of just one amino acid can result in allergies, low energy, sluggish digestion, poor resistance to infection, and premature aging. Wheatgrass contains three main digestive enzymes—amylase, protease, and lipase—to break down carbohydrates, proteins, and fats.

Wheatgrass juice is very rich in chlorophyll, which helps the blood carry oxygen to all cells. It is very similar to the hemoglobin molecule of human blood. Chlorophyll cleanses the liver, tissues, and cells and purifies the blood. Wheatgrass juice helps remove toxic heavy metals from the blood such as lead, mercury, and aluminum. Chlorophyll is a great detoxifier because it breaks up impacted matter in the colon and helps fight infection. It's vital to digestion, aids in mental clarity, and acts as a defense against anaerobic bacteria.[598]

Chlorophyll in wheatgrass also stimulates peristalsis, the muscle movement necessary for natural elimination. In addition, it assists the lining of the intestines by neutralizing toxic substances and facilitating easy elimination by its mild diuretic effects. Chlorophyll in wheatgrass also increases the functions of the heart and affects the vascular system. It raises the basic nitrogen exchange and is therefore a tonic that cannot be compared with any other nutrient.[599] [600]

Finally, wheatgrass has been called "the king of alkaline foods" because of its highly alkalizing effect. Wheatgrass juice has been used clinically to treat digestive disorders such as ulcerative colitis and irritable bowel syndrome. A clinical double-blind study on wheatgrass therapy for ulcerative colitis showed regular wheatgrass juice therapy significantly reduced symptoms.[601]

Further, wheatgrass contains compounds called P4D1 (a protein) and SOD—superoxide dismutase (an antioxidant enzyme), which have been shown to reduce cellular corrosion and mutation. P4D1 also helps regenerate RNA and DNA (human genetic material) that can be damaged by electromagnetic radiation (computers, cell phones, etc.) and X-rays. SOD also protects human cells from constant attacks by free radicals that hide out in chemical additives in food and the polluted environment.[602]

Why I'm Wild About Wheatgrass

I'm wild about using wheatgrass because wheatgrass aids with the following:

1. **Reduces inflammation.** P4D1 helps reduce symptoms of and suppresses pancreatitis, stomatitis, and inflammation of the oral cavity and dermatitis.[603]

2. **Has anti-cancer properties.** P4D1 is able to attack cancer cells by helping make the walls of the cancerous cells more open to attack by the body's white blood cells.[604]

3. **Facilitates oral health.** Swishing wheatgrass in the mouth kills bacteria that cause gingivitis and bad breath. Some holistic dentists have seen great reduction of bleeding gums by soaking gauze in wheatgrass and applying it directly to the affected areas.[605]

Drink a Shot

Because wheatgrass is very fibrous and difficult to digest if eaten, it is best juiced from living grass. Freeze-dried processed powder forms are not as effective as juicing. If you are going to juice fresh wheatgrass, you have to grow it. Don't shake your head; I promise you don't need a green thumb, and it practically grows itself. Go to www.wheatgrasskits.com, and you will be sent everything you need to grow and juice your own USDA-Certified Organic, non-GMO wheatgrass. If you are following a gluten-free diet, have no fear: wheatgrass does not contain the gluten found in wheat plants.

An entire tray of wheatgrass is ready to juice in less than ten days. I recommend starting a second tray at day five, and you will never run out of it. There's nothing more refreshing than a shot of wheatgrass. I have one almost every day. For some people, it has an acquired "earthy" taste, so I recommend mixing a shot or two in a glass of carrot juice with a touch of refreshing ginger. Or put your freshly squeezed shot of wheatgrass in your morning smoothie. Most salad dressings are filled with unhealthy chemicals and preservatives. Make your own using wheatgrass! A shot of wheatgrass, lemon, and a pinch of garlic powder makes a nutritious, power-packed, great-tasting salad dressing.

To use as a daily whole-food multivitamin, wheatgrass doesn't have to cost you a lot of time. Spend a half hour on the weekend and juice enough wheatgrass to fill an ice cube tray and freeze it. Then during those hectic weekdays, simply put a wheatgrass ice cube into water or your favorite juice. In the evening, you can even add a wheatgrass ice cube to your favorite mixed alcoholic beverage. Now you can tell everyone you have "a healthy drinking habit." One ice cube tray will last two weeks. Fill up two trays, and you have enough for a month.

Toss your multivitamins into the toilet; they end up there anyway! A shot of wheatgrass gives your body all the whole-food nutrients it needs without the chemicals and toxins most multivitamins contain. If you're not interested in growing and juicing your own wheatgrass, you can have freshly squeezed juice shipped to your front door by going to www.dynamicgreens.com.

The ABCs of Choosing a Supplement

As the formulator of several supplements currently sold in thirty countries, I believe there is a need for supplementing lousy eating habits. What I don't believe in is putting faith in unregulated manufacturers that don't make safety, purity, and potency a priority. I'm also against all the chemicals, dyes, and preservatives used in most supplements. I am a strong advocate of taking herbal, homeopathic vitamins, minerals, probiotics, and krill oil supplements, as long as they are derived from a whole-food, natural source. To find good-quality supplements sold by a good manufacturer, follow the ABCs: Absorption, Balance, and Certification.

A—Absorption

A whole-food, natural nutritional product is the best way to ensure absorption and assimilation. Taking a chewable tablet is better than swallowing pills. Digestion begins in the mouth. We were designed to chew our food—our fruits, vegetables, and other plants. Why would we not chew our nutritional supplements? Your great-grandmother never swallowed a vitamin pill, nor did she drink her vitamins. The nutrition she received every day came from what she chewed. That was also true of the generations before hers and so on.

Think about when you first swallowed a pill. How did it feel? Very unnatural. In fact, swallowing a pill doesn't come naturally. That task has to be learned. Many adults still have a hard time gagging down pills. How hard was it to learn how to chew? You never learned to chew because it's inherent to your survival. The best way to absorb your whole-food nutritional supplements is to chew them. Because whole-food chewable options are not yet mainstream, you may have no other choice but to take your supplements in pill or liquid source.

If you choose pills, stay away from tablets or compressed pills containing binders, fillers, waxes, shellac, or added artificial colorings. Never take pills that contain gelatin, which is created by boiling the skin, tendons, and ligaments of animals. Gelatin capsules sometimes contain harmful properties due to animal origin. Since many animals are given antibiotics and eat foods that contain pesticides, these toxins can show up in gelatin capsules. Instead of gelatin, look for capsules with vegetable or plant cellulose or veggie caps, as these offer better absorption. To ensure you are getting whole-food sources, which are also better absorbed, look for words in parentheses in the ingredients list, such as *leaf*, *fruit*, *extract*, *plant*, *stem*, *root*, or *seed*. This tells you that the source is naturally derived. If you see a chemical listed next to the ingredient, it's synthetic. For liquid products look for "cold processed" because when whole-food liquids are pasteurized (heated), they lose most of their potency. Avoid the preservatives sodium benzoate and potassium sorbate. Instead look for liquid products that use a natural preservative such as citric acid or Natamax. Stay away from salts that are often added to increase the stability of the nutrient including acetate, bitartrate, chloride, gluconate, hydrochloride, nitrate, and succinate. If you see any of these words on the label, they are counterfeits and will decrease absorption.

B—Balance

If you look at nature, fruits, vegetables, legumes or nuts, or other plants do not contain massive amounts of vitamins, minerals, enzymes, or amino acids. Only in pill form do you find hundreds and thousands of milligrams. In nature, it's about balance, not mega doses! As we discussed, Dr. Linus Pauling, the "godfather of vitamin C," recommended everyone take 3,000 milligrams of vitamin C every day. Considering an orange has approximately 30 milligrams, the equivalent is eating up to 100 oranges each day! More is not always better, and as we've discussed in this chapter, mega doses can lead to serious disease and even death. It's about *balance* not *dosage*. It's best to supplement your diet with a whole-food, plant-based supplement. Don't panic if you don't see milligrams listed. If it's truly a whole food, you may not see any amounts listed, but instead you'll see a "proprietary" fruit or vegetable blend listed. Keep in mind that many fruits and vegetables contain trace and macro minerals in parts per million (ppm), including calcium, iron, boron, manganese, zinc, vanadium, sodium, and copper. With nature it's not about seeing thousands of milligrams on the label; it's about finding the proper natural balance that man-made nutrients simply don't offer.

The body is a unique traffic director. When it requires more of a specific nutrient, it will take it from the food you eat. For example, men need more zinc than women because their prostate gland is dependent on this mineral. So when a man eats shellfish, his body will take the high zinc content and bring it to the prostate. Females, on the other hand, are more prone to having thyroid gland dysfunction. Since the thyroid needs iodine for optimal health, when a woman eats shellfish, its iodine content is what her body will absorb, not the zinc.

Don't get caught up in the "numbers" game and how much RDA you've been brainwashed into believing you need. Choose whole-food, plant-based supplements with the proper *balance* of nutrients. With nature, a little goes a long way!

C—Certification

What you see on the label isn't always what you get in the bottle. Manufacturers are not held accountable for delivering what their label promises. In February 2015, the New York State attorney general announced that testing found four major retailers were selling supplements that didn't contain *any* of the ingredients they claimed. Walmart, Walgreens, Target, and GNC used cheap fillers like powdered rice, asparagus, and even houseplants! In addition, they found that the ginseng supplements sold at Walgreens, contained only powdered garlic and rice. Walmart's memory-enhancing herbal product, ginkgo biloba, actually contained powdered radish and wheat. Perhaps they lost their memory during the formulation process? It looks like they also forgot what the words "wheat- and gluten-free" on their label means. Next up . . . Target's St. John's wort and valerian root products all tested negative for the herbs they have listed on the labels. GNC, the nation's largest health-supplement chain, sold products with unlisted ingredients like peanuts and soybeans, potentially life threatening if you have allergies.[606] Sound a little out of control? Well, it is. Because the nutritional supplement industry is not regulated, it's important to find an honest manufacturer who is accountable; otherwise you could be buying supplements made in someone's garage.

When choosing any dietary supplement, look for a product that is certified as cGMP, which means it has passed Current Good Manufacturing Practice regulations. This certification is given by an organization called the National Products Association (NPA) and ensures a stringent series of tests have been passed, and that proper design, monitoring, and control of manufacturing processes and facilities have been evaluated. Adherence to the cGMP regulations assures the identity, strength, quality, purity, and safety of all the ingredients. It also makes sure the nutritional labels are accurate and prevents contamination, mix-ups, deviations, failures, and errors of the formula. You can see if your manufacturer is certified by visiting www.npainfo.org.

Also look for the United States Pharmacopoeia (USP) or British Pharmacopoeia (BP) designation on the label. This means that the vitamin isolates are the highest quality you can buy, and are the most easily dissolved in the digestion process. These organizations are nongovernmental and set the official standards for health-care products. USP and BP set widely recognized protocols for the quality, purity, strength, and consistency of dietary supplements in more than 130 countries. The USP- and BP-verified marks found on a product's label also indicate the ingredients will break down and release into the body within a specified amount of time and do not contain harmful levels of specified contaminants. USP and BP verification assures the products have been made using sanitary and well-controlled procedures. To find manufacturers that use these standards, visit www.usp.org.

Discoveries: Hundreds of nonbiased studies show the dangers of synthetic vitamin and mineral supplements. Most supplements on the market are created in labs using the same chemicals found in nail-polish remover, silver polish, gasoline, paint, etc. On the contrary, natural, whole-food vitamins and minerals are not toxic to the body. These nutrients, created by nature, aid in the prevention of disease and increase a person's life span.

Instincts: The human body requires an array of whole-food nutrients—from vitamin A to zinc—to maintain normal function. This is what fuels the muscles, organs, bones, and brain. Centuries ago, a person didn't go to the drugstore to purchase vitamins in a bottle. He or she got everything the body needed from nature. Multivitamins contain approximately thirty ingredients, a miniscule amount compared to the many *hundreds* of nutritional compounds found in plants that work in harmony to protect us from chronic disease. Ask yourself, "Should I be consuming chemicals, binders, fillers, and dyes or whole-food ingredients from nature?" Trust your instincts.

God: The human body was not created in a laboratory. Why should your nutritional products be?

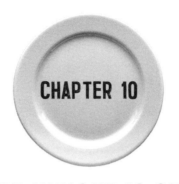

CHAPTER 10

YOUR WEIGHT IS OVER
THE SKINNY ON DIETS

"Now there are more overweight people
in America than average-weight people.
So overweight people are now average.
Which means you've met your New Year's resolution."

—Jay Leno

With so many different types of diets and weight-loss options to choose from, it's no wonder Americans spend $46 billion on diet products a year. On my radio show, I've been asked to weigh in and throw down the gauntlet on which diet works and which philosophy is most sound. What I have to say is, "They ALL work!" Whether it's eating for your blood type, Atkins, Paleo, Keto, Zone, South Beach, Vegan, Nutrisystem, Weight Watchers, or any variation that exists now or in the future, if you stick to the program, you will experience a weight loss.

One of the main reasons why so many types of diets work is because they all have one thing in common—they change a person's routine. They all promote eating *different* foods in *different* ways at *different* times. Whether it's eating grapefruits, eating steak three times a day, changing your portion sizes, or going 100 percent vegan, when you mix up your daily routine, you will alter your metabolism and change your blood glucose levels and your body's pH, which in turn can lead to a weight loss. Unfortunately, most of the time, the results can be temporary.

If you've tried one of the many hundreds of weight-loss plans or followed a fad diet, you know this to be true. The majority of you lost the most weight in the first thirty days, continued to lose weight in month two, and only lost a minimal amount of weight after day ninety. By the fourth month, you reached a plateau and became frustrated, which made you walk away from the diet you were on that "was" working. So here we are back to square one surrounded by a multibillion-dollar weight loss industry that just isn't working!

What are we supposed to do? Continue buying tickets to ride a merry-go-round of fad diets? The word "diet" comes from the Greek word diatia, which means "way of living." The reason most people achieve such poor results when trying to lose weight is because they are not addressing the true meaning of the word diet. Changing your *routine* leads to initial weight loss, but changing your *way of living* is what brings permanent weight loss. Once and for all, I hope to set the record straight about what we are doing wrong about keeping our weight in check. This chapter reveals the three obstacles of permanent weight loss, and they have nothing to do with exercise.

Is There a Skinny Gene?

So many people blame genetics for their weight problem. In fact I've heard it used as a rationalization to remaining overweight, with people saying, "Oh, my parents were fat, so I inherited it from them." This is plain false. Your genes have nothing to do with why you can't fit into your jeans! Your parents may be overweight because they are still part of the modern-day culture. In the year 1900, less than 5 percent of the population was considered overweight, compared to today's 70 percent. Back then there were no grocery stores, and people had to rely on the fresh produce from their pesticide-free gardens. When they ate animals, they were hormone- and antibiotic-free that they, or someone in their family, killed for dinner. Our ancestors didn't have cars, so they had to walk to their destinations. Today most of us sit behind a desk all day or stand behind a cash register. Instead of having our own garden to gather food from, people today go to drive-through restaurants for lunch, consume processed frozen foods for dinner, and top it off with sugar-laden cookies, cakes, and ice cream for dessert. Then at night we sit on the couch, watch TV, and snack on fattening pretzels and potato chips. None of these behaviors existed hundreds of years ago. Stop blaming your great-grandparents' parents for your weight problems. When my patients finally come to accept that they can no longer blame their genes, they ask me about an exercise regimen, assuming this will make all the difference. Unfortunately that's just another wives' tale.

In the 1970s, one of the best-selling books was Jim Fixx's *The Complete Book of Running*. Fixx is credited with helping start America's fitness revolution, popularizing the sport of running and demonstrating the health benefits of regular jogging. He was trim and lean and his muscular legs adorned the cover of more than one million books sold. He was the epitome of good health and shared how running could help you lose weight and gain a healthy heart. He made running the biggest thing since sliced bread. Leading cardiologists across the country happily endorsed Fixx's book and encouraged their patients to take up running for a healthier heart.

Unfortunately, at the young age of fifty-two, Jim Fixx died while running along a country road . . . from a massive heart attack. Although Jim was a big believer in running, he was not an advocate of healthy eating. His story is proof positive that exercise alone is not the key to a healthy body. An autopsy revealed that all three of his coronary arteries were damaged by arteriosclerosis (plaquing of the arteries), the underlying cause of heart attacks. Mr. Fixx's left coronary artery was 99 percent blocked and his right coronary artery was 80 percent blocked.[607]

Poor diet is a contributing factor to arterial plaque. Fixx was known for his bad eating habits. Ultra-marathoner Stan Cottrell, a friend of Fixx, appeared with him at a conference and stated, "Just before Fixx went in to speak, he stuffed himself with four donuts and said, 'I didn't have time for breakfast.'"[608 609]

Don't Count Calories, Make Your Calories Count

Fad diets come and go, but the most popular diet of the last century is calorie counting. It's become the standard methodology for people wanting to lose weight. But even as far back as 1924, prominent medical doctor Dr. Phillip Norman questioned the value of calorie counting: "The conception of the calorie has retarded logical and rational reasoning in regard to diet, more so than any single other factor."[610] The problem with a calorie-counting diet is that it can put your body into a "famine" mode that causes you to gain back your original weight and sometimes even more. This is why calorie-counting diets are often referred to as "yo-yo diets." By definition, a calorie is a measurement of heat. It's the amount of heat required to raise the temperature of one kilogram of water through one degree Celsius. A calorie is *heat!* If heat caused weight gain, everyone living at the southern hemisphere would be obese. But actually they're leaner.[611]

The biggest calorie-counting organization in the world is called Weight Watchers. They've been having people count calories for more than fifty years! Interestingly in 2011 David Kirshaw, CEO of Weight Watchers, said in a *Time* magazine interview, "Calorie counting has become unhelpful. When we have a 100-calorie apple in one hand and a 100-calorie pack of cookies in the other, to view them as being 'the same' makes no sense."[612] For Weight Watchers to make a statement like that really puts into perspective the lack of success calorie counting has when it comes to losing weight and keeping it off. Calorie counting diets simply do not work! It also means having to become a mathematician, and that takes the enjoyment out of eating. If you eat the right wholesome foods, you don't have to count calories.

Fruit: The Big Sugar Controversy

Fruit gets a bad rap because it contains sugar (aka fructose). There are many health advocates that recommend totally eliminating fruit from the diet. They believe that fruit creates a sugar overload that can lead to obesity, heart disease, and type 2 diabetes. In my opinion, that's taking things way too far. Fruit is an important part of the diet. Yes, it is true that fruit contains sugar, but so do vegetables. One cup of sweet potatoes contains 6 grams of sugar yet it's the perfect food option for diabetics. One stalk of broccoli contains 2.6 grams of sugar. The reason eating sweet potatoes and broccoli won't spike your blood sugar is because they contain a lot of fiber, which buffers out the sugar content. When deciding which fruit to eat, it's important to look at the glycemic index (GI). A glycemic index measures how the fruit you eat will affect your blood sugar levels. The best way to keep your blood sugar in balance is to eat fruits that have higher fiber content and a lower GI.

Instead of reaching for grapes and bananas, opt for fruits high in fiber that have a lower GI, like apples and blueberries. Even though these fruits are still high in sugar (blueberries have a whopping 15 grams of sugar per cup!), because of their fiber content, the natural fruit sugar is released slowly into the body and won't cause any unhealthy sugar spikes. In spite of their high sugar content, blueberries can actually help normalize blood sugar levels and reduce your risk of diabetes by 23 percent.[613] What about the most commonly eaten fruit in the world, the apple? How can this fruit, which is *loaded with sugar*, be attached to the claim, "An apple a day keeps the doctor away"? Because an apple is chock-full of antioxidants, vitamins, and minerals and contains lots of fiber. This fiber, called pectin, buffers out the apple's fructose, keeping you from having an insulin spike. People who eat five or more apples per week are less likely to develop diabetes than those who don't eat apples.[614] However, you should never peel apples because most of that sugar-buffering fiber comes from the skin.

Glycemic Guide to Eating Fruits

Eat all the *green light* fruits you want, limit your *yellow light* fruits, and consider the *red light* fruits as an occasional candy treat.

Green Light (low glycemic fruits)	Yellow Light (medium glycemic fruits)	Red Light (high glycemic fruits)
Apples, Tangerines, Pears, Blueberries, Grapefruit, Oranges, Strawberries, Raspberries, Blackberries, Cherries, Peaches, Plums, Cranberries, Elderberries, Gooseberries, Tangerines, Boysenberries	Mangos, Kiwis, Grapes, Figs, Papaya, Apricots, Cantaloupes, Honeydew Melon, Pomegranates, Bananas	Watermelon, Pineapples, Dates, Raisins, Candied Fruits, Concentrated Fruit Juices

Exercise Makes Losing Weight Difficult!

Say what? After the most respected running guru of our time died of a heart attack, sedentary people had a hard time believing that exercise was important. The truth is exercise *is* important and necessary for a healthy body, but if you want to lose weight, changing your diet is far more effective. It takes five hundred jumping jacks to burn off 100 calories. However, eliminating one soda subtracts 150 calories. Which has a greater impact? Considering the average person consumes three to five sodas every day, it seems pretty obvious that you can't spend every day doing four thousand jumping jacks to erase your lousy dietary choices.

I've been a member of a gym for most of my adult life. I am not anti-exercise! I am, however, against working out as being *the* weight-loss solution. Most exercise gurus will tell you to exercise and *burn burn burn* the calories you eat, if you want to lose weight. That is not true.

If you are a member at the gym, I'm sure you've seen Hank (I never asked his name but he looks like a Hank). He's that overweight guy running on the treadmill or stationary bike who sweats so profusely that it ends up all over the machine and sometimes splatters on the person next to him. (I stopped running on the empty treadmill next to Hank.) Hank is always at the gym. He's so dedicated! Week after week, month after month, I would see sweaty Hank painfully running on the treadmill. Unfortunately he's still carrying the same weight. Maybe you're like Hank? You exercise and lose a pound or two, but it comes right back. So you increase the minutes you spend on the treadmill, or you increase the incline, thinking that might help. Have you noticed, however, that the more you exercise, the hungrier you get? That's because exercise actually stimulates hunger. This causes you to crave more food and eat more, which in turn negates the weight-loss benefits of exercise. The truth is, exercise makes losing weight more difficult!

In 2009 the peer-reviewed journal *PLoS ONE* published a study of 464 overweight women who didn't exercise regularly. Women were placed into four groups. Three of the groups were asked to work out with a personal trainer for 72 minutes, 136 minutes, and 194 minutes per week, respectively, for six months. Women in the fourth group were the controls—they maintained their normal daily activity routines. None of the women in any of the groups changed their dietary habits. The women in all four groups, including the control group, lost weight! Those who exercised with a trainer several days a week for six months did not lose significantly more weight than the control subjects did. The study found that most of the women who exercised ate more than they did before they started the experiment. Those who exercised intensively with a trainer did not lose more weight than those who didn't because none of the four groups changed their eating habits.[615]

The *Journal of Obesity Research* published a study conducted by a Columbia University team, which showed a pound of muscle burns approximately six calories a day in a resting body, compared to two calories that a pound of fat burns.[616] This means that if you worked out enough to burn off 10 pounds of fat, you would be able to eat only an extra forty calories per day, about the amount in a teaspoon of butter, before beginning to gain the weight back. So, if after a vigorous workout you drank a 20-ounce bottle of Gatorade (130 calories), your hard workout would be futile because the caloric expenditure from the workout and your caloric intake becomes a wash. As you can see, because your body is starving after a workout, a vicious cycle ensues. That old wives' tale "lose weight by burning more calories than you eat" is wrong. No matter how many jumping jacks you do or how long you ride that stationary bike, exercise alone simply will not work! You can't outrun your fork. That's why exercise is not on my top three ways to lose weight.

Ask a hundred people if they would like to lose some weight and eighty-five will tell you they do. Ask them if they have dieted or exercised and lost weight but gained it all back, and most of them will sigh and answer "Yes." There are three obstacles keeping people from losing weight *and keeping it off*: Eating too many white foods, lack of deep restorative sleep, and being exposed to obesogens (chemicals that cause weight gain!). Think of these three pillars as your permanent weight loss tricycle. Your eating habits are just one wheel. You can't accelerate and move forward without the other two.

Obstacle #1: White Foods

While so many fad diets have come and gone, for almost three decades I've recommended the same eating plan for my patients. It has helped thousands balance their blood sugar, increase their energy levels, and lose unwanted pounds. You too can achieve this by simply living by the mantra, "If it's white, keep it out of sight!" When I say white, I'm referring to foods that are white in color and have been processed and refined like milk, flour, rice, pasta, bread, crackers, cereal, and anything sweetened with table sugar or high-fructose corn syrup. There are a few natural exceptions to this rule: cauliflower, garlic, mushrooms, parsnips, onions, potatoes, bananas, turnips, coconut, white fish, and white poultry meat. All the other white foods contain a high concentration of simple carbohydrates that will make your blood sugar spike and then drop, causing you to overeat and gain weight.

Think of white foods as the "bad carbs," loaded with public enemy number one—sugar! The average person consumes 150 to 170 pounds of refined sugar every year![617] That is *a lot* of sugar—especially when you compare it to how much we consumed in the past. Fewer than one hundred years ago, the average intake of sugar was only about 4 pounds per person per year. That's a 4,000 percent increase in sugar consumption today. Sugar is a major cause of our obesity epidemic. If you are not one to add table sugar to your food or beverages, you're still consuming too much sugar. This sweetener can be hidden in foods like canned or jarred tomato sauce (15 grams of sugar per half-cup serving), granola bars (12 grams of sugar), Greek yogurt (17 to 33 grams of sugar per 8-ounce serving), and Vitamin Water (one 20-ounce bottle has about 32 grams of added sugar)! Also stay clear of processed grains like pasta because, even though you won't see a lot of "sugar" listed on the label, it increases your blood sugar and triggers a release of insulin.

Less-processed "good carbs" are more satisfying to the cells of your body and are therefore more filling than refined carbs. The bad foods make portion control very difficult because they do not satiate well. The more you eat, the more you gain. By eating more whole grains like brown rice, oats, barley, rye, and quinoa, you are getting a great source of fiber, which creates a slower absorption rate and keeps you feeling full longer. For people suffering from celiac disease or a gluten allergy, the best choice is buckwheat. Because it is neither a grain nor related to wheat, buckwheat is gluten-free and safe for those with celiac disease or gluten sensitivities. You can use buckwheat in place of wheat flour to make pancakes and pasta. In fact, buckwheat noodles are a popular cuisine in Japan. If you want to sweeten your coffee, tea, or if a recipe requires sugar, you can use pure raw honey, organic coconut sugar, organic maple syrup, yacón syrup, stevia, or lo han guo (a natural sweetener made from the monk fruit).

Can You DIG This?

Ever wonder why people get hungry shortly after eating at a Chinese restaurant? That's because most of the dishes are served with white rice. White rice is brown rice that has been completely stripped of its bran and germ layer, reducing its fiber and nutrient content. Simple sugars and other unnatural ingredients are also added to white rice for taste. Not only does brown rice contain more filling fiber, but it also has two times as much manganese and phosphorus as white rice, three times more iron, three times as much vitamin B3, four times the vitamin B1, and ten times the vitamin B6. That's why white rice is on the list of white foods you should steer clear of.

White Foods to Avoid:

- white bread
- pasta, unless it's whole grain
- white rice
- white flour, and products made with it such as cookies, crackers, cake, pretzels, doughnuts, bagels, and muffins
- potatoes and potato chips
- corn and corn chips
- popcorn
- sugar and products containing sugar
- sugar-sweetened soft drinks
- sugar-cured meats (e.g., cured ham)
- salt (processed)

BREAD: Slicing Through the Myths

Bread has gotten such a bad reputation. Many of the latest fad diets have labeled bread public enemy number one. Actually, it's the white flour used to make bread, pasta, cakes, and cookies that should be avoided. Why is white flour so unhealthy? For that answer, let's look at how it's made.

First, they take whole wheat and remove the outer layer of bran. This bran is repackaged and sold at health food stores for people to use when they get constipated—often from eating too many cakes and cookies and too much bread! They also remove the germ, which they sell back to you in health food stores as wheat germ. This wheat germ is chock-full of disease-fighting phytosterols, vitamins, and fiber. Once they remove all this good stuff, they grind the rest into a powder, bleach it, add synthetic (fake) inorganic vitamins, and sell it to you as "enriched" flour. Unfortunately, these synthetic vitamins added to white flour products don't get absorbed into the blood's cells as effectively as they would from a whole grain (see chapter 9).

Another negative attribute of bread is gluten. In fact, going "gluten-free" is considered by most diet experts to be the best thing you can do to optimize your health. Gluten is a family of proteins found in grains like wheat, rye, spelt, and barley. People suffering from Celiac disease need to avoid gluten. Their immune system attacks the gluten particles but also ends up attacking the lining of the gut. Approximately 2.4 million Americans have celiac disease.[618] Some people have gluten sensitivity and should also eliminate it from their diet. You can tell if you have gluten sensitivity by listening to your body. If you eat things like whole grain pasta, bread, or cereal and often feel run down and tired, or get a stomachache with bloating or diarrhea afterward, then cut back or eliminate gluten. But for all the rest of you, which is the majority, completely boycotting gluten and whole grains is not necessary.

Whole-grain bread and pasta are actually good for you. They offer fiber, healthy plant-based protein, vitamins, minerals, and a variety of phytochemicals that help to improve your health. Whole grains have all of the parts of the original kernel—bran, germ, and endosperm—in the original proportions. In refined grains, the bran and germ are stripped away, so stay away from this option. Look for the word "whole"—either whole grain or whole wheat. Also, make sure the grain is one of the first three ingredients listed on the label. Look for products with a "whole grain" stamp from the Whole Grains Council, which ensures there's at least half a serving of whole grains inside.

I find it puzzling that dietitians and authors of digestive health books are telling people to completely eliminate whole grains from their diet. Whole grains have many digestive benefits. Their fiber content keeps bowel movements regular, which can help ward off constipation, diarrhea, leaky gut syndrome, and diverticulosis. Whole grains also contain lactic acid, which promotes the growth of "good bacteria" in the large intestine.[619]

These organisms aid digestion, promote better nutrient absorption, and can even help improve the immune system.

Whole grains, particularly wheat, contain phenolic acids, a type of antioxidant with documented cancer-inhibiting properties.[620] Whole grains also help lower triglycerides and prevent your body from absorbing "bad" cholesterol that can contribute to heart disease. In fact, research published by the Harvard School of Public Health shows that people who eat two to three servings of whole grain products daily are 30 percent less likely to have a heart attack or die from heart disease compared to those who eat less than one serving per week.[621] This includes whole wheat, oats, brown rice, barley, quinoa, rye, buckwheat, and millet.

If you're concerned about your weight, the bread of choice is rye. *The Nutrition Journal* published a study in 2009 that showed eating a breakfast that includes rye bread can help you decrease your hunger for eight hours.[622] Another study published in May of 2016 in *PloS One Medical Journal* found that whole-grain rye toast also lowers blood sugar surges.[623]

A year later, in May of 2017, the *British Medical Journal* published research that analyzed 100,000 subjects over a twenty-five-year period. They discovered that participants with the highest intake of gluten had a rate of heart disease significantly lower than those with the lowest intake of gluten. After adjustments for consumption of refined grains, eating gluten was associated with a 15 percent *lower risk* of developing coronary heart disease. They concluded, "The avoidance of gluten may result in reduced consumption of beneficial whole grains, which may affect cardiovascular risk. The promotion of gluten-free diets among people without celiac disease should not be encouraged."[624] When was the last time you heard anything *good* about whole grains that contain gluten? The latest food fads make them out to be the culinary equivalent of Satan!

Eating whole grains daily, such as brown rice or whole-wheat bread, reduces colorectal cancer risk by 17 percent for every 90-grams-per-day of whole grains that are eaten. This was the finding of a report by the American Institute for Cancer Research and the World Cancer Research Fund.[625]

For those of you avoiding gluten but also taking probiotic supplements for your digestive health, I have some bad news for you. More than half of the top-selling probiotic supplements contain gluten. Even supplements that have "gluten-free" on the label can contain gluten, according to the

Celiac Disease Center at Columbia University. In 2015, their team of scientists analyzed twenty-two of the bestselling probiotic supplements from Amazon and several national retail chains. They then subjected the products to a type of laboratory test known as liquid chromatography-mass spectrometry. They found twelve of the supplements—or roughly 55 percent—contained detectable levels of gluten. Eight of these twelve products carried gluten-free claims on their labels.[626] Unless you have Celiac disease or gluten sensitivity, whole-grain bread (containing gluten) can be a healthy addition to your diet.

My White-Loss Story

I eat great. I eat pure. I avoid dairy and made the choice not to eat red meat more than twenty-five years ago. I eat organic herbs, vegetables, and fruit and even grow my own! I exercise at least three times a week. But in spite of all that, for several years I remained around 15 pounds overweight. I am not a lover of sweets. In fact, I can probably count on one hand how many desserts I've eaten in my lifetime. My one big weakness is popcorn. I love it! In fact, coming home and making some air popped organic popcorn was a nightly ritual for me. I believed that watching a movie without popcorn was sacrilegious! Popcorn is loaded with fiber and is low in calories, and if you don't salt or pour butter on it, it's a great healthy snack—so I thought. I would eat an entire tub of popcorn in one sitting.

Popcorn is considered a high glycemic index (GI) food. As we discussed previously, those foods that have a higher GI are more likely to cause your blood-sugar levels to spike after you eat them. One day I made the decision to eliminate my vice and stop eating popcorn. To my astonishment, I lost 5 pounds the first week, simply by not eating a giant bowl of popcorn every night! After six weeks, I had lost the full 15 pounds! That was seven years ago, and the pounds have never come back. Did I eliminate popcorn from my life? Absolutely not. It's still my favorite snack. I just eat it in moderation. Now, I enjoy a bowl of air popped organic popcorn three times a month. After you remove the foods listed in the previously mentioned White Foods to Avoid list and lose the desired weight, having an occasional bowl of popcorn, pasta, or even a cookie (just *one*) is not going to kill you.

Simple Food Swaps

We are creatures of habit and tend to gravitate toward what we are used to. As motivational guru Zig Ziglar said, "If you do what you always did, you'll get what you always got." A needed change does a body good. I promise, it's not that difficult. It just takes doing a few simple food swaps.

Commercial table salt is very heavily processed, which is why it's white. It typically contains 97.5 percent to 99.9 percent sodium chloride. Meanwhile, high-quality unrefined salts like Hawaiian black volcanic and Himalayan salt are only 87 percent sodium chloride. Plus these healthier salt options contain up to 84 minerals and trace elements, including calcium, magnesium, potassium, copper, and iron. These minerals help to satiate your cells. Eating processed table salt void of these nutrients makes you want to eat more. This is why fast food restaurants use so much table salt. It makes you crave more of their food. Instead of using processed white flour in your recipes, go with almond flour, coconut flour, buckwheat flour, or quinoa flour. Rather than using white processed sugar, choose healthier alternatives like coconut sugar, monk fruit (aka lo han guo), xylitol (made from birch bark), or stevia. By doing some simple food swaps, you can still enjoy the foods you love without compromising flavor.

Sample No White Food Meal Plan.

Below are a few meal suggestions. For more detailed recipes and health tips, visit my website: DrDavidFriedman.com

---

BREAKFAST CHOICES (pick one):

- Two scrambled eggs with spinach and avocado
- Organic multigrain oatmeal
- Buckwheat pancakes with yacón syrup (a natural sweetening agent that research shows can curb appetite and reduce fat)[627] [628]
- Whole grain cream-of-wheat cereal (with unsweetened almond milk)

Add to the above two slices of organic turkey bacon or a slice of cantaloupe.

LUNCH CHOICES (pick one):

- Green leafy salad with 6 ounces grilled organic chicken (extra-virgin olive oil-based vinaigrette dressing)
- Turkey, tomato, and avocado on rye
- Butternut squash soup
- Veggie burger (whole wheat bun)
- Baked sweet potato with cinnamon

Add to the above some steamed veggies with herbs.

SNACK CHOICES (pick one):

- A handful of nuts—almonds, cashews, macadamia nuts
- ½ cup of fresh fruit—blueberries, strawberries, apples, oranges
- One apple dipped into 2 tablespoons organic almond butter
- Vegetables dipped into 4 tablespoons of hummus
- Smoothies (Blend one banana and blueberries with almond or cashew milk.)

DINNER CHOICES (pick one):

- Grilled wild-caught fish (6 ounces)
- Grilled organic chicken with spices and herbs (6 ounces)
- Grilled scallops over baby spinach, topped with lemon vinaigrette
- Whole wheat pasta (4 ounces) with red clam sauce
- Vegetable stir fry (use extra-virgin olive oil)

Add to the above ½ cup of steamed broccoli or asparagus or a medium sweet potato.

DESSERT CHOICES (pick one):

- Poached pears
- Baked apple
- Coconut yogurt with slivered almonds
- Mango sorbet. Blend frozen, peeled, and cubed mangos, add honey or yacón syrup with lime juice. Freeze for 45 minutes or until almost solid.

Obstacle #2: Lack of Restorative Sleep

In November 2006, a sixteen-year study of almost seventy thousand women was conducted at Case Western Reserve University in Cleveland. Those who slept five hours or less a night were 30 percent more likely to gain more than 30 pounds compared to those who slept longer.[629]

A lot of research has been conducted on how a lack of sleep contributes to obesity. A study from June 2012, published in the *American Journal of Human Biology*, showed that sleeping less than six hours increases a person's Body Mass Index (BMI), leading to obesity.[630] But the most impressive research comes from Brigham and Women's Hospital in Boston, which found that disrupted sleep patterns raise blood sugar levels and slow the body's metabolic rate, or the rate at which the body burns calories while at rest. That particular study, published in April 2012, analyzed sleep behaviors in a completely controlled laboratory environment by mimicking jet lag and typical shift work sleep deprivation. In addition to controlling how many hours of sleep each participant achieved, researchers also controlled other lifestyle factors, including activities and diet. The evidence showed short or poor-quality sleep is linked to an increased risk of obesity.[631]

While several factors can be contributed to the rise in obesity, when we look at our sleep patterns, we see some compelling correlations. In 1960 American adults averaged 8.5 to 9 hours of sleep per night, and the obesity rate was less than 12 percent. Today adults average 6.5 to 7 hours of sleep, and the obesity rate has climbed to 33 percent. Children averaged 9 to 10 hours of sleep in 1960, the ideal amount needed to support their growing cells. Less than 3 percent of children were considered obese during this time. Today children average just 8 hours of sleep, and the obesity rates for children and adolescents in the United States has escalated to a disturbing 17 percent![632] Of course sitting for hours on end playing video games (including at night when they are supposed to be sleeping) also contributes to the childhood obesity epidemic as well.

Is the rise in obesity and lack of sleep just a coincidence? "No!" says Dr. Michael Breus, aka "The Sleep Doctor." Dr. Breus's best-selling book, *The Sleep Doctor's Diet Plan: Lose Weight Through Better Sleep*, shares how not sleeping is a major cause of the obesity problem afflicting the nation. A regular and favorite guest on my radio show, Dr. Breus, clinical psychologist and board-certified sleep expert, revealed to my listeners how a good night's rest can keep us from getting fat.

"Not sleeping prevents us from losing weight. As we become more sleep deprived, our hormones go crazy," Dr. Breus explained. "Specifically, those hormones that affect appetite and metabolism. Two of the big culprits are ghrelin and leptin. Ghrelin is a hormone I call the GO hormone because it tells you to *go* eat. I call leptin the STOP hormone because it tells you to *stop* eating when you're full. When you're sleep deprived, you have more GO hormone and less STOP hormone."

Dr. Breus also says, "Sleep deprivation affects the metabolism. This is your body's way of conserving energy. The more sleep deprived you are, the slower your metabolism."[633]

Another hormone that rises when you are sleep deprived is cortisol. The body releases this hormone in response to stress, and it is a major contributor to fat accumulation in the abdomen. Cortisol also increases blood sugar levels and raises blood pressure. When you are stressed, you crave "good mood food" like sweets, carbs, and fattening foods because they increase your serotonin levels—a neurotransmitter that makes you feel good. But this *temporary* happiness can lead to a *permanent* weight gain, especially around the mid-section. The most dangerous form of fat is belly fat (also known as visceral fat). This type of fat is stored when cortisol levels are too high, causing your cells to become resistant to insulin, which puts you at a higher risk for high blood pressure, diabetes, heart attacks, strokes, and premature death. Belly fat is also a precursor to a disease called nonalcoholic fatty liver disease, which is considered the most common cause of chronic liver disease in the United States.[634]

Human growth hormone (HGH) is also secreted by the pituitary gland during deep sleep. HGH stimulates growth and cell reproduction and regeneration. Studies have shown that obese adults have lower levels of HGH than normal-weight adults. They also have a relative decrease in muscle mass, and, in many instances, decreased energy and quality of life.[635]

Dr. Breus shared how a lack of sleep can have a profound effect on our HGH levels. "The more sleep deprived you become, the less stage 3 and stage 4 sleep you get," he explained. "These stages create physically restorative sleep where HGH is secreted. HGH is one of the things that tells your body whether you should be storing fat or using it as energy."

He makes a very important point. Imagine coming home from work and instead of turning your car off and shutting down the engine, you put the car in park and leave its engine running. All night long that car engine would be burning fuel. The same holds true when your body doesn't shut down at night. All night long it is burning fuel. When you wake up the next morning your body will crave more fuel, i.e., food.

We are magnificent beings, innately wired to be self-sufficient. Once our bodies are deprived of fuel, they go through a feast or famine response and will crave an overabundance of food and store it as fat for later use. Sleep deprivation makes our bodies constantly crave more fuel (ghrelin), stops the hormone that tells us that we're full (leptin), and lowers the hormone that helps convert fat to fuel (HGH), which puts stress on the body (cortisol), which, in turn, produces dangerous belly fat. This hormonal roller coaster not only causes weight gain but also accelerates the aging process and causes wrinkles, memory loss, weakness, gray hair, and diminished libido. You have the ability to combat all of these things by simply getting a good night's rest. Many of you may already sleep eight hours, but do you really get eight hours of deep, restorative, healing sleep? Many people close their eyes but end up tossing and turning throughout the night.

Research published in the *American Journal of Epidemiology* showed alarming numbers on just how little sleep we get each night. Women get, on average, just 6.3 hours of sleep per night, and men sleep only 5.6 hours.[636]

Can You DIG This?

Sleep deprivation affects 2.9 billion people worldwide. In America, people spend $23 billion a year trying to get a better night's sleep. That's more than they spend on any other ailment, making sleeplessness the biggest epidemic facing the nation today. Sleeping less than seven hours per night doubles your risk of dying, and sleeping less than six hours quadruples your risk of dying.[637 638]

Why are people so sleep deprived? One man that is partially to blame is Thomas Edison! That's right, the genius who invented the light bulb. Our body is biologically programmed to be active during daylight hours and shut completely down when it's dark out. Before the invention of the light bulb, our ancestors slept ten to twelve hours every night in pure darkness.

At night, the pineal gland of the brain produces a hormone called mela-tonin, aka "hormone of darkness." Melatonin creates the body's day/night circadian rhythm, including the timing with which other hormones are released. Melatonin stimulates HGH secretion,has a role in regulating ghrelin, and affects cortisol levels, which are all dependent on the body's circadian cycle. [639] [640] [641] This explains why shift workers who sleep during the day tend to gain weight more than workers who sleep at night.[642] A Harvard University study showed that sleeping, eating, and being active at times that are at odds with the body's normal circadian cycle increases the risk of diabetes and obesity.[643]

How to Sleep Better

Dark and cool! Any light in the bedroom confuses your circadian center of the brain into believing that it's daytime, and this results in less melatonin release. Items producing any light can affect your sleep, including a night-light, TV, stereo display, alarm clock, cell-phone charger, and even that streetlight shining through the windows. If you want to get a deep sleep, make your room as dark as possible. Consider using blackout curtains or eyeshades. Temperature also affects your sleep. How comfortable you feel determines how long you will sleep. The body sleeps best in a cooler setting (between 65 and 72 degrees). If it's above or below this, the body will have a harder time reaching good-quality rapid-eye-movement (REM) sleep, the stage in which you dream. Beware of memory foam mattresses and pillows because they tend to produce heat. Experts from the Ameri-can Academy of Sleep Medicine say a bedroom should be thought of as a cave—dark and cool.

Quiet. Make sure your bedroom is quiet, free from noise or other distrac-tions. If you have a bed partner who snores or if you snore, try using a cervical pillow. This will help open the airway, similar to what tilting back the head accomplishes during CPR. If you are a light sleeper and noises keep you awake (birds, animals, crickets, rain, or traffic sounds), try using foam earplugs.

No food or alcohol before bedtime. Eating within two to three hours before bedtime can be a recipe for weight gain and a restless night. Digesting food while sleeping causes the blood sugar to increase for a longer period because there's no activity to utilize the sugar. This makes more of the calories you eat turn into fat. Restrict drinking fluids, including alcohol, close to bedtime to prevent nighttime bathroom awakenings. Many people think alcohol is a sedative. That's true. It will put you to sleep faster; however, it causes more nighttime awakenings. Don't use any caffeinated products six hours before bedtime. This includes chocolate, coffee, tea, sodas, and energy drinks. Some over-the-counter pain relievers also contain caffeine.

Top-10 Sleep-Inducing Foods

One of the biggest obstacles I hear from patients trying to lose weight is snacking at night. People come home from work, sit in front of their TV or computer, and go for the comfort foods. Snacking doesn't have to be fattening. Eating certain foods in the late afternoon or early evening can actually help you fall asleep, increase the quality of sleep and promote weight loss.

1. **Almonds:** These are at the top of my list of healthy and relaxing snacks. They contain magnesium, which promotes sleep and aids in muscle relaxation. Almonds also offer a great source of protein, which can help maintain a stable blood sugar level and promote deeper sleep by turning off your adrenaline-awake cycle and promoting a rest-and-digest cycle. Unsweetened almond milk is also a great late-night beverage.
2. **Walnuts:** This nut offers a great source of tryptophan, a sleep-enhancing amino acid that helps make serotonin (your "feel good" hormone) and melatonin, the "body clock" hormone that sets your sleep-wake cycles. Additionally, University of Texas researchers found that walnuts contain their own source of melatonin, which may help you fall asleep faster.
3. **Bananas:** Bananas offer an excellent source of magnesium and potassium, which help relax overstressed muscles. They also contain tryptophan, a precursor for serotonin, which helps the body regulate appetite, sleep patterns, and mood.

4. **Cherries:** Eating cherries or drinking an eight-ounce glass of cherry juice will help you fall asleep faster and stay there. Cherries naturally increase the body's supply of melatonin. You can also eat one serving of dried cherries as a healthful, sleep-inducing snack.

5. **Oatmeal:** Oatmeal is rich in calcium, magnesium, phosphorus, silicon, and potassium—all known to support sleep. Add some bananas or almonds.

6. **Flaxseeds:** Rich in omega-3 fatty acids, flaxseeds help relieve stress and help you relax before bedtime. Sprinkle some flaxseeds on that evening oatmeal or eat a tablespoon separately.

7. **Turkey:** Packed with tryptophan, this lean meat can help you relax and fall asleep. A lean ground turkey lettuce wrap makes a great nighttime snack. Chopped water chestnuts and fresh herbs (such as cilantro and basil) make for some great added flavoring to this low-calorie, sleep-inducing snack.

8. **Chamomile tea:** This is a great bedtime tea because it has a mild sedating effect, which helps turn off restless minds and bodies.

9. **Honey:** You would think having something sweet in the hours before bedtime would keep you awake, but the glucose in honey tells your brain to turn off orexin, a neurotransmitter that's linked to alertness and wakefulness. Drizzle a little in your chamomile tea.

10. **Hummus:** A popular dish that originated in the Middle East, hummus has a texture and consistency similar to peanut butter. Several ingredients are used in making hummus, but the primary ingredient is chickpeas (also known as garbanzo beans), which are high-protein legumes. Other ingredients of hummus include lemon juice, fresh garlic, paprika, and olive oil. Tryptophan, phenylalanine, and tyrosine are the amino acids found in hummus that can promote good-quality sleep and uplift a person's mood. Put a few tablespoons on celery sticks, and you have a healthy, sleep-inducing snack!

Obstacle #3: Obesogens

Another reason people struggle so much with their weight is because of chemicals called obesogens. These are chemicals, either natural or man-made, that take control of your metabolic systems, causing weight gain. They come from compounds found in certain plastics, in pesticides and fungicides, in soy and sweeteners, and in the hormones that are injected into our livestock. These obesogens increase appetite and disrupt normal development and lipid metabolism, all of which can lead to obesity. They create an imbalance of hormones such as growth hormone, insulin, and cortisol. People exposed to obesogens may also suffer from a deficiency or change in the ratio between androgen and estrogen sex steroid levels, which normally modifies the fat balance in the body. This can lead to lowered growth hormone secretion, unbalanced cortisol levels, and increased resistance to insulin.[644] Obesogens can be found in makeup, water bottles, nonstick pans, microwave popcorn, and even your shower curtain. In fact, the average person is exposed to over 100 obesogens every day! Additionally, obesogens have been correlated with heart disease, diabetes, obesity, and high cholesterol.[645]

The Most Common Obesogens

High-fructose corn syrup (HFCS) is a leading cause of obesity, especially in children. This is the most common food and drink sweetener on the market. This obesogen wreaks havoc on the insulin and appetite regulating hormones, fooling you into thinking you're hungry, even if you are not. This increase in appetite leads to fat production.[646] HFCS is cheaper than sugar, thanks to the government's farm bill corn subsidies. Products with HFCS are sweeter and cheaper than products made with cane sugar. This allows the average soda size to go from 8 ounces to 20 ounces with no additional costs to the manufacturers. In June 2004, the *Journal of Clinical Endocrinology & Metabolism* showed that ghrelin, the hormone that makes you feel hungry and tells you to eat, was not suppressed after eating HFCS.[647] In May 2009, the *Journal of Clinical Investigation* showed that participants assigned to a high-fructose drink gained more visceral fat compared to the group with a high-glucose drink. In other words, a high fructose intake is more likely to create abdominal fat than sugar. Abdominal fat is considered the most dangerous fat because it's associated with increased risk of type 2 diabetes and cardiovascular diseases.[648]

Bisphenol-A (BPA), a synthetic estrogen primarily used to harden plastics, has been shown to increase insulin resistance. BPA is found in plastic food and beverage containers, canned foods, baby formulas, bottle tops, and water supply lines. Some dental sealants and composites also contain BPA. The United States produces 6 billion pounds of BPA annually, and it's detectable in 93 percent of Americans. This chemical is also found in thermal paper items including receipts, event and cinema tickets, labels, ATM receipts, and airline tickets.[649] Pregnant woman should never touch their eyes, nose, or mouth after handling these thermal-paper products! The American Chemistry Council petitioned the FDA to phase out the chemical from plastic baby bottles due to the health dangers associated with ingesting the chemical. In July 2012, the FDA finally made it official: BPA can't be used in plastic baby bottles and cups.[650]

When you put a thermal-imaging receipt from a cash register into your wallet, it contaminates your currency with BPA. This makes the paper money you handle a secondary source of exposure.[651] That means you are getting a dosage of the female hormone estrogen from your money. In addition to BPA being linked to health problems such as cancer, infertility, and breast cancer, it has also been shown to be a major contributor to the obesity epidemic.[652]

Pesticides used to destroy pests that feed on fruits and vegetables are linked to obesity, diabetes, and other morbidities.[653] The average American is exposed to ten to thirteen pesticides every day, and 90 percent are endocrine disrupters, which have been linked to obesity.

Pharmaceutical drugs can contain obesogens. Some antidepressants, known as selectively serotonin reuptake inhibitors (SSRIs), are linked to causing obesity because they affect food intake and lipid accumulation, which leads to obesity.[654] Actos, Avandia, and Thiazolidinedione are diabetic drugs that improve insulin sensitivity but also make people fat.[655]

Perfluorooctanoic acid (PFOA) is a surfactant used in nonstick cookware. PFOA has been detected in the blood of more than 98 percent of the general U.S. population.[656] It is a potential endocrine disruptor linked to obesity.[657]

Hormones such as estrogen, progesterone, and testosterone are being used to increase the weight of cattle. When you eat the cattle, these same substances may increase the weight in YOU! A study in the *International Journal of Obesity* from researchers at ten different universities, including Yale

University School of Medicine and Johns Hopkins University, found that the use of steroid hormones in meat production and on conventional dairy farms could be contributing to obesity.[658]

Antibiotics in chicken and farmed fish. Because chicken and farmed fish are kept in small pens/cages, antibiotics are often used to help them fight off infection and grow larger. These antibiotics are obesogens.

Can You DIG This?

So many weight-loss clinics, diet books, and experts contend that the primary reason people can't lose weight is because they eat too many calories. That is not true. Adults have actually been eating steadily fewer calories for almost a decade, despite the continued increase in obesity rates, according to research published in the *American Journal of Clinical Nutrition*. They analyzed trends since the 1970s and found that among adults, average daily energy intake rose by a total of 314 calories from 1971 to 2003 and then fell by 74 calories between 2003 and 2010.[659] That is a lot less calorie consumption, enough to warrant a considerable drop in obesity. No matter how few calories you consume, being exposed to more obesogens will make it more difficult to weigh less.

How to Avoid Obesogens

- Use eco-friendly alternatives to plastic bottles for hot or cold liquids. Aluminum BPA-free sports water bottles are also available.
- Stay clear of plastic containers with the number 3 or 7 on the bottom, which may leach BPA. Instead look for the numbers 1, 2, 4, 5, and 6, which are unlikely to contain BPA.
- Keep water bottles cool (warm temperatures increase BPA leaching) and never microwave plastic.
- Eat organic produce; avoid processed foods in plastic or shiny gloss exterior containers.
- Eat grass-fed, free-range, or wild-caught chicken and fish.
- Avoid nonstick pans and prepackaged foods.
- Eat fewer canned foods. Instead go for fresh or frozen. For instance, tuna can be found in pouches that do not contain BPA.

- Avoid artificial sweeteners.

Artificial Sweeteners' Sweet Deception

The most popular chemicals that are linked to causing obesity are, by far, artificial sweeteners. They're everywhere! Americans spend $67 billion per year on artificial sweeteners, which is more than they spend annually on beauty products, coffee, and pets combined! Food and drink manufacturers market these sweeteners with slogans like "guilt-free," "no calories," and "zero carbs." Unfortunately America has been duped, and the truth may come to you as no sweet surprise. Anything that is labeled "artificial" means it's created by chemists in a laboratory. These sugar alternatives are formulated with an array of toxic chemicals that lead to imbalances in the body and have been linked to ailments like depression, arthritis, Alzheimer's disease, Parkinson's disease, and even cancer. In spite of the public becoming aware of this information, it's a risk many are willing to take in order to trim down those unwanted pounds. Sadly there is no concrete evidence showing that these sugar substitutes help people lose weight. In fact, studies suggest quite the opposite. Restaurants and grocery stores offer us a colorful rainbow assortment of blue, yellow, and pink packets. Let's examine the three most popular.

Aspartame

The most popular is the blue packet—aspartame—a sweetener used in more than six thousand consumer items, including soft drinks, yogurt, chewing gum, salad dressings, and even multivitamins. Aspartame, sold as NutraSweet and Equal, was first discovered in 1965 by a scientist at G.D. Searle and Company. Aspartame was discovered inadvertently while a chemist was formulating an anti-ulcer drug. He accidentally discovered its sweet taste when he licked his finger to turn the page. The tip of his finger had been contaminated with aspartame, which created a sweet taste. This sweet chemical would end up making more money being sold as a sweetener than it ever would have as an ulcer medication. Searle's early tests of aspartame showed that consuming high levels produced tumors in the brains of experimental rats and epileptic seizures in monkeys and was converted by animals into formaldehyde![660] In spite of these dangerous side effects, the FDA approved aspartame as a dry-food additive in 1974.

Many scientists reviewed the data, including renowned brain researcher John Olney from Washington University in St. Louis. Olney was appalled after learning aspartame caused brain tumors in rats, and he petitioned the FDA for a public hearing. Dr. Olney proved that aspartic acid (one aspartame component) caused microscopic holes in the brains of rats after eating the substance. Consumer Action for Improved Foods and Drugs also petitioned for a public hearing because the product caused epileptic seizures in monkeys and possible eye damage. Aspartame includes phenylalinine, which causes phenylketonuria (PKU) in a small number of susceptible children, and methyl alcohol, a dangerous neurotoxin.

In 1975 an FDA inspector conducted a routine review of the Searle's testing facilities and found many violations. This report led the FDA commissioner to put together a Special Commissioner's Task Force to review Searle's labs. In December of 1975, this task force reported serious problems with Searle's research on aspartame. Eleven landmark studies were conducted in a manner so blatantly flawed, it exposed serious doubts about aspartame's safety and cast possible criminal liability for Searle.[661] The U.S. attorney for Chicago sought a grand jury review of the monkey seizure study. This U.S. attorney let the statute of limitations run out and then ended up joining Searle's law firm. Fast-forward five years to October 1980. The FDA's public board of inquiry finally evaluated aspartame's safety and found that the chemical caused an unacceptable level of brain tumors in animal testing. Based on that fact, the board ruled that aspartame should not be allowed into the food supply. This ruling uncovered fifteen years of regulatory deception by the FDA and the Searle drug company.

In November 1980, shortly after the public board of inquiry's ruling, Ronald Reagan became president. In January of 1981, just as Reagan was taking office, he stated at a sales meeting that one of his top priorities was to get aspartame approved by the end of the year. He appointed Dr. Arthur Hull Hayes as FDA commissioner. Hayes had aspartame approved as a food ingredient within six months! Two years later, the FDA approved aspartame for soft drinks. Hayes was later exposed for accepting corporate gifts, ended up leaving the FDA, and went to work with Searle, as their senior medical advisor. In 1985 corporate giant Monsanto (yes, them again!) purchased Searle and all the rights to NutraSweet (aspartame's trademarked name). Searle's lawyer, Robert Shapiro, became president of Monsanto! Are all these revolving doors making you dizzy?

Shortly after the FDA approved aspartame for soft drinks, more than ten thousand complaints about the artificial sweetener began to flood into the FDA's office.[662] The most common of the complaints reported people experiencing nausea, dizziness, blurred vision, headaches, and seizures after ingesting aspartame. The FDA contacted the Centers for Disease Control (CDC) to review the complaints, and the center found that the symptoms in approximately 25 percent of the complainants had stopped and then restarted, corresponding with their having stopped and then restarted consuming aspartame. Proof at last! The CDC's findings were given to the FDA, but the report was discounted. Why would the FDA disregard a report from the agency it solicited for help to investigate? The day the FDA received the CDC report, Pepsi-Cola had just launched a media campaign announcing they had switched to aspartame. The Pepsi announcement and aggressive marketing made NutraSweet a household name. By 1995 human brain tumors like those in the animal studies increased by 10 percent and even some previously benign tumors turned malignant. Searle along with the FDA's deputy commissioner belittled this new data and said aspartame posed no health problems. In 1997 this very same FDA official became vice president of clinical research for . . . here we go again . . . Searle![663]

To this day, more complaints on aspartame's adverse reactions as a food additive have been received. In February of 1994, the U.S. Department of Health and Human Services released the listing of adverse reactions reported to the FDA. Aspartame accounted for more than 75 percent of all adverse reactions reported to the FDA's Adverse Reaction Monitoring System (ARMS). The FDA lists ninety-two official side effects from aspartame, ranging from anxiety, arthritis, and weight gain to death. However, it is still legally used in our food![664]

Aspartame's main ingredient, phenylalanine, can interfere with proper mental function and wreak havoc on the nervous system. In diet soft drinks, it can act as a neurotoxin that triggers degenerative diseases. Throughout the 1980s, actor Michael J. Fox did commercials for Pepsi, and, in the latter years of his contract, he promoted exclusively Diet Pepsi. And throughout this period, he became an avid consumer of the company's diet cola. He would later be one of the youngest people in history to develop

Parkinson's disease. (It is a disease that normally is known to afflict people over fifty.) Why did he get this disease at such an unprecedented young age of twenty-nine? N-methyl-D-aspartate (NMDA) receptors in the brain are responsible for the neurotoxicity associated with Parkinson's disease. Aspartate is one of the main components that is released when aspartame is metabolized, and it directly affects the NMDA receptors. Therefore, regular intake of aspartame will cause damage to those receptors and may possibly lead to Parkinson's disease. Alzheimer's is also connected to high exposures of this chemical.[665]

During one of my morning health segments on Lifetime Television, I conducted a two-part feature exposing the dangers of artificial sweeteners. I wanted to share the connection to Michael J. Fox's Parkinson's disease with his diet-soft-drink consumption, but after the legal team at Lifetime Television reviewed the script, it excluded that part of the segment. They were concerned there just wasn't enough proof, and, of course, that meant possible legal repercussions. I refused to sit back and allow such an important part of this feature to get the axe. So I forwarded the powers that be a plethora of evidence, including compelling research conducted by James Bowen, M.D., and Arthur M. Evangelista, former FDA investigator, showing aspartame is a powerful neurotoxin.[666] I included "Evidence File #6: Aspartame & Parkinson's Disease" submitted by Mark D. Gold with the Aspartame Toxicity Information Center.[667] [668] After reviewing this research and more, I was given the thumbs up by the legal team at Lifetime and my segment aired to rave reviews. I received hundreds of letters from viewers with the same theme. I'll share one with you:

Dear Dr. Friedman,

For over a year I've suffered from debilitating dizziness, fatigue, and memory loss. My doctor had me get a CTscan, MRI, and blood work, but none of these gave him anything to help diagnose my condition. While I sat in front of my TV with my morning cup of coffee sweetened with aspartame, there you were giving me the answers to the severe health issues that had been afflicting my life. The chemicals causing fatigue, dizziness, and memory loss were going into my system as I watched your segment. Little did I know, I had been poisoning

my body every morning! [After your segment] I poured that cup of coffee in the sink and have never touched artificial sweeteners again. All my symptoms are gone, and I've never felt better in my life! Thank you for waking me up that morning.
　　—Sarah B.

Splenda

Now it's on to the yellow packets, sucralose, commonly sold as Splenda. It is claimed to be "the safest" artificial sweetener, even though there have been no major studies proving its safety. Before sucralose was approved as a sugar substitute, it was an insecticide. How is this insecticide-turned-sugar substitute created? First they start with real sugar, which is chemically modified with chlorine to make it calorie-free. Then acetone, a chemical used in nail-polish remover, is added as a buffer. Benzene, a toxic carcinogen found in gasoline, is added to the mix. By the way, benzene is listed as one of the EPA's "most dangerous chemicals."[669] Then they throw in a little toluene, a chemical used in glues and paints, and mix it with methanol, a poisonous wood alcohol also used in antifreeze and windshield washer fluid.[670] But we mustn't forget the ingredient I love to *death* . . . formaldehyde! That's right; this is the same chemical used to embalm dead bodies. For those who start their day off using sucralose, this puts a new meaning to the term "killer cup of coffee."

The safety of sucralose was in question before the FDA approved the chemical for human consumption. The longest human study conducted was a four-day trial focusing on sucralose and how it affects tooth decay but not the long-term health effects on humans. The FDA claims that more than a hundred animal studies on sucralose were reviewed proving it to be safe, but what they fail to mention is that the side effects they discovered, which seemingly got swept under the corporate carpet, include:

- increased male infertility by interfering with sperm production and vitality
- brain lesions
- enlarged and calcified kidneys
- decreased red blood cells—a sign of anemia—at levels above 1,500 milligrams/kilograms/day

- spontaneous abortions in nearly half the rabbit population given sucralose, compared to zero aborted pregnancies in the control group
- a 23 percent death rate in rabbits given sucralose, compared to a 6 percent death rate in the control group.[671]

Saccharin

Pretty in pink packets—not so much. Saccharin, commonly sold as Sweet'N Low, is an artificial sweetener linked to causing cancer in animals in the 1960s and 1970s. It had a warning label just like cigarettes do today. Saccharin is a coal tar derivative and has no food value whatsoever. Think about it: were we designed to eat something derived from *coal*?

Many chemicals are used in the formulation of saccharin, one of them being ammonia. That's right—ammonia, the same stuff you use to clean your toilet. Saccharin is used in many items, including over-the-counter drugs! The recommended daily dosage of chewable aspirin or acetaminophen tablets for a school-age child is equivalent to the same amount of saccharin contained in one can of a diet soft drink. A group of companies that market low-calorie foods and beverages petitioned to have saccharin removed from the EPA's list of cancerous chemicals. In 2000 the National Toxicology Program (NTP) determined that saccharin should no longer be listed as a potential cancer-causing agent because the initial studies were primarily conducted on animals and not humans. In 2001, the FDA reversed its position on saccharin, declaring it completely safe for human consumption.[672]

Despite the ruling, many scientists still believe the chemical is carcinogenic. Some of today's leading scientists got together and argued to the National Toxicology Program, a division of the National Institute of Environmental Health Sciences, that declaring saccharin safe would "result in greater exposure to this probable carcinogen in tens of millions of people, including children. If saccharin is even a weak carcinogen, this unnecessary additive would pose an intolerable risk to the public."[673] Epidemiologist Richard Clapp, associate professor of Boston University's Department of Environmental Health, who co-signed the letter to the NTP, stated, "With numerous studies suggesting that saccharin may cause cancer in humans, we should be extremely cautious." Another co-signer, Samuel Epstein, M.D., professor of environmental medicine at the School of Public Health, University of Illinois Medical Center, Chicago, wrote, "In light of the many animal *and human studies* clearly demonstrating that saccharin is carcinogenic, it is astonishing that the NTP is even considering delisting saccharin."

Other scientists maintained that saccharin increases the risk of cancer, including Emmanuel Farber, M.D., Ph.D., professor of pathology at Jefferson Medical College and chairman of the National Academy of Sciences' 1978 panel that concluded that saccharin is a carcinogen; William Lijinsky, former director of the Chemical Carcinogenesis Program at the National Cancer Institute at Frederick; and cancer epidemiologist Devra Davis, director of the Health, Environment, and Development Program at the World Resources Institute. In this document, they cited six studies of humans, including a large National Cancer Institute study, which found an association between artificial sweetener consumption and bladder cancer, especially in heavy consumers of diet foods.[674] These efforts were futile; the multibillion dollar saccharin industry prevailed.

Healthful Sugar Substitutes

Lo han guo is a natural sweetener derived from the monk fruit and is three hundred times sweeter than sugar but with none of the calories.[675] Because of its low glycemic index, it's a great choice for diabetics. Lo han guo is also great for cooking and baking because it's very stable under high temperatures.

Coconut sugar is derived from the coconut palm tree. It is a rich source of vitamins and minerals including potassium, magnesium, B3, B6, zinc, and iron. It contains a fiber called inulin, which slows glucose absorption and lowers its glycemic index.[676]

Stevia is another great sugar alternative that has been used for more than 1,500 years in South America. It's 100 percent natural and virtually calorie free!

Xylitol is a low-calorie, diabetic-friendly, delicious sugar alternative extracted from the birch tree. Xylitol also helps reduce cavities and has received official endorsements from several national dental associations, making it the ideal sugar alternative for chewing gums and candy.

Most of these healthful sugar alternatives are available at health food stores or can be purchased online. In conclusion, look to nature, not chemists, for your sweetener.

Chemicals Galore: The Perils of Diet Soda

The "guilt-free" rationale of diet sodas because of their low-calorie, artificial sweetener content makes people wrongfully believe that there is no limit to how many they can consume. Just because something is "calorie-free" doesn't make it an effective weight-loss product. The bitter truth is that soft drinks containing artificial sweeteners don't aid in weight loss. On the contrary, they have been linked to obesity and many diseases. Stop drinking them! People use artificially sweetened drinks because they believe sugar is so fattening. Actually, a teaspoon of sugar contains only 16 calories. That's it! The equivalent of the amount of calories you'd get after eating a cup of mushrooms, a cup of cucumbers, or ¼ cup of green beans. While there are a plethora of health concerns associated with consuming sugar, a small amount is *not* going to make you fat; however, a *minimal* amount of artificial sweeteners *can* make you fat. Beverages that contain artificial sweeteners do not make you skinny nor do they have any value whatsoever!

Diet Soft Drinks Cause Obesity!

America spends $21 billion on diet soft drinks. All this money is being spent on an elaborate money-making hoax! These diet drinks actually contain chemical sweeteners that stimulate appetite and contribute to obesity. A study at the University of Texas Health Science Center at San Antonio found that participants who drink two or more diet soft drinks daily have a ballooning waist circumference 500 percent greater than those who drank none. This eight-year study showed that diet soft drinks *increase the risk of obesity* by 41 percent for every soft drink ingested.[677] Considering the average diet-soft-drink consumer will have five sodas per day, this creates a 200 percent increased risk of obesity from the very beverage that people have been fooled into believing is keeping them from gaining weight. I'm not an advocate of drinking regular sodas but they are actually the lesser of two evils. You are far better off drinking regular soda than diet soft drinks if you are concerned about your weight. Many people believe that diet soft drinks will keep their blood sugar in check. If that's you, it might surprise you to learn that drinking just one diet soda per day puts you at a 67 percent higher risk of getting type 2 diabetes and 36 percent increased risk of developing metabolic syndrome, a group of risk factors linked to obesity, heart disease, diabetes, and stroke.[678] Don't be fooled into believing that because they contain "no sugar" they are diabetic-friendly drinks.

I had a patient named Beth who weighed 373 pounds and was upset because she kept gaining weight no matter what she tried. She told me she drank eight diet soft drinks every day! In fact, every time I treated her she would be sipping from an open can of diet cola. I told her that her beverage was one of the reasons she was gaining weight.

She replied, "That can't be true. Why would the FDA allow the label to say 'zero calories' if diet soft drinks were fattening?"

Finally I had to use some tough love. I pulled out her chart and showed her that six months prior when I first examined her she had weighed 335 pounds. I asked her how she could possibly fathom eight diet sodas per day benefiting her if she has gained 38 pounds in six months? She finally "got it" and agreed to break the habit. Eight weeks later she had lost 16 pounds. Within five months of getting off the diet sodas, she lost another 46 pounds! Keep in mind, she did not add any exercise to her regimen nor did she change her eating habits. By simply not poisoning her body with artificial chemicals, her hormones balanced, her appetite decreased, and she stopped craving and eating as much food. A year after being off diet sodas, Beth lost a total of 146 pounds!

Diet Soft Drinks Are Addictive

When you drink diet soft drinks the pancreas releases insulin because the brain has been signaled that something sweet is on the way. When left unsatisfied, the addiction part of the brain kicks in, very similar to other addictions like cigarettes, alcohol, and even drugs. In other words, the human brain continues to chase the "high" these artificial sweeteners cause, which constantly teases the brain, making it crave more. In a 2008 study, women who drank water that was alternately sweetened with sugar and Splenda couldn't tell the difference—but their brains could. Functional MRI (fMRI) brain scans revealed that even though both drinks lit up the brain's reward system, the sugar did so more completely. This makes the brain keep telling the body to get ready for sugar but doesn't get the reward it expects, so it craves even more. Study author Martin P. Paulus, M.D., a professor of psychiatry at the University of California, San Diego, suggests that diet soda might be addicting because artificial sweeteners have positive reinforcing effects similar to alcohol and even drug abuse.[679] Diet soft drinks create physical and psychological cravings.

Diet Soft Drinks Can Cause Heart Attack and Stroke

One of the most ludicrous things I have ever seen is Diet Coke's The Heart Truth® campaign. On their website it states:

> The Heart Truth® is a national awareness campaign, sponsored by the National Heart, Lung, and Blood Institute (NHLBI), part of the National Institutes of Health, U.S. Department of Health and Human Services. They have partnered with NHLBI to raise awareness about heart disease in women and equip them to take action against risk factors.[680]

If that were true, they would tell women to STOP DRINKING DIET COKE! As Diet Coke cans and advertisements are adorned with a heart-flag logo, giving woman the impression that the beverage is "heart healthy," it's time they were told the truth: diet soft drinks increase the risk of heart disease and stroke.

For ten years, researchers at University of Miami and Columbia University in New York followed more than 2,500 people and discovered those who drank diet soda every day had a 61 percent higher risk of stroke and heart attack than those who did not consume the beverage. This information was presented at the American Stroke Association's International Stroke Conference in Los Angeles.

Interestingly, some studies also suggest a link between vascular problems and caramel-containing products. Caramel is the ingredient that gives the dark color to sodas such as Diet Coke.[681] Research from the Multi-Ethnic Study of Atherosclerosis found that people who drank diet soda every day had a 36 percent greater risk of developing metabolic syndrome and a 67 percent greater risk of developing diabetes. Both of these conditions greatly raise the odds of having a stroke or heart attack.[682]

D*iscoveries:* Fad diets will help you lose weight; the problem is keeping it off. We need to change our lifestyles and not just our eating routines.

I*nstincts:* You can't blame your grandparents for having fat genes. If you look at history, only in recent times have we suffered from an obesity epidemic. What is causing this "modern-day" problem? Does your gut really tell you that your grandparents are to blame? We eat more fattening, enzyme-altering, and hormone-disrupting chemicals in our food and beverages; we live a more sedentary lifestyle; we make lousy food choices; and sleep more poorly today than any time in history. Evidence supports contributing factors to the obesity epidemic, including consuming chemicals, eating *white foods* like flour and refined sugar, and not getting enough restorative sleep.

G*od:* Many people trying to lose weight consume artificial sweeteners every day, yet their weight problem remains. These same people spend billions of dollars on fad diets, shakes, and fat burners, many of which ironically call for the use of such chemicals. Our bodies reject these sweeteners, rebelling against them in the form of weight gain. When consuming artificial sweeteners, the pancreas releases insulin and this causes the brain to remain unsatisfied, making you crave sugar and carbs. We simply were not designed to ingest the chemicals sold in tiny packets of blue, pink, and yellow.

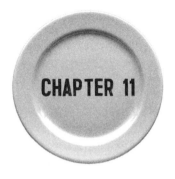

CHAPTER 11

THE FOOD AND NUTRITION POLICE
WHAT HAPPENED TO FREEDOM OF CHOICE?

"The ten most dangerous words in the English language
are 'Hi! I'm from the government, and I'm here to help.'"
—Ronald Reagan

It was Monday, June 16, 2003. I stopped at a gas station, swiped my credit card, and received a message that it was declined. How strange! I went into the gas station and handed the clerk another credit card. That one was also declined! I called the credit card company, and I was told that a freeze had been placed on my cards. What? Since I spent all the money I had in my wallet on gas, I stopped at an ATM machine at the grocery store to withdraw some cash. I received an odd message: "Insufficient funds." My heart sank when I checked my account and read: ZERO! Had I been robbed? Was I victim of identity theft? I immediately drove to my bank, and the vice president informed me that my assets had been frozen, and I could not withdraw a dime or write any checks. Clearly, a big mistake had been made. I asked him who demanded an asset freeze. I was told it was the FTC (Federal Trade Commission).

When I returned to my office, a sheriff was waiting for me. He handed me a civil summons. Turns out the company of an all-natural aloe vera–based wellness product I was selling in my office was being sued by the Federal Trade Commission for "selling an unapproved drug." I later learned that the FTC and a SWAT team of armed U.S. marshals raided the company's California headquarters and manufacturing plant and seized all the company's assets, records, and computers, as well as the cars, houses, and belongings of the CEO and president. More than six hundred employees were escorted out of the buildings and sent home. Computers were confiscated as evidence.

I called David Newman, the FTC attorney whose name was listed on my summons, to tell him a terrible mistake had been made. If the company had done something wrong, I was not an owner, held no corporate position, and was not a stockholder. I was just an independent distributor, similar to an Avon representative. I had no input on how the company operated its business. Mr. Newman told me that the FTC had decided to go after the company and its top two independent distributors (one being me) to make an example out of us. Their witch hunt was called "Operation Cure All," a coordinated effort between the Food and Drug Administration (FDA) and various state attorney generals to crack down on unscrupulous marketers, preying on sick and vulnerable consumers. The FTC's guerilla warfare attacks on hundreds of companies selling "unapproved drugs" would bring the government hundreds of millions of dollars in seized assets.

The FTC had not issued a single warning letter to me, nor had I received a cease and desist. As a doctor, I am legally allowed to share the benefits of diet, homeopathic remedies, herbal supplements, vitamins, minerals, teas, and tinctures. I learned that I was included because I had recorded an audio that covered some of the science and health benefits of these natural ingredients. Sharing health benefits of a natural product *outside my office* is considered illegally promoting an unapproved drug. Once that happens, the FTC has legal grounds to freeze a person's assets and issue a fine. The audio I recorded simply shared some of the science and health benefits of the aloe vera–based product. By FTC guidelines, distributing a third-party resource is deemed illegal. In other words, if I share the health benefits of aloe vera with a hundred of my patients, it's within my scope of practice, but recording a CD with this same message that a distributor or customer shares with a hundred people is against federal law!

Why would the FTC freeze the assets of someone who is merely promoting a nutritional product? They say it's so the people they go after can't flee the country. In actuality, they freeze assets as a way to paralyze people's ability to hire a top-notch lawyer to defend them. After the FTC freezes someone's assets—rarely does anyone get their day in court—they issue a press release to the media to discredit the "guilty party" by contacting his local news stations, magazines, and newspapers, so his entire community knows what a scam artist he is for promoting a natural product and claiming it enhances people's health. This person now gets portrayed as a snake-oil salesman who deceived poor, innocent victims. When the FTC had my local newspaper and television news run the story, it tarnished my impeccable reputation.

Before I continue, I'll share what the FTC defines as an "unapproved drug." Any nutritional or whole-food product that claims to "cure, treat, prevent, or diagnose a disease." The FTC definition of a disease is diverse and includes everything from the common cold, arthritis, obesity, and hemorrhoids to osteoporosis, urinary tract infection, and depression. An example of something deemed an "unapproved drug claim" is a calcium manufacturer stating that its product may help prevent osteoporosis (yes, even the word *may* is not allowed). If a calcium supplement label had this claim, the FTC could come in and shut down the manufacturer, freeze its assets, and fine them millions of dollars. Ironically, the FTC is okay with Tums being sold as a calcium supplement and using the URL www.osteoperosis.com, but it considers it illegal for a nutritional company to market its calcium product using this disease name. Are you curious why the FTC allow the makers of Tums to use the word *osteoporosis*? Follow the money . . . Tums is owned by Big Pharma giant GlaxoSmithKline. Drug companies can make this "drug claim," but a calcium supplement, being their competition, cannot.

Okay, back to my misadventure . . . I spent the next sixty days responding to the FTC's complaint. Because I was being included in the overall company lawsuit, I had to defend the company's claims and sales materials. I submitted hundreds of studies that included third-party, peer-reviewed, double-blind scientific research showing the health benefits of the product's whole-food ingredients. I forwarded sworn affidavits from doctors and patients who had shared their testimonials. I also included before-and-after blood work, leaving no doubts of the powerful, health-enhancing properties of the product (blood never lies). I was certain that once the FTC saw this proof, it would realize this was all a big misunderstanding.

After the FTC read my rebuttal, what my lawyer told me that day would finally reveal to me just how corrupt the system is. He said the FTC was impressed with how much effort I had put into proving that the health claims that were made were accurate; however, because I did such a great job illustrating how the product might indeed help prevent and even reverse disease, I had just sealed my coffin! Come to find out, if a nutritional product is *proven* to help cure or prevent a disease, then it must be sold as a pharmaceutical product and go through a lengthy, stringent, and expensive drug-approval process. My lawyer said, because I went out of my way to *prove the efficacy* of the aloe product, I simply *proved their case*, which meant an even bigger fine would be issued.

Without getting my day in court to plead my case, I was told by my lawyer that I had no choice but to sign a permanent injunction not admitting to any guilt but agreeing to pay $1 million as "restitution." Why restitution? The FTC said it was to compensate all the poor, innocent victims who were scammed and duped into believing the product could enhance their health, because only drugs can do that. A very small percentage of this "restitution" pot is actually sent to these "victims." In fact, independent distributors, health-food stores, retail stores, gyms, hair salons, and even doctors' offices considered victims of these so-called fraudulent products are excluded from receiving monetary restitution, because according to the FTC, these venues are simply "part of the Ponzi scheme." The FTC is penalizing these innocent victims they pretend to protect!

Not only was my stellar reputation as a doctor, author, educator, and researcher blemished, but legal fees and "consumer redress" cost me my life savings and every penny of my retirement. The manufacturer of the aloe vera product was eventually sued by the FTC for $120 million dollars, which caused them to close their doors for good.

The saddest part is the FTC did not receive one complaint about the product that I was being chastised for selling in my office. NOT ONE! The product worked! In fact, the FTC received thousands of calls, letters, emails, and faxes from satisfied customers, begging them not to take the product off the market. However, customer testimonials are considered illegal. If you have high cholesterol and took a natural tea that helped lower it, wouldn't you want to share this great news with others? Sharing this testimonial on a website, through social media, in a brochure, or even in front of a group is considered by the FTC to be illegal, and you and the manufacturer of the product could be sued for promoting an "unapproved drug." Testimonials are perfectly legal for any other product sold on the market. In fact most consumers rely on product reviews before making a purchase. However, if any food or nutritional product has testimonials on its efficacy for curing or preventing any disease, it's 100 percent illegal.

If not a single unhappy consumer complaint, then who complained to the FTC? For that answer, follow the money. Big Pharma! When news circulates around the internet, TV, and radio about anything natural that can help cure, treat, or prevent cancer, diabetes, heart disease, or even toenail fungus (seriously), Big Pharma loses money. More than 800,000 satisfied customers took the aloe vera product I had endorsed, with sales of more than $22 million per month. It had an astounding 86 percent repurchase rate—a statistic that would make even McDonald's envious! In spite of the company's no questions asked, unconditional sixty-day money back guarantee, the company only received less than one-tenth of 1 percent of the product returned (and most of these were unopened bottles). The money that Americans spent on this alternative wellness product translated into hundreds of millions of dollars on lost doctors' visits and prescription drugs. When consumers spend money on a *wellness* product, it means less money is being spent on *sickness* care. Diabetics taking this product sent reports sharing how they were able to reduce and in some cases even eliminate their insulin use. In fact, a family member of mine with diabetes was able to cut his insulin by 80 percent! His doctor told him that he had never seen anything like it in his twenty-five-year career.

On my radio show, I interviewed Neal Barnard, M.D., founder and president of the Physicians Committee for Responsible Medicine (PCRM). He's one of America's leading advocates for health, nutrition, and higher standards in research. He is the author of the book *Dr. Neal Barnard's Program for Reversing Diabetes*. In this book, he shares unequivocal proof that a nutritional approach and plant-based diet can help people cut their blood sugar, improve their insulin sensitivity, and reduce and even eliminate their need for medication. How can Dr. Barnard write and speak about this on TV and radio and not be labeled a quack snake-oil evangelist and sued by the FTC? Why wasn't I able to share how a plant-based, whole-food nutritional product helped diabetes? Because Dr. Barnard put his research and opinions in a book, this makes his statements protected by the first amendment.

Can You DIG This?

When it comes to diet and nutrition, freedom of *speech* exists in this country only in book form. In the chapters of a book, authors can legally recommend nutritional products and a diet that can cure, treat, and prevent disease. An author is within his legal rights to write, "An apple a day helps keep the doctor away." However if this author owns or works for an apple company that uses this same phrase on a label, website, or in any marketing materials, the FTC would consider that an unapproved drug claim, because it implies eating the fruit makes you less likely to need medical care. The FTC could come in with guns, shut down the apple company, and seize its orchards, as if it were an illegal marijuana field.

I wasn't the only one being accused of promoting an "unapproved drug. . . ."

Cereal Shakedown

"Heart-healthy diets rich in whole grain foods can reduce the risk of heart disease. Regular consumption of whole grains as part of a low-fat diet reduces the risk for some cancers, especially cancers of the stomach and colon." General Mills, the maker of Cheerios Toasted Whole Wheat Grain Cereal, posted these words on its website, aired a similar-sounding television commercial, and printed a box that said, "helps lower cholesterol."

In 2009, in reaction to General Mills's advertising launch, the FTC took action, saying the cereal was being marketed as a drug, because it was promoted for the use in the prevention, mitigation, and treatment of disease. Cheerios was indeed considered a drug under section 201(p) of the Act [21 U.S.C. § 321(p)] because it is not recognized as safe and effective for use in preventing or treating hypercholesterolemia (high cholesterol) or coronary heart disease. General Mills was told it was in violation of the Federal Food, Drug, and Cosmetic Act (FDCA). Therefore, the product couldn't be legally marketed with these claims in the United States without an approved new drug application.[683]

Cheerios contains whole-wheat grains, which evidence shows may lower cholesterol, but saying so on a Cheerios box or a company website makes it an unapproved-drug claim! The benefits of whole grains is well documented. But according to the government, if these claims are used to promote a cereal, the product is considered a nonapproved drug.

General Mills responded with a seven-page rebuttal, similar to the one I submitted during my debacle. In this letter dated May 14, 2009, General Mills presented several peer-reviewed scientific studies proving their claims were truthful and not misleading.[684] General Mills wrote: "These factual statements about the clinical trial results simply convey useful information to consumers and do not constitute or reveal intent by General Mills to market Cheerios as a drug." What General Mills didn't understand (and which I learned the hard way) was that, according to the government, if the statements are true, and eating Cheerios really did lower cholesterol, the product, by definition, is considered a drug! General Mills ended up surrendering and changing its Cheerios label in order to avoid having the product taken off the market or having to go through a drug-approval process.

Hundreds of leading corporations have also been reprimanded by the FTC and FDA for selling an "unapproved drug." Below are just a few examples:

GNC: Ordered to pay $2.4 million penalty to settle FTC charges for having made unsubstantiated nonapproved drug claims for forty-one products.[685] GNC also settled a previous lawsuit filed by the FTC for nonapproved drug claims and were fined $600,000.[686]

QVC: This TV network was ordered to pay $7.5 million to settle charges that it aired deceptive claims for three dietary supplements.[687] Among the illegal drug claims, the FTC found QVC guilty of stating an energy-enhancing supplement could "significantly increase energy, strength, or stamina in consumers who recently had surgery, are recovering from illness, or suffer from various conditions, such as fibromyalgia, chronic fatigue syndrome, and cancer." Had QVC stated the product would increase energy, stamina, and strength for truck drivers, this claim would be perfectly legal! Just the insinuation that a natural product can positively affect someone with a "disease" is against the law.

POM Wonderful LLC: POM Wonderful, a pomegranate juice product, lost a lawsuit with the FTC, even after presenting competent and reliable scientific evidence that supported the consumption of pomegranate juice by saying that pomegranate supports prostate health and reduces the risk of prostate cancer. A judge ruled that this was a drug claim. POM Wonderful did something most Davids would never do—sued Goliath! POM Wonderful LLC filed suit against the FTC in September 2010, seeking a declaratory judgment that their requirements violated statutory and constitutional law. David lost. In 2015 the U.S. Court of Appeals upheld claims of false advertising by POM Wonderful LLC, ruling the government could prohibit the pomegranate juice maker from all disease claims.[688]

Airborne Health, Inc.: This organization was ordered to pay $30 million to settle FTC charges that it did not have adequate evidence to support its advertising claims that the immune booster could help prevent colds. All evidence presented that showed their product indeed worked merely proved the FTC's case that Airborne was being sold as a non-approved drug.[689]

Dannon: Activia and DanActive yogurts were being sold as treatments for medical disorders and disease. The product had spokesperson and actress Jamie Lee Curtis stating that Activia could help improve digestive health. The company was ordered to pay $45 million in damages![690]

Tropicana: The FTC put the squeeze on Tropicana's claims. Tropicana was charged by the FTC for making nonapproved drug claims that their orange juice could promote a healthy heart and reduce the risk of strokes. A consent agreement was reached for any future actions.[691]

Nu Skin International, Inc: This organization was fined $1.5 million for nonapproved drug claims for its dietary supplements.[692] The FTC said the fat-loss, muscle-maintenance, and glucose-regulating product Nu Skin sold was without scientific evidence to support its claims, i.e., didn't pass the drug-approval process.

Revlon, Inc: The FTC went after Revlon for unsubstantiated health claims regarding an anti-cellulite body complex and some anti-aging products. Revlon signed a consent agreement that it would no longer make any nonapproved drug claims or face a fine.[693]

Hypocrisy, Not Health

Hundreds of companies have been reprimanded, sued, and closed down because they are selling products that the government deems to be deceptive and/or not proven to work. None of the above companies, by the way, produced a product that made anyone sick or die—unlike the FDA-approved weight-loss drug, fen-phen, which was considered safe. This *approved* anti-obesity treatment prescribed to millions in the early to mid-'90s caused serious heart-valve damage and a deadly lung condition called primary pulmonary hypertension. No armed agents showed up at the drug company's door and seized any of its property nor did any of the owners, executives, or distributors have their assets frozen. But the FTC did send in an armed SWAT team to shut down an all-natural elderberry juice factory, for the crime of selling an "unapproved drug."[694]

The FDA approved the arthritis medication Vioxx. After 140,000 cases of serious heart disease and 60,000 *deaths*, its maker, Merck, finally took the deadly drug off the market. Evidence of a cover-up was documented in the *Wall Street Journal*, citing internal company e-mails and marketing materials, which revealed two thousand scientific studies that showed an increased risk of heart attacks and strokes after the use of Vioxx.[695] The government ignores a proven conspiracy to cover up something that *caused* deadly heart attacks and strokes yet spends taxpayers' money to hunt down Tropicana because it says its orange juice *could help prevent* heart attacks and strokes? And it attacks Dannon Yogurt because it claimed the product helps aid digestion?

The federal government constantly ignores complaints about dangerous side effects (including death) from people taking pharmaceutical drugs but will come down hard on nutrition and food products making "false and misleading" claims to cure, treat, or prevent a disease—even when these situations haven't caused one customer complaint! Yet the FDA has no qualms about approving drugs with side effects that it knows causes birth defects, liver damage, cancer, heart disease, and strokes. Hundreds of similar examples exist.

Let's look at one more involving the popular pain-relieving drug Celebrex. After massive public pressure, the FDA finally decided Pfizer, the maker of the drug, was making false and misleading claims. The FTC, whose job it is to prosecute companies that produce unsubstantiated and misleading health claims, took absolutely no action against Pfizer.

I'm not implying that all claims by nutrition and food corporations are legit. Many companies out there are making false and misleading health claims not backed by science. But why should we allow organizations like the FDA and FTC, the same groups that regulate toenail fungus medications, to govern the protocols of our breakfast cereals and herbal teas? The FTC and FDA allow Big Pharma to make outlandish health claims for drugs. For example, the anti-depressant drug Prozac is touted to help with depression, but a common side effect of the drug is *depression* and *suicidal thoughts*! The drug Tamiflu is allowed to claim it helps prevent the flu, but common side effects of the drug include fever, chills, muscle aches, and sinus drainage—flu-like symptoms! So if you get the flu after taking Tamiflu, the drug company can just blame it on the "side effect," and not the drug's lack of efficacy. But Airborne is fined $30 million for a natural product with no cold-like side effects that actually helps fight the ailment? Airborne works! I know dozens of friends, family members, and patients who use it when they travel on airplanes. When they don't use it, they get the sniffles from breathing in everyone's recirculating air. When using Airborne, people don't get the sniffles. What harm is the company doing other than affecting the deep pockets of Big Pharma? In the eyes of the government, Airborne is criminal!

Big Fat Lie

In 2003, the government labeled obesity a "disease." Why on Earth would they do that? Because that meant all diet products stating they aid in weight loss would be considered, by the definition of the law, a "nonapproved drug." How convenient. Now only an approved obesity drug could legally make fat-loss claims. This decision brought with it an avalanche of money to the FTC because now they were allowed to sue weight-loss products for millions of dollars. The FTC launched "Operation Big Fat Lie," a nationwide law enforcement sweep against companies making false weight-loss claims in national advertisements. Operation Big Fat Lie was designed to stop deceptive advertising and provide refunds to consumers harmed by unscrupulous weight-loss advertisers; encourage media outlets not to carry advertisements containing bogus weight-loss claims; and educate consumers to be on their guard against companies promising miraculous weight loss without diet or exercise.

The FTC has made more than a hundred enforcement actions against weight-loss companies. Below are a few that have been sued and/or ridiculed in the media; some even shut down.

- Xenadrine EFX: $12.8 million settlement
- One-a-Day WeightSmart: $3.2 million settlement
- TrimSpa: $1.5 million settlement
- CortiSlim and CortiStress: $12 million settlement
- Medifast Inc.: $3.7 million settlement

The above companies presented evidence that their products worked, including thousands of satisfied user testimonials, all of which were deemed "illegal" by the FTC. They simply could not produce the rigorous substantiation and double-blind studies they required. And even if they could, their products would have to be relicensed as pharmaceuticals. Yes, if a natural product claims to help with obesity, it is, by definition, an unapproved drug! Are "approved weight-loss drugs" that go through the stringent government approval process more safe and effective? No. Here are some weight-loss drugs that were granted approval and deemed *safe* by the FDA:

- **Sibutramine (Meridia)** causes increased risk of heart attacks and strokes.
- **Fenfluramine/Dexfenfluramine (Redux)** is associated with heart valve problems and death.
- **PPA (phenylpropanolamine)** is linked to bleeding strokes.
- **Xenical (orlistat)** and the over-the-counter version Alli may lead to serious liver damage and death!
- **Qnexa (renamed Qsymia)** is correlated with kidney stones, pancreatitis, birth defects (such as cleft lip or palate), cognitive impairment, and metabolic acidosis—a known risk factor for heart arrhythmia.

Okay, so they are associated with dangerous side effects—at least they helped people lose weight—or do they? Actually, the effectiveness of

FDA-approved weight-loss drugs are not impressive. These drugs lead to an average weight loss of only about 10 pounds more than what would occur without the drugs, according to the U.S. Department of Health and Human Services and the National Institute for Health and Disease Prevention.[696]

Many of the natural weight-loss products deemed by the FDA to be unapproved drugs have far better results without the life-threatening side effects. What I find ironic (or strategic) is, at the same time the government classified obesity as a disease, it was also funding the American Dairy Association's "Drink Milk and Lose Weight" campaign. Coincidence? Unlike private companies that sell diet pills, the government makes billions of dollars from the dairy industry (remember more money is spent on antibiotics for cattle than humans). The FTC didn't require any scientific proof that milk causes weight loss. Had it not been for a relentless pursuit by a physician's advocacy group against the dairy industry for deceptive advertising, we would still be seeing these bogus unsubstantiated "drug claims" made by the dairy industry. It was proven that no supporting evidence exists whatsoever of any weight-loss benefits from drinking milk.[697][698] In fact, double-blind research shows quite the opposite—those who drink the most milk, gain the most weight.[699]

Why didn't the FTC come in with guns and freeze the dairy industry's assets and defile it in the media? Follow the money! Unless we as a nation do something, the FTC will continue to sue and degrade decent companies, doctors, experts, and product formulators who create any type of entrepreneurship products that take money away from Big Pharma.

Drugs from Nature

Around 70 percent of all new drugs created, produced, and introduced by Big Pharma in the past twenty-five years have been derived from natural products, according to a study published in the *Journal of Natural Products*.[700] Natural remedies aren't a profit center for Big Pharma, so many drugs start off using natural ingredients, add synthetic components, and mix it with proprietary chemicals. Then additional pharmaceuticals are mixed in, which causes side effects that make it necessary for a person on the drug to be monitored by a doctor, therefore, requiring a prescription. Then they inflate the price by ten to fifteen times, and there you have it—an "approved drug" that is allowed to make preventative and cure claims.

Take, for example, red rice yeast, referred to in Japan as a *koji*, meaning "grain or bean overgrown with a mold culture." It's a food preparation tradition going back to 300 BC.[701] Red rice yeast contains an active ingredient called monacolin K, which suppresses the production of LDL cholesterol. Many clinical trials have found that red yeast rice is effective in reducing cholesterol in subjects with high LDL levels. In fact, double-blind studies show it decreases cholesterol levels by 30 percent in only eight weeks![702] I've recommended red rice yeast to my patients with high cholesterol and always see astounding results.

Statin drugs like lovastatin lower circulating total cholesterol and LDL cholesterol. The active ingredient in red rice yeast and statin drugs are so similar, chemical analysis shows that lovastatin and monacolin K are identical.[703] Merck & Co patented lovastatin and now sells it under the brand-name Mevacor.

For thousands of years, red rice yeast has been freely used in the world to help lower cholesterol for millions of people. But now it's considered an illegal "nonapproved drug" because it competes with Big Pharma. Red rice yeast can be purchased for $10 for a month's supply. Statin drugs can cost up to $600 per month! Because red rice yeast contains similar properties of a prescription drug, it is now subjected to being regulated as a drug. The FDA has gone after companies for selling red rice yeast products and removed them from the marketplace because they affect cholesterol levels, which only a "drug" can legally claim.[704]

Can You DIG This?

How does the FDA make money? For the first eighty-six years of the FDA's existence (1906–1992), all of the FDA's funding came through the U.S. Treasury and tax dollars. Unfortunately, in 1992, that all changed. A law was passed that new drug applications that the FDA is responsible for overseeing and approving will be paid for by drug companies. That's right. Drug companies pay the FDA directly to have a drug reviewed. Therefore, Big Pharma has become a valuable money maker for the FDA.[705] Since the drug companies are paying the agency that regulates them, do you think, *just maybe*, there could be a "you scratch our back, we'll scratch yours" scenario going on? Or *just maybe*, there could be some paid-for motivation on the part of the FDA to go after its nature-based competitors? According to Elaine

Feuer, criminologist and author of *Innocent Casualties: The FDA's War Against Humanity*, the answer is a resounding "Yes!" Feuer documents the FDA's suppression of nutrients and alternative treatments that are successfully used to treat serious illnesses in other countries. In America we are denied our constitutional right of freedom of choice in health care.[706]

Last, let's look at the most commonly used drug in the world—aspirin. It's used to treat an array of conditions like fever, inflammation, headaches, back pain, and hardening of the arteries, and is widely used to keep blood from over clotting. At the first sign of a heart attack, if you chew an aspirin, it can save your life! Don't give Big Pharma a pat on the back for this wonder drug. Those kudos go to Mother Nature—a tree called the white willow. The bark and leaves of the tree contain a compound called salicin, which was synthesized in laboratories into acetylsalicylic acid, which is today's scientific name for aspirin. If a company selling white willow bark makes any of the health claims that the makers of aspirin do, it's considered illegal. In fact, if a manufacturer puts on its label that white willow can help relieve a headache or reduce inflammation, that's an illegal drug claim! The FTC could come in and freeze the company's assets, fine them, and degrade it in the media as snake-oil salesmen!

More than 100,000 people die annually from "approved drugs" in America. That's more deaths than from fires, airline accidents, and murders combined.[707] Natural products labeled as "nonapproved drugs" have *safely* helped cure, treat, and prevent disease for thousands of years! No need to **D.I.G.** anymore. The dirt is rather obvious.

THE MILLIONAIRE WITHIN
INVEST WISELY IN YOUR HEALTH

*"Healing is a matter of time, but it is
sometimes also a matter of opportunity."*
—Hippocrates

Every year hundreds of millions of people play the lotto, gamble, and invest their money in the stock market, hoping to become rich. And while we stay busy chasing the buck, most of us don't realize when looking into the mirror each day, we're looking at someone who is already a multi-millionaire. That's right. According to medical research published by the Indiana School of Medicine, your body is worth $45 million! Use this itemization the next time you see your accountant:

- bone marrow = $23 million dollars, based on 1,000 grams at $23,000 per gram
- DNA = $9.7 million (at $1.3 million per gram)
- antibodies = $7.3 million
- one lung = $116,000
- one kidney = $182,000
- heart = $57,000
- 32 fertile eggs = $224,000

- 12 sperm donations a month for 23 years = $250,000 (Guys, don't quit your day job!)

Now let me ask you: if you had a Rolls Royce worth half a million dollars, would you fuel it up with regular gas, fail to change the oil, and ride on deflated tires? Of course not. You'd make sure it was tuned up properly and all the factory recommendations were followed to a tee. Similarly, your $45-million body has requirements for it to function at an optimal level, yet research shows that Americans don't take care of their bodies as well as they might a luxury automobile.[708]

Medical experts have long recognized the relationship that diet plays on disease. From what your mother ate when you were in the womb to your diet during infancy to old age, the food you consume determines your health (or lack thereof). In 1988 Dr. C. Everett Koop, the former surgeon general of the United States, announced, "Diet-related diseases account for 68 percent of all deaths."[709] While that didn't make media headlines like the election of Sonny Bono as the new mayor of Palm Springs, it was the first time the government openly acknowledged the diet–disease connection. Dr. Koop's statement was profound! Sixty-seven deaths out of a hundred are a result of not eating properly and failing to supplement. Walk outside your front door and look at ten homes in your neighborhood. Seven of them will have occupants who will die from diseases linked to poor diet and lack of proper nutrition, translating to hundreds of millions of people that would be alive today if they simply fueled their bodies properly. Americans spend $2.5 trillion per year on health care. That's *trillions* with a T. Why do they call it "health care" anyway? It should be called sick care! It's used when people get sick as opposed to wellness care for preventative measures and maintaining a healthy body.

Success magazine published a Gallup poll asking people what they defined as the meaning of "being successful." Six out of ten responded "good health" as being synonymous with success over anything else. Then why is the United States the unhealthiest developed country on the planet?

- Diabetes has doubled since 1997.
- Heart disease and high blood pressure now affect 54 million people. That's more than the entire population of Florida, Georgia, Alabama, North Carolina, and South Carolina combined.

- Every forty-five seconds, someone in the United States has a stroke.
- Obesity is at an all-time high. Obesity is such an epidemic that it's now classified as a disease.

So many people worry about losing their homes, their 401k, and money in the stock market. But there is a much greater recession taking place with your biggest asset: your body! If you eat too much of the wrong foods, which results in developing diabetes, you just lost $315,000.00 (the price of a healthy pancreas). If you smoke cigarettes, deduct your internal net worth by $232,000.00 (the price of your lungs). And so on. Even when the housing bubble popped, we didn't see this kind of financial devastation taking place. After reading the previous chapters, don't think that a life of hamburgers, French fries, and diet soft drinks have sealed your fate. Don't beat yourself up. There's nothing like right now to practice self-forgiveness and make a commitment to incorporate some, if not all, of the good health practices that I hope you have discovered throughout this book. It's never too late to make a change and undo any damage that has been done. Think of your old habits as if they were an image on an Etch A Sketch. Just shake it, and the slate is clean. If the way you are eating, supplementing, or dieting needs some shaking up, too, then go ahead and clean the slate. Give yourself a "do over."

Perhaps you've heard about the smoker who had clear lungs years after quitting, or the asthmatic turned personal trainer. Or what about the formerly obese marathon runner? How about the quadruple-bypass patient who got healthy by changing his lifestyle and diet? The reason this is possible is because cells, organs, and blood vessels of the human body are wired for self-rejuvenation. Every day 50 trillion human cells die and get replaced. After humans ingest chemicals, drugs, and toxins, they go to the liver, which acts as a detoxifying garbage disposal. The liver's life span on the chemical-warfare front is short lived. In less than a year, the human liver will renew itself and start anew.

- Then there's your blood. Every 120 days, new blood cells are formed. These transport oxygen to all of our body parts. The cells of your intestines renew every three days. So if you've eaten hamburgers every week for twenty years—you get a do over!

- The epidermis, or surface layer of the skin, is renewed every twenty days. So if you've been using sun protection with dangerous cancer-causing chemicals, you get a do over!
- The alveoli of the lungs (air exchanging cells) completely regenerate every year. That means if you stop smoking today—your lungs get a do over!
- Within ten years all of your bones are renewed.
- In twenty years you have a brand-new heart.

Now, while all of these things should give you some peace of mind, I must stress one especially vital element that will ensure your do over really sticks, and with which the healthiest meal or exercise regimen can never compete—a positive, committed mind-set. This book, while geared toward exposing you to the corruptions, lies, practices, technologies, and foods that are detrimental to your health, is also about changing your mind about how you currently live and how you want to live. It is my hope that you feel better about the future of your diet, nutrition, and health and confident in your choices moving forward. Don't blame yourself for the past; empower yourself for the future. *Dis-ease* is not something that necessarily happens *to us*, it is something that can happen *because of us*. Knowing you possess the power, plan *your* do-over.

Turn Back the Clock

If the only party you host on your birthday is a pity party, consider this: your real age is meaningless. What they say is true: age *is* just a number. It's your biological age that counts, and more and more doctors are realizing this fact. I know a woman who was forty and pregnant with her first child. She noticed the words "geriatric pregnancy" written across the paper file that held her health history. Needless to say, this woman, who was a Pilates practitioner, an experienced runner, never smoked a day in her life, and ate organic *everything* . . . was mortified. When she confronted her doctor, he assured her that her label was just a formality, and that he has seen pregnant women in their twenties whose bodies were decades older than hers. When she took a test to find out her biological age, this "geriatric" woman discovered she was twenty-nine! She went on to have two more healthy babies after that. And, at the age of forty-five, she ran the New York City marathon.

Dr. Michael Roizen and Dr. Mehmet Oz created a wonderful test, similar to what the woman above took, that calculates a person's real age, based on lifestyle, genetics, and medical history (www.sharecare.com/static/realage-oz). It's amazing how much all of these factors, plus many others, like daily stress, contributes to the body's aging clock. Think of all the U.S. presidents we've seen who have taken office looking like movie stars, only to leave office like haggard white-haired old men. Then watch those former presidents regain their youthful looks after some time away from the White House.

I had the honor of interviewing Dr. Roizen at the prestigious Cleveland Clinic, where he is chief wellness officer. During my interview, which aired on Lifetime Television, Dr. Roizen explained that aging and life span have many determining factors, and genes have little to do with it. That means you can't blame your great-grandparents. The human body has the ability to control its genes like a light switch. It can be turned on or off. For instance, changing your diet, adding an exercise regimen, and even daily meditation or yoga can turn on a gene named GSTM1 (glutathione S-transferase mu 1). This health-enhancing gene produces a protein in the body that destroys prostate, breast, and colon cancer. Dr. Roizen said, "If you change your bad habits today, within three years it will be like you never had those bad habits."[710]

Can You DIG This?

Your first stop on your do over can be taking the RealAge test for yourself to see how your biological age compares to your real age. Then adjust your eating and lifestyle habits and take the test again in six months—you'll add years to your life and life to your years! While millions rely on plastic surgery to look younger, the body has its own fountain of youth within. By adopting a more healthful lifestyle and eating habits, you can rejuvenate your skin, decrease the growth of gray hairs, remove belly fat, and stabilize blood sugar and blood pressure. You have the power to keep your $45-million body in shape and earn interest on that balance.

Imagine a Life Without Drugs

It's sad how so many people rely on long-term drugs for their health care. In fact, the average sixty-year-old takes at least five prescription drugs on a daily basis. For more than thirty years, physician and nutrition expert and best-selling author John A. McDougall, M.D., has been teaching optimal body renewing and better health through a plant-based diet. As I shared in chapter 7, Dr. McDougall is the founder and medical director of the nationally renowned McDougall Program. During this highly successful live-in program, followers of the McDougall Program have experienced a broad range of dramatic and lasting health benefits such as weight (fat) loss and the reversal of serious illness, such as heart disease, diabetes, and cancer without the use of drugs! In fact, many people enter the program with a lengthy list of prescription drugs they're taking, and within just a few days, leave without ever needing them again. During my interview with Dr. McDougall, I asked how the body can respond so quickly. "It's like a cigarette smoker that stops his last cigarette; he breathes again within twenty-four to forty-eight hours," he explained. "Or that hard-core drunk that can't get off the living room floor; he stops the booze, and the body immediately begins to recover. The same applies to food. When you stop giving grease, oil, and fat to people and fuel the human body with what it was designed to live on, the results are as close to a miracle as possible, because the human body *is* a miracle. It *wants* to be healthy and not sick. When you feed people well, their blood pressure drops, their blood sugar balances, their cholesterol drops, and their bowels move."[711]

What can you do today to help you eliminate your dependence on drugs? Simply replace foods known as "degenerating" with foods that are "rejuvenating" to the body. When a healthy cell dies, it gets replaced with the food choices you make. Eating unhealthy (degenerating) foods creates unhealthy and sick cells. This is what can lead to a lowered immune system and an accelerated aging process. Eating foods that regenerate the body will allow you to reverse these negative effects. Regenerating foods promote *life* while degenerating foods encourage death.

Foods that cause unhealthy degeneration:
- sugar
- caffeine
- white flour
- refined carbohydrates
- processed foods

- artificial sweeteners, colorings, and additives
- alcohol
- fatty and processed meats
- vegetable and hydrogenated oils
- fried food
- genetically modified foods

Foods that cause healthy regeneration:
- fruits
- vegetables
- bean and lentils
- seeds, nuts, and grains
- sea vegetables
- wheatgrass
- extra-virgin olive oil
- organic grass-fed poultry
- fish containing omega-3 fatty acids: sardines, wild-caught salmon, tuna, herring, cod, mackerel

Motivation guru Zig Ziglar said it best: "If you do what you always did, you'll get what you've always got!" For those of you who are overweight, sick, tired all the time, or taking medications to help you poop better, sleep better, have sex better, lower your blood pressure, blood sugar, and increase your hormones, remember that your body was designed to be healthy on its own, but only with the right fuel.

Conquering Stumbling Blocks

Throughout my twenty-eight years in practice, I've heard countless reasons as to why people experience failure on their pathway toward wellness. Excuses are merely nails used to build a house of failure. And, in my opinion, doing that isn't giving you the credit you deserve. If your attitude isn't in the right place, nothing can be achieved. Quit selling yourself short! You *can* conquer stumbling blocks and give yourself the do over you deserve.

First off, tell that little voice inside your head to go away. I believe that in life we live by two factors: what we desire and the reason we don't have it. Sadly, too many of us get stuck on the reasons we don't have what we want. The difference between *try* and *triumph* is a little UMPH! If you want to tap into the healing potential of your body and enjoy its healthy *uses*, get rid of all your *excuses*! The following are some tips to beat the most popular stumbling blocks I hear from my patients.

Excuse #1: I'd love to eat better, but cooking healthy meals takes time, and I have kids, a full-time job, and a house to clean.

Response: See, you're already doing a good job keeping your job, having great kids, and managing to clear out at least some of the dust. What's one more thing? A solution is to cook on the weekends and store food to eat during the week. If there's two of you, make dinner for six, and you'll have leftovers. It takes fifteen minutes to grill several chicken breasts. Because most grocery stores offer precut veggies, it takes no time to create a grilled chicken salad or a stir-fry. You can use the leftovers to make chicken salad or chop them up to roll into romaine lettuce leaves and create your own wraps. Another easy meal to prepare that will last all week is soup. The options are endless! Invest in a slow cooker, which makes an enormous amount of leftovers that you can refrigerate or freeze for later use. There are hundreds of options for soups, stews, chili, sandwich fillings, etc. (www.allrecipes.com). Start with chicken broth; add a little wine, garlic, and vegetables. That's it! Also, make sure you check out my website for healthy and easy-to-make recipes (www.DrDavidFriedman.com).

Another terrific tool that helps pangs of boredom is called the Spiralizer, which enables you to turn veggies such as squash, eggplant, carrots, and zucchini into pasta shapes. Adding a variety of sauces and protein such as shrimp or organic free-range chicken allows you to create a new "pasta" dish every day (www.spiralizer.us).

Excuse #2: Times are tough, and I just can't afford to purchase healthier choices, like organic foods.

Response: This may seem like a good excuse, but eating unhealthy cheaper foods can cost you tenfold the money in medical expenses and drugs in the long run. But is eating well really *that much more* expensive? The answer is "No." Avoiding toxic additives like high-fructose corn syrup, MSG, aspartame, and genetically modified ingredients will not break the bank. You can save money by cutting out the middle man and seeking out local farms and farmers' markets. If you are unemployed and at rock bottom, it's even possible to live entirely on an organic diet using government subsidies. *Foodstamped* (www.Foodstamped.com), a 2011 documentary, chronicles a family who eats a 100 percent organic diet on just $40 a week.

Further, organic brown rice, when purchased in bulk, can be economical and versatile, as it can be used in many types of meals. Healthy organic almonds, cashews, flax, or sunflower seeds are available for a very low price—especially when you bag them yourself. Certified organic eggs are cheap, considering how many meals a regular carton of twelve eggs can provide. But seeing is believing, so let's crunch some numbers:

Table 12.1: Comparing the costs of organic versus nonorganic produce

Average Cost of Fruit

	Organic	Non-Organic
Banana	0.80/lb.	0.70/lb
Apples	$4.49—3 lbs.	$3.99—3 lbs.
Strawberries	$4.49—16 oz.	$3.99—16 oz.
Oranges	$4.99—4 lbs.	$4.49—4 lbs.
Total	$14.77	$13.18
$1.60 = difference in organic vs. non-organic fruit		

Average Cost of Vegetables

	Organic	Non-Organic
Carrots	$1.99/3 lbs., 0.89/lb.	$1.89/3 lbs., 0.89/lb.
Broccoli	$2.49/lb.	$1.99/lb.
Celery	$.99/lb.	$.89/lb.
Total	$5.47	$4.77
70¢ = difference between organic and non-organic vegetables		

* These prices were in effect at a local farmers' market, Wilmington, North Carolina, on September 12, 2017.

Excuse #3: I eat out a lot, and it's impossible to eat healthy, especially at fast-food restaurants.

Response: There are healthy choices you can make, even at fast food restaurants. From McDonald's to Kentucky Fried Chicken (KFC), you can choose healthier options. For example, go easy on the condiments. Two tablespoons of mayonnaise adds a whopping 190 calories, 140 milligrams sodium, and 22 grams of fat. The same amount of ketchup gives you 30 calories, 380 milligrams of sodium, and 32 grams of sugar! Instead squeeze a few small drops (1/4 of a standard foil ketchup packet) directly on the top part of the bun. Putting ketchup right on top brings the flavor to your taste buds more quickly, and you won't even notice the difference in volume. There are several websites and smart phone apps that can guide you toward the best menu items to choose from when you find yourself pressed for time and in the drive-through line. My favorite resource is www.helpguide. org. Here are a few examples of how to eat healthier at fast food restaurants:

The Big Burger Chains

Less-healthy choices	More-healthful alternative
Fried chicken sandwich	Grilled chicken sandwich
Fried fish sandwich	Veggie burger
Salad with toppings, such as bacon, cheese, and ranch dressing	Garden salad with grilled chicken and low-fat dressing
Breakfast burrito with steak	Egg on a whole-wheat muffin
French fries	Plain baked potato or a side salad
Milkshake	Almond milk parfait
Chicken "nuggets" or tenders	Grilled chicken strips
Adding cheese, extra mayo, and special sauces	Limiting cheese, mayo, and special sauces. Try lemon and salsa instead.

The Big Fried Chicken Chains

Less-healthy choices	More-healthful alternative
Fried chicken, original or extra-crispy	Skinless chicken breast without breading
Teriyaki wings or popcorn chicken	Honey BBQ chicken sandwich
Caesar salad	Garden salad
Chicken and biscuit "bowl"	Mashed potatoes
Adding extra gravy and sauces	Limiting gravy and sauces

The Big Taco Chains

Less-healthy choices	More-healthful alternative
Crispy shell chicken taco	Grilled chicken soft taco
Refried beans	Black beans
Steak chalupa	Shrimp ensalada
Crunch wraps or gordita-type burritos	Grilled "fresco" style steak burrito
Nachos with refried beans	Veggie and bean burrito
Adding sour cream or cheese	Limiting sour cream or cheese

Subs, Sandwich, and Deli Choices

Less-healthy choices	More-healthful alternative
Foot-long sub	Six-inch sub
High-fat meat such as ham, tuna salad, bacon, meatballs, or steak	Lean meat (roast beef, chicken breast) or veggies
The "normal" amount of higher-fat (cheddar, American) cheese	One or two slices of lower-fat cheese (Swiss or mozzarella)
Adding mayo and special sauces	Adding low-fat dressing or mustard instead of mayo
Keeping the sub "as is" with all toppings	Adding extra veggie toppings
White bread or "wraps,"	Whole-grain bread or taking the top slice off your sub and eating it open-faced

Excuse #4: I've just eaten something I shouldn't have, so I might as well go all the way.

Response: We are human. We have desires. Don't punish yourself for an entire day when you overindulge. All of us have gotten lost while driving a car. Do we say, "Oh well, I'm lost. I might as well just keep driving more off course"? No! We do our best to get back on route to our desired destination. And we eventually do! This same attitude is necessary when you find yourself off course, eating things you know you shouldn't have.

Excuse #5: I want to eat healthier, but my spouse is a die-hard hamburger and greasy French fry lover.

Response: Cooking healthfully for one is not easy. You may have to cook two different meals and "trickle" some of the good stuff into your spouse's unhealthy meals. Kim Barnouin, sidekick on my radio show, is the author of the *New York Times* best-selling Skinny Bitch series. She is a devout vegan who won't eat any animal products—period! However, her husband doesn't share the same views. She told me she will occasionally sneak things on his plate and after he tries many of the whole-food, plant-based meals she makes, he's hooked. This allows her to cook many healthy vegan-friendly dishes for her spouse between his meat and onion ring cravings. It doesn't have to be "all or nothing." Keep in mind, if you can get your spouse to agree to eat healthfully just three days out of seven, that's 468 healthful meals each year!

Excuse #6: I am addicted to sweets! I just can't live without them!

Response: A little sugar every now and then is not going to kill you. It's the *daily* sugar habit that puts you into jeopardy. If you can't go an entire day without sugar, there are many healthful, low-calorie alternatives to satisfy your sweet tooth, without compromising your health. My two favorites are Xylitol and coconut sugar. Xylitol is a naturally derived sweetener from the birch tree and approved as a sugar substitute for diabetics. Xylitol tastes sweeter than sugar and can be used in place of sugar in recipes. Coconut sugar is a low-calorie, all-natural sweetener from the fruit of the coconut plant. It's a great source of fiber and also contains the minerals iron, zinc, calcium, and potassium, as well as antioxidants that may also provide some health benefits.

If you need to reach for that occasional candy to satisfy a sweet tooth, go for the unsweetened dark chocolate. Organic cocoa (80 percent) contains an ingredient called theobromine, which has been shown to benefit cardiac health. Cocoa also reduces cortisol, the stress hormone, and contains antioxidants called flavonoids. All in moderation, of course! Don't go overboard.

Excuse #7: I exercised, so I have earned the right to splurge.

Response: Burning off a lot of calories will leave the body hungry, so give it something wholesome. Exercising tears down muscle—and what you feed yourself determines how those muscles build back up (i.e. you are what you eat). Do you want those muscle fibers replaced with the contents of a hamburger and a shake from McDonald's? Exercise doesn't give you the leeway to indulge like you think. For example, a three-mile fast-paced run that takes thirty minutes will burn approximately 300 calories (based on a 135-pound woman). That's about the equivalent of three-quarters of one Starbucks blueberry muffin. If you were to eat that entire muffin, you'd not only gain back that 300 calories you just burned but also will have consumed seventy-five additional depleting calories. However, eating a grilled chicken salad brings you the same 300 calories. Which do you think turns to fat? That 300-calorie blueberry muffin or a lean 300-calorie grilled chicken salad? Don't splurge just because you've exercised; eat sensibly.

Excuse #8: "I can eat it because it's 'fat free.'"

Response: The fact that you see "fat free" might actually cause you to eat more of it! When people believe their food is more healthful, they tend to eat more of it, which ends up packing on additional calories. The food industry knows this and their marketing teams use buzz words like *fat free* and *zero guilt* to entice you to eat more of what they sell. But since removing fat also removes much of the flavor, many companies replace fat with sugar. The manufacturers use the label as a smoke screen to give an otherwise unhealthful food, like jelly beans, an aura of health. Of course jelly beans are never made with fat; they're pure sugar, which turns to fat. Be careful not to fall for the fat-free trap.

Excuse #9: "I can't let food go to waste."

Response: Ask yourself one question: do you want it to go to waste or to your waist? When you eat out at a restaurant and start to feel full—stop eating! That's your body telling you something. Take the hint! If you aren't able to take home a doggie bag, then let the waitress throw the rest in the trash. If you are cooking at home, make only enough food for everyone to have one portion. If you do have leftovers put them in the fridge or freezer for another day.

Excuse #10: "I'm always hungry!"

Response: If that's the case, your food choices might be the culprit. Remember the Lay's potato chips slogan, "Bet you can't eat just one"? That's a safe bet! Processed foods like potato chips, tortilla chips, and French fries are empty calories that don't make you feel full, so your brain keeps sending signals: "Feed me more!" Research conducted at the University of California, Irvine, found the fat in these types of foods triggers a biological mechanism that likely drives gluttonous behavior.[712] Hunger pangs can be a sign of dehydration. One glass of water shut down midnight hunger pangs for almost 100 percent of the dieters studied in a University of Washington study.[713] You might need water, not food. And when you are legitimately hungry, go for water anyway, before eating. It will make you fuller. A salad before a meal or a cup of broth will also fill up your tummy, which is a great trick when there isn't a completely healthful main course on the way.

When you want to nosh between meals, reach for a handful of almonds. This source of protein offers filling fiber and contains the most nutrients in comparison to all other nuts. Another food item to turn to when you are hungry is a slice of organic rye bread. Compared to other grains, rye is rather unique because of how slowly it gets absorbed into the body. That means you stay fuller longer. Rye is also chock-full of essential vitamins and minerals not found in other types of bread. An interesting Finland study published in the *American Journal of Clinical Nutrition* showed that people who eat rye turn on a gene that prevents diabetes, lowers cholesterol, reduces inflammation, and improves blood sugar. Consumption of fiber-rich rye bread can also aid in digestion and ease constipation.[714]

I follow a "flexitarian diet." Flexitarian is a marriage of two words: *flexible* and *vegetarian*. I eat an 80 percent whole-food, plant-based diet and 20 percent wild-caught fish, organic chicken, and eggs. I stay away from beef, dairy, and pork. At my biological age of fifty-two (my RealAge® is thirty-five), I am proud to say I've been blessed with great health and energy to do everything I want in life. I don't take any prescription or over-the-counter drugs. My blood pressure, heart rate, cholesterol, and weight are perfect! During my last annual physical, my doctor told me most patients my age are taking medications for pain, cholesterol, high blood pressure, or diabetes. Having the proof that hard work, commitment, and knowledge of what it takes to build a *wellness care* regimen instead of being part of society's *sickness care* program of drugs and their associated side effects is rewarding beyond compare! I hope by reading this book, you will use these tools to experience the same joy. Go ahead. Shake it up. Use your do over!

ABOUT THE AUTHOR

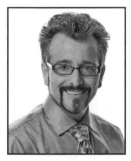 Dr. David Friedman is a #1 National Best-selling author, Doctor of Naturopathy, Chiropractic Neurologist, and Clinical Nutritionist. He is a Board Certified Alternative Medical Practitioner (AMP), Board Certified in Integrative Medicine (BCIM), and a registered Naturopathic Diplomate (RND). He's a former teacher of neurology and a contributing writer for many leading health and fitness magazines. He's been a guest on over a hundred syndicated radio and television shows and his best-selling audio-book, "America's Unbalanced Diet," has sold over a million copies, helping to raise awareness about the unhealthy foods people are consuming. His patients include A-list celebrities, movie stars, and sports icons, many who travel across the country to see him because they trust no one else. As the health expert for Lifetime Television's syndicated morning show and host of To Your Good Health Radio, millions of people have enjoyed his weekly, cutting-edge features, offering solutions to everyday health and wellness issues.

Dr. Friedman's memberships include:

- Naturopathic Medical Association
- Academy of Integrative Health & Medicine
- American Dietetic Association
- American Association of Drugless Practitioners
- Academy of Nutrition and Dietetics
- American Holistic Health Association
- World Public Health Nutrition Association
- Foundation for Chiropractic Education and Research

To receive updated information and to join Dr. Friedman's online community, please visit www.DrDavidFriedman.com and enter your name and email—it's free.

ACKNOWLEDGMENTS

First and foremost, I want to thank all the magnificent and brilliant minds that have challenged me over the years to question the status quo. Health advocates including Dr. T. Colin Campbell, Dr. Stephen Sinatra, Dr. John McDougall, Dr. Neal Barnard, Dr. Joseph Mercola, Dr. Earl Mindell, Dr. Barry Sears, Dr. David Katz, Dr. Mark Hyman, and John Robbins. These are just a few of the brilliant minds and mentors that have inspired me and whom I've also had the pleasure of interviewing on my radio show. I'm not a conformist to any one set of rules and some of the authors I admire, many whom I consider close friends, do not share the exact views I do. But that's okay. If we all shared the same viewpoints, I wouldn't have written this book. I pride myself in exploring all *differences of opinions* because there have been many times in my life when I thought I made up my mind, only to later change it by 360 degrees. When someone says, "It's my way or the highway" that usually motivates me to press the accelerator and move on.

I am infinitely grateful and appreciative to everyone at Turner Publishing for seeing the true potential of this book to change and transform lives. Thank you for allowing me the creative freedom to make every chapter come alive without pulling out the chopping block. Special thanks goes to Harvey Diamond for writing the foreword and for mentoring me on the steps needed to bring this manuscript from A to Z. You authored the #1 best-selling health book in history, yet you still remain genuine and *touchable*. I also give thanks to my "Chew On This!" sassy co-host, and *New York Times* best-selling author Kim Barnouin (*Skinny Bitch*). We've been referred to as "The Dynamic Duo of Due Diligence" and it's been such a joy working with you over the years.

My sincere gratitude goes to Jack Canfield (co-author of *Chicken Soup for the Soul, Success Principles*, and featured teacher in *The Secret*). Being mentored by an author that has sold over half a billion books was like a little league baseball player getting batting tips from Mickey Mantle! After brainstorming with you in your living room, my book took on a totally new dynamic and dimension, including the title, for which I have you to thank. You are a humble man with a servant's heart and a huggable soul.

A big shout-out goes to my wonderful editor Michele Mastrisciani for seeing the big picture, reshaping my words without changing them, and being a "compartmentalizing" extraordinaire! Jon O'Neal, for overseeing the editing process. Thanks also goes to Larissa Henoch for the wonderful illustrations, Yahor Shumski and Madeline Cothren for your help with the cover design, and Kelley Blewster, my line editor, for playing devil's advocate and challenging me to present *even more* evidence to back up every statement. Thanks also goes to Carol Rosenberg for your organizational skills and help with the many references used throughout the book.

Kudos to Jeffrey Herman, truly the *who's who* of literary agents. Thanks for believing in me and my vision and presenting my book with such passion. It's such an honor to have you on my team. And Steve Harrison, what can I possibly say to express my gratitude except to use the words of an OBGYN whose patient just had triplets, "You over delivered!" While most men prefer to keep driving instead of stopping to ask for directions, thanks to your Quantum Leap road map, I found my way.

To my incredible publicist Barbara Teszler, thank you for helping me get my message out to the masses. You have tenacious focus and are the queen of the "follow through"! A big fist bump to photographer extraordinaire Daniel J. Hadley (aka "Rembrandt with a camera"). A very special shout-out goes to Lisa Votta for encouraging me to stop using "my plate is too full" excuse and put my fingers on the keyboard and begin this journey. Continuing appreciation goes to my assistant Kristine Movizzo for helping to connect with and build lasting relationships that would eventually lead to all the pieces of this book coming together. You're a gem and I'm forever grateful.

And heartfelt gratitude and commiseration to all my loyal radio listeners. Over the past fifteen years, many of you have written to me and shared your wonderful testimonials after hearing something that inspired and changed your life. That's truly the greatest reward of all. I also give thanks to my mother, who instilled in me that "never give up" mentality and how if I keep jumping high enough, I could reach the sky. Most importantly, I give thanks to God, my pilot. Only after I gave the steering wheel to Him did I make it through the turbulent times in my life.

REFERENCES

1. Dave Asprey interview. 2015. "Bulletproof Diet." *To Your Good Health Radio*, air date: 5/21/15 http://radiomd.com/show/to-your-good-health-radio /item/31195-the-bulletproof-diet-get-leaner-healthier-smarter.

2. Hubisz, John. 2003. "Middle-School Texts Don't Make the Grade." *Physics Today* 56 (5): 50–54. scitation.aip.org/content/aip/magazine/physicstoday /article/56/5/10.1063/1.1583534.

3. Lesser, Lenard I., and Cara B. Ebbeling, et al. 2007. "Relationship Between Funding Source and Conclusion Among Nutrition-Related Scientific Articles." *PLoS Med* 4 (1): e5. doi:10.1371/journal.pmed.0040005. journals.plos.org /plosmedicine/article?id=10.1371/journal.pmed.0040005.

4. Consensus. NIH.gov. 1994. "Optimal Calcium Intake." *NIH Consensus Development Conference Statement June 6–8, 1994* 12 (4): 1–31. Accessed May 2, 2016. consensus.nih.gov/1994/1994optimalcalcium097html.htm.

5. Skinner, Halcyon G., and Gary G. Schwartz. 2008. "Serum Calcium and Incident and Fatal Prostate Cancer in the National Health and Nutrition Examination Survey." *Cancer Epidemiology, Biomarkers & Prevention* 17 (9): 2302–5. doi:10.1158/1055-9965.EPI-08-0365. cebp.aacrjournals.org /content/17/9/2302.full.

6. Bolland, Mark J. 2010. "Effect of Calcium Supplements on Risk of Myocardial Infarction and Cardiovascular Events." *BMJ* (July): 341. c3691. www.bmj.com /content/341/bmj.c3691.

7. Miller, Edgar R. III, and Roberto Pastor-Barriuso, et al. 2005. "Meta-Analysis: High-Dosage Vitamin E Supplementation May Increase All-Cause Mortality." *Annals of Internal Medicine* 142 (1): 37–46. doi:10.7326/0003-4819-142-1-200501040-00110. annals.org/article.aspx?articleid=718049

8. Vitamin D Council. "Vitamin D Council." Accessed May 2, 2016. www.vitamindcouncil.org.

9. Michaud, Dominique S. 2006. "Vitamin D and Pancreatic Cancer Risk in the Alpha-Tocopherol, Beta-Carotene Cancer Prevention Cohort." *Cancer Research* 66 (20): 9802–3. doi:10.1158/0008-5472.CAN-06-3193. cancerres.aacrjournals.org /content/66/20/9802.full.

10. Ross, A. Catharine, and Christine L. Taylor, et al., eds. 2011. *Dietary Reference Intakes for Calcium and Vitamin D*. Washington, DC: National Academies Press, pp. 403–56. http://www.ncbi.nlm.nih.gov/books/NBK56058/.

11. Brody, Jane E. 1998. "Taking Too Much Vitamin C Can Be Dangerous, Study Finds." *New York Times*. April 9. Accessed May 2, 2015. www.nytimes.com /1998/04/09/us/taking-too-much-vitamin-c-can-be-dangerous-study-finds.html.

12. Brady, Paul. "Can You Text on a Plane? A Guide to In-Flight Phone Use." *CN Traveler*. May 25, 2016. http://www.cntraveler.com/stories/2014-06-16/everything-you-need-to-know-about-using-a-cell-phone-on-a-plane.

13. Cumming, Robert G. 1994. "Case-Control Study of Risk Factors for Hip Fractures in the Elderly." *American Journal of Epidemiology* 139 (5).

14. Michaelsson, Karl. 2014. "Milk Intake and Risk of Mortality and Fractures in Women and Men." *BMJ*. 349:g6015. October 28.

15. Feskanich, D., W.C. Willet, M.J. Stampfer, G.A. Colditz. 1997. "Milk, Dietary Calcium, and Bone Fractures in Women: A 12-Year Prospective Study." *American Journal of Public Health*. 87 (6): 992–7.

16. Kunz, C., et al. 1990. "Human-Milk Proteins: Analysis of Casein and Casein Subunits by Anion-Exchange Chromatography, Gel Electrophoresis, and Specific Staining Methods." *The American Society for Clinical Nutrition*. 51 (1): 37–46.

17. American Chemical Society (ACS). "Gulf of Mexico has greater-than-believed ability to self-cleanse oil spills." ScienceDaily. ScienceDaily, 8 April 2013. www.sciencedaily.com/releases/2013/04/130408152733.htm.

18. Ferris, Robert. 2017. "Much of the Deep-water Horizon oil spill has disappeared because of bacteria." CNBC. June 26. http://www.cnbc.com/2017/06/26/much-of-the-deepwater-horizon-oil-spill-has-disappeared-because-of-bacteria.html.

19. Hibbeln, J.R., et al. 2007. "Maternal Seafood Consumption in Pregnancy and Neurodevelopmental Outcomes in Childhood." *Lancet* 369 (9561): 578–85.

20. Julvez, J., et al. 2016. "Maternal Consumption of Seafood in Pregnancy and Child Neuropsychological Development: A Longitudinal Study Based on a Population with High Consumption Levels." *American Journal of Epidemiology* 183 (3): 169–82.

21. Engle, Ralph L., Jr. *Archives of Internal Medicine* 112 (1963): 87. archinte.jamanetwork.com/issue.aspx?journalid=71&issueid=15492.

22. Freedman, Neal D., et al. 2010. "Association of Meat and Fat Intake with Liver Disease and Hepatocellular Carcinoma." *Journal of the National Cancer Institute*. 102 (17): 1354–65.

23. Bauer, Brent. 2014. "Buzzed on Inflammation." *Mayo Clinic Health Letter* (online edition) February. Accessed May 2, 2016. healthletter.mayoclinic.com/editorial/editorial.cfm/i/163/t/Buzzed%20on%20inflammation/.

24. Fiorenza, Luca, and Stefano Benazzi, et al. 2011. "Molar Macrowear Reveals Neanderthal Eco-Geographic Dietary Variation." *PLoS ONE* 6 (3). doi:10.1371/journal.pone.0014769. www.ncbi.nlm.nih.gov/pmc/articles/PMC3060801/?report=classic.

25. Philosophical Transactions of the Royal Society of London. 1991. "Hominoid Dietary Evolution." *Biological Science* 334 (1270): 199–209.

26. Eaton, S. Boyd, and Melvin Konner, 1985. "Paleolithic Nutrition—A Consideration of Its Nature and Current Implications." *New England Journal of Medicine*. 312:283–289.

27. Zaraska, Marta. 2016. "How Humans Became Meat Eaters." *The Atlantic* February 19. https://www.theatlantic.com/science/archive/2016/02/when-humans-became-meateaters/463'05/.

28. Cavalieri, Paola, and Peter Singer, eds. 1993. *The Great Ape Project*. New York, NY: St. Martin's Griffin.

29. World Heritage Enyclopedia. "Hunter-Gatherer Diet." *World Public Library*. Accessed May 2, 2016. worldlibrary.org/articles/Hunter-gatherer_diet#cite_note-94.

30. Bijal, T. 2004. "Chimps Shown Using Not Just a Tool but a 'Tool Kit.'" *National Geographic News* October 6. Accessed January 1, 2010. news.nationalgeographic. com/news/2004/10/1006_041006_chimps.html.

31. McBrearty, Sally, and Nina G. Jablonski. 2005. "First Fossil Chimpanzee." *Nature* 437 (September): 105–8. doi:10.1038/nature04008. www.nature.com/nature /journal/v437/n7055/full/nature04008.html.

32. Pickrell, John. 2003. "Chimps Belong on Human Branch of Family Tree, Study Says." *National Geographic News* May 20. Accessed May 2, 2016. news. nationalgeographic.com/news/2003/05/0520_030520_chimpanzees.html.

33. Gohkman, David, and Eitan Lavi, et al. 2014. "Reconstructing the DNA Methylation Maps of the Neandertal and the Denisovan." *Science* 344 (6183): 523–7. doi:10.1126/science.1250368. Accessed May 3, 2016. http://science.sciencemag.org/content/early/2014/04/16/science.1250368.

34. Helmuth, H. 1998. "Body Height, Body Mass and Surface Area of the Neanderthals." *Zeitschrift für Morphologie und Anthropologie* 82 (1): 1–12. PMID 9850627. https://www.jstor.org/stable/25757530?seq=1#page_scan_tab_contents.

35. Froehle, Andrew W., and Steven E. Churchill. 2009. "Energetic Competition Between Neandertals and Anatomically Modern Humans." *PaleoAnthropology* 96–116. http://paleoanthro.org/media/journal/content/PA20090096.pdf.

36. National Institutes of Health. 1998. "Clinical Guidelines on the Identification, Evaluation, and Treatment of Overweight and Obesity in Adults." *NIH Publication* 98 (4083). http://www.nhlbi.nih.gov/guidelines/obesity/ob_gdlns.pdf.

37. Health Discovery. "Ideal Body Weight for Men." Accessed May 2, 2016. http://www.healthdiscovery.net/links/calculators/ideal_bw_men.htm.

38. Alper, Joe. 2003. "Rethinking Neanderthals." *Smithsonian* June. Accessed May 2, 2016. http://www.smithsonianmag.com/science-nature/rethinking-neanderthals-83341003/?no-ist.

39. Richards, Michael P., and Paul B. Pettitt, et al. 2009. "Neanderthal Diet at Vindija and Neanderthal Predation: The Evidence from Stable Isotopes." *PNAS* 97 (13): 7663–66. doi: 10.1073/pnas.120178997. http://www.pnas.org /content/97/13/7663.full.

40. Mills, Milton R. 2009. "The Comparative Anatomy of Eating." *VegSource* November 21. Accessed May 2, 2016. http://www.vegsource.com/news/2009/11/ the-comparative-anatomy-of-eating.html?fb_comment_id=10150163352344400_ 23918443#f332bf1f8c.

41. Ibid.

42. Koop, C. Everett. 1985. "The Heimlich Maneuver." *Public Health Reports* 100 (6) November-December: 557. http://www.ncbi.nlm.nih.gov/pmc/articles /PMC1425324/?page=1.

43. Mills, Milton R. 2009. "The Comparative Anatomy of Eating." *VegSource* November 21. Accessed May 2, 2016. http://www.vegsource.com/news/2009/11/the-comparative-anatomy-of-eating.html?fb_comment_id=10150163352344400_23918443#f332bf1f8c.

44. Fiorenza, Luca, et al. 1979. "The Effect of Meat Protein on Colonic Function and Metabolism." *The American Journal of Clinical Nutrition* 32 (October): 2094-2101.

45. Windey, K., V. De Preter, K. Verbeke. 2012. "Relevance of Protein Fermentation to Gut Health." *Molecular Nutriton and Food Research*. 58: 184–96.

46. Martin, Laura J. 2011. "Eating Meat May Raise Colon Cancer Risk." *WebMD* May 23. Accessed May 2, 2016. http://www.webmd.com/colorectal-cancer/news/20110523/eating-meat-may-raise-colon-cancer-risk.

47. Centers for Disease Control and Prevention. "Centers for Disease Control and Prevention." Accessed May 2, 2016. http://wwwnc.cdc.gov.

48. Buzby, Jean C., and Tanya Roberts, et al. 1996. "Bacterial Foodborne Disease: Medical Costs and Productivity Losses." *Agricultural Economic Report* AER-741 (August): 93. http://www.ers.usda.gov/publications/aer-agricultural-economic-report/aer741.aspx.

49. Cordain, Loren, and Janet Brand Miller, et al. 2000. "Plant-Animal Subsistence Ratios and Macronutrient Energy Estimations in Worldwide Hunter-Gatherer Diets." *The American Journal of Clinical Nutrition* 71 (3) (March): 682–92. http://ajcn.nutrition.org/content/71/3/682.full

50. Ghose, Tia. 2012. "Caveman Diet Secret: Less Red Meat, More Greens." *LiveScience* October 25. Accessed May 2, 2016. http://www.livescience.com/24302-stone-age-diet.html.

51. Ibid.

52. Diamond, Jared. 2003. *The Rise and Fall of the Third Chimpanzee: How Our Animal Heritage Affects the Way We Live*. London, England: Vintage Books.

53. Macko, S. A., and G. Lubec, et al. 1999. "The Ice Man's Diet as Reflected by the Stable Isotopic Composition of His Hair." *FASEB Journal* 13 (3) (March): 559–62. http://www.fasebj.org/content/13/3/559.full.

54. Hall, Stephen S. 2007. "Last Hours of the Iceman." *National Geographic News* (July). Accessed May 2, 2016. http://ngm.nationalgeographic.com/2007/07/iceman/hall-text.

55. Rossella, Lorenzi. 2011. "Iceman Had Bad Teeth." *Discovery News* (June). Accessed May 2, 2016. http://news.discovery.com/history/oetzi-iceman-bad-teeth-110615.html.

56. Spindler, Konrad. 1995. *The Man in the Ice: The Discovery of a 5,000-Year-Old Body Reveals the Secrets of the Stone Age*. 1st ed. New York City, NY: Harmony Books.

57. Tu, Jean-Louis. "Lesson of the Pottenger's Cats experiment: Cats are Not Humans." *Beyond Vegetarianism*. http://www.beyondveg.com/tu-j-l/raw-cooked/raw-cooked-1h.shtml. Accessed May 2, 2016.

58. Freston, Kathy. 2011. "Shattering the Meat Myth: Humans Are Natural Vegetarians." *Huffington Post*. November 17, 2011.

59. Henry, Amanda G., and Alison S. Brooks, et al. 2010. "Microfossils in Calculus Demonstrate Consumption of Plants and Cooked Foods in Neanderthal Diets (Shanidar III, Iraq; Spy I and II, Belgium)." *PNAS*. (November) Accessed May 10, 2016. http://www.pnas.org/content/108/2/486.

60. Ibid.

61. Ibid.

62. Mercola, Joseph. 2009. "The Milk Myth: What Your Body Really Needs." *Dr. Mercola* (July 18). http://articles.mercola.com/sites/articles/archive/2009/07/18 /the-milk-myth-what-your-body-really-needs.aspx.

63. Holick, M. 1995. "Environmental Factors That Influence the Cutaneous Production of Vitamin D." *American Journal of Clinical Nutrition* 61(3 Suppl): 638S–645S.

64. John Dobbing et al. 1994. "A warm chain for breastfeeding." *The Lancet* 344 (November 5, 1994).

65. Brewin, B. 1994. "What is Truth?" *The Lancet* 343 (June 11, 1994).

66. USDA. 2012 "Profiling Food Consumption in America." USDA.gov. Accessed May 3, 2016. www.usda.gov/factbook/chapter2.htm.

67. Stuebe, Alison. 2009. "The Risks of Not Breastfeeding for Mothers and Infants." *Rev Obstet Gynecol* 2 (4): 222–31.

68. John Dobbing et al. 1994. "A warm chain for breastfeeding." *The Lancet* 344 (November 5, 1994).

69. Henry G. Bieler. 1969. *Food Is Your Best Medicine*. Random House (May 1969), p. 213.

70. National Dairy Council. Home page. Accessed May 3, 2016. www.nationaldairycouncil.org.

71. American Dairy Association and Dairy Council. Home page. Accessed May 3, 2016. http://www.adadc.com.

72. Women's Health Initiative. U.S Department of Health and Human Services. Accessed March 2013. https://www.nhlbi.nih.gov/whi/whywhi.htm.

73. International Osteoporosis Foundation: Facts and Statistics. https://www.iofbonehealth.org/facts-statistics.

74. Ziadé, Nelly. 2014. "Osteoporosis-Related Mortality: Time-Trends and Predictive Factors." *European Medical Journal of Rheumotology* 1:56-6.

75. Axe, Josh. 2016. "The Truth about Pasteurization." https://draxe.com/pasteurization-homogenization-raw-milk/.

76. Weinsier, R. 2000. "Dairy Foods and Bone Health: Examination of the Evidence." *American Journal of Clinical Nutrition* 72 (3): 681–9.

77. Recker, R. 1985. "The Effect of Milk Supplements on Calcium Metabolism, Bone Metabolism, and Calcium Balance." *American Journal of Clinical Nutrition* 41:254.

78. Nilas, L. 1984. "Calcium Supplementation and Post-Menopausal Bone loss." *British Medical Journal* 289:1103.

79. Abelow, B. 1992. "Cross-Cultural Association Between Dietary Animal Protein and Hip Fracture: A Hypothesis." *Calcific Tissue Int* 50:14–8.

80. Campbell, T. Colin. 2006. *The China Study*. Texas: BenBella Books. 205.

81. Hurley, Jayne, and Stephen Schmidt. 1993. "Getting a Little Culture." *Nutrition Action Healthletter* (June). Accessed May 10, 2016. https://www.highbeam.com/doc/1G1-13175659.html.

82. Feskanich, D., et al. 1997. "Milk, Dietary Calcium, and Bone Fractures in Women: A 12-Year Prospective Study." *American Journal of Public Health* 87 (6): 992–7.

83. Owusu, W., et al. 1997. "Calcium Intake and the Incidence of Forearm and Hip Fractures Among Men." *Journal of Nutrition* 127 (9):1782–7.

84. Kaiser Permanente. 2011. "Elderly Women Who Break a Hip at Increased Risk of Dying Within a Year." *Archives of Internal Medicine* (September 26). Accessed May 13, 2016. https://share.kaiserpermanente.org/article/elderly-women-who-break-a-hip-at-increased-risk-of-dying-within-a-year/.

85. Cumming, R. G., et al. 1994. "Case-Control Study of Risk Factors for Hip Fractures in the Elderly." *American Journal of Epidemiology* 139:493–503.

86. Tucker K. L., M. T. Hannan, H. Chen, et al. 1999. "Potassium, Magnesium, and Fruit and Vegetable Intakes Are Associated with Greater Mineral Density in Elderly Men and Women." *American Journal of Clinical Nutrition* 69 (4): 727–736. New, S.A., S. P. Robins, M. K. Campbell, et al. 2000. "Dietary Influences on Bone Mass and Bone Metabolism: Further Evidence of a Positive Link Between Fruit and Vegetable Consumption and Bone Health?" *American Journal of Clinical Nutrition* 71(1): 142–151.

87. Ross, A. Catharine, and Christine L. Taylor, et al. 2011. "Dietary Reference Intakes for Calcium and Vitamin D." Institute of Medicine, Food and Nutrition Board. National Academy Press. Accessed May 10, 2016.

88. Holick, M. 1995. "Environmental Factors that Influence the Cutaneous Production of Vitamin D." *American Journal of Clinical Nutrition* 61 (3 Suppl): 638S–645S.

89. Stamp, T. 1987. "Comparison of Oral 25-Hydroxycholecalciferol, Vitamin D, and Ultraviolet Light as Determinants of Circulating 25-Hydroxyvitamin D." *Lancet* 1 (8026):1341–3.

90. Sheard, N. F. 1993. "Cow's Milk, Diabetes, and Infant Feeding." *Nutrition Review* 51:79–89.

91. Joint WHO/FAO Expert Consultation. 2002. "Diet, Nutrition and the Prevention of Chronic Diseases." WHO Technical Report Series. Geneva, January 28–February 1.

92. Campbell, T. Colin, and Thomas M. Campbell. 2006. *The China Study*. Dallas, TX: Benbella Books.

93. Reichelt, K. L., and A-M Knivsberg, et al. 1991. "Probable Etiology and Possible Treatment of Childhood Autism." *Brain Dysfunction* 4:308–19.

94. Dohan, F. C., and J. C. Grasberger. 1973. "Relapsed Schizophrenics: Earlier Discharge from the Hospital After Cereal-Free, Milk-Free Diet." *American Journal of Psychiatry* 130:685–8.

95. New Scientist Magazine. 1991. "Fuss over Fat Leads to Rethink on Publicity." *New Scientist* 129 (1759):17. Accessed May 10, 2016. https://www.newscientist.com/article/mg12917592-800-fuss-over-fat-leads-to-rethink-on-publicity/.

96. Seely, Stephen. 1991. "Is Calcium Excess in Western Diet a Major Cause of Arterial Disease?" *International Journal of Cardiology* 33 (2): 191–8.

97. Moss, Margaret. 2002. "Does Milk Cause Coronary Heart Disease?" *Journal of Nutritional & Environmental Medicine* 12 (3): 207–16.

98. Luc MD, Djoussé, and James S. Pankow, et al. 2006. "Influence of Saturated Fat and Linolenic Acid on the Association Between Intake of Dairy Products and Blood Pressure." *Hypertension* (June).

99. Oski, Frank A. 2010. *Don't Drink Your Milk.* Ringgold, GA; TEACH Services, Inc.

100. Oster, Kurt A. 1983. *The XO Factor: Homogenized Milk May Cause Your Heart Attack.* Utah: Park City Press.

101. Hoard's Dairyman, the *National Dairy Farm Magazine*, April 10, 2004, p. 268. Accessed May 10, 2016. http://www.rense.com/general51/pus.htm.

102. Adkinson, R. W. 2001. "Implications of Proposed Changes in Bulk Tank Somatic Cell Count Regulations." *Journal of Dairy Science.* 84 (2): 370–4.

103. Kalter, R. J., R. Milligan, W. Lesser, W. Magrath, and D. E. Bauman. 1984. "Biotechnology and the Dairy Industry: Production Costs and Commercial Potential of the Bovine Growth Hormone." Research Bulletin, Department of Agricultural Economics, Cornell University.

104. Michael Satchell "The Next Bad Beef Scandal?" *U.S. News & World Report*, September 1, 1997.

105. "Antimicrobials Sold or Distributed for Use in Food-Producing Animals." *Food and Drug Administration Department of Health and Human Services* 2010. https://www.fda.gov/downloads/ForIndustry/UserFees/AnimalDrugUserFeeActADUFA/ucm277657.pdf.

106. Raymond, Richard. "Antibiotics and Animals Raised for Food." *Food Safety News.* January 7, 2013 http://www.foodsafetynews.com/2013/01/antibiotics-and-animals-raised-for-food-lies-damn-lies-and-statistics/#.WOZ3zlMrLJN.

107. Ingersoll, Bruce. 1989. "Milk Found Tainted with Wide Range of Drugs." *Wall Street Journal*, December 29.

108. Epstein, Samuel F. 2007. *What's in Your Milk?* Indiana: Trafford. February. p. 155.

109. Moss, Michael. 2010. "While Warning about Fat, U.S. Pushes Cheese Sales." *New York Times*, November 6. Accessed May 8, 2016.

110. Ibid.

111. "U.S. Government Calls for End to Dairy Weight Loss Ads." *Washington Post*, May 12. Accessed May 3, 2016. http://www.washingtonpost.com/wp-dyn/content/article/2007/05/12/AR2007051201248.html?hpid=sec-health.

112. Harvard T. H. Chan School of Public Health. Home page. Accessed May 3, 2016. www.hsph.harvard.edu/news.

113. Campbell, T. Colin, interview with author. 2012. "Forks over Knives" *To Your Good Health Radio*, April 4. http://toyourgoodhealthradio.com/forks-over-knives/.

114. Jovana, K. 2009. "The Milk Debate." *American Society of Nutrition* (August 8). http://www.nutrition.org/asn-blog/2009/08/the-milk-debate/.

115. Berkey, C. S., H. R. H. Rockett, W. C. Willett, G. A. Colditz. 2005. "Milk, Dairy Fat, Dietary Calcium, and Weight Gain A Longitudinal Study of Adolescents." *Archives of Pediatrics and Adolescent Medicine* 159 (6): 543-50.

116. Stein, Rob. 2005. "More Milk Means More Weight Gain." *Washington Post*, June 7. http://www.washingtonpost.com/wp-dyn/content/article/2005/06/06 /AR2005060601348.html.

117. Cohen, Robert. 1995. "Advice from Doctors to Doctors: Townsend Medical Letter." NotMilk.com, May. Accessed May 10, 2016. http://www.notmilk.com /deb/townsend.html.

118. Knip, M., et al. 2010. "Dietary Intervention in Infancy and Later Signs of Beta-Cell Autoimmunity." *New England Journal of Medicine* 363 (20):1900–8.

119. Høst, A. 1994. "Cow's Milk Protein Allergy and Intolerance in Infancy: Some Clinical, Epidemiological, and Immunological Aspects." *Pediatric Allergy and Immunology* 5 (5 Suppl.).

120. Mead, Nathaniel. 1994. "Cow's-Milk Allergy Is a Risk Factor for the Development of Functional Gastrointestinal Disorders in Children." *Natural Health*, July.

121. Verge, Charles F., and Neville J. Howard, et al. 1994. "Environmental Factors in Childhood IDDM: A Population-Based, Case-Control Study." *Diabetes Care* 17 (12): 1381–89.

122. Harlan, D. M., and M. M. Lee. 2010. "Infant Formula, Autoimmune Triggers, and Type 1 Diabetes." *New England Journal of Medicine* 363 (20): 196–3.

123. Scott, F. W. 1990. "Cow Milk and Insulin-Dependent Diabetes Mellitus: Is There a Relationship?" *American Journal of Clinical Nutrition* 51(3): 489–91.

124. Verge, Charles F. MBBS, et al. 1994. "Milk and Type 1 Diabetes." *Diabetes Care*. 17:1381–1389, 1488–1490.

125. Schmidt, Michael A. 1996. *Healing Childhood Ear Infections: Prevention, Home Care, and Alternative Treatment*. Narayana Publishers.

126. American Academy of Allergy Athsma and Immunology. "Food Allergy." AAAAI. org. Accessed May 3, 2016. http://www.aaaai.org/conditions-and-treatments /library/at-a-glance/food-allergy.aspx.

127. Barclay, Elizabeth. 2012. "A Nation of Meat Eaters: See How It All Adds Up." *NPR*, June 27. http://www.npr.org/sections/thesalt/2012/06/27/155527365 /visualizing-a-nation-of-meat-eaters

128. Davis, Brenda, and Vesanto Melina. 2003. *The New Becoming Vegetarian*. Healthy Living Publications. pp. 57–58.

129. BBC News. 2005. "Red Meat 'Linked to Cancer Risk.'" *BBC News*, June 15. Accessed May 10, 2016. http://news.bbc.co.uk/2/hi/health/4088824.stm.

130. Pattison, D. J., et al. 2004. "Dietary Risk Factors for the Development of Inflammatory Polyarthritis: Evidence for a Role of High Level of Red Meat Consumption." *Arthritis & Rheumatism* 50 (12): 3804–12.

131. Lang, Susan. 1996. "Eating Less Meat May Help Reduce Osteoporosis Risk." *Cornell Chronicle* 28 (13) November 14.

132. Robbins, John. 1987. *Diet for a New America*. Tiburon, CA: HJ Kramer, p. 172, citing the *American Journal of Clinical Nutrition*.

133. "Dietary Reference Intakes for Energy, Carbohydrate, Fiber, Fat, Fatty Acids, Cholesterol, Protein, and Amino Acids." Food and Drug Administration, Institute of Medicine of the National Academies, 2005. https://www.nal.usda.gov/fnic/.

134. "Elephant Basics." 2015. National Elephant Center Fellsmere, FL. http://www.nationalelephantcenter.org/learn/.

135. Robbins, John. 1987. *Diet for a New America.* Tiburon, CA: HJ Kramer.

136. Schwarzenegger, Arnold. 1981. *Arnold's Bodybuilding for Men.* Ontario: Fireside.

137. Martin, William Forrest, and Nancy Rodriguez. 2002. "High Protein Diets Cause Dehydration, Even in Trained Athletes." *The Federation of American Societies for Experimental Biology,* April 22.

138. Craig, W. J., and A. R. Mangels. 2009. "Position of the American Dietetic Association: Vegetarian Diets." *Journal of the American Dietetic Association* 109 (7): 1266–82. doi:10.1016/j.jada.2009.05.027. PMID 19562864.

139. Craig, W. 1994. "Iron Status of Vegetarians," *American Journal of Clinical Nutrition* 59 (Sup): 1233S–37S. Virginia Messina and Mark Messina. 1996. *The Dietitian's Guide to Vegetarian Diets: Issues and Pallications.* Gaithersburg, MD: Aspen Publishers.

140. "Vegetarian Diets for Children: Right from the Start." The Physicians Committee for Responsible Medicine (PCRM). Accessed May 10, 2016. http://milk.procon.org/view.answers.php?questionID=000848.

141. Messina, M. P. H., R. D., Virginia, and Mark Messina. 1996. *The Vegetarian Way: Total Health for You and Your Family.* New York City, NY: Harmony. p. 102.

142. Mozafar, A. 1997. "Is There Vitamin B12 in Plants or Not? A Plant Nutritionist's View." *Vegetarian Nutrition: An International Journal* 1: 50–52.

143. McDougall, John A. 2007. "Vitamin B12 Deficiency—The Meat-Eaters' Last Stand." *The McDougall Newsletter* 6 (11) November. Accessed May 10, 2016.

144. CDC. "Coronary Heart Disease and Stroke Deaths—United States, 2009." Centers for Disease Control and Prevention. Accessed May 10, 2016. http://www.cdc.gov/mmwr/preview/mmwrhtml/su6203a26.htm.

145. Preis, S. R., et al. 2010. "Dietary Protein and Risk of Ischemic Heart Disease in Middle-Aged Men." *American Journal of Clinical Nutrition* 92 (5): 1265–72.

146. Sinha, R., et al. 2009. "Meat Intake and Mortality: A Prospective Study of Over Half a Million People." *Archives of Internal Medicine* 169 (6): 562–71.

147. Jakobsen, M. U., et al. 2009. "Major Types of Dietary Fat and Risk of Coronary Heart Disease: A Pooled Analysis of 11 Cohort Studies." *American Journal of Clinical Nutrition* 89 (5): 1425–32.

148. Fraser, G. E., 2009. "Vegetarian Diets: What Do We Know of Their Effects on Common Chronic Diseases?" *American Journal of Clinical Nutrition* 89 (5): 1607S–12S.

149. Larsson S. C., J. Virtamo, A. Wolk. 2011. "Red Meat Consumption and Risk of Stroke in Swedish Men." *American Journal of Clinical Nutrition* 94:417–421. 21653800.

150. Larsson, S. C., J. Virtamo, and A. Wolk. 2011. "Red Meat Consumption and Risk of Stroke in Swedish Women." *Stroke: A Journal of Cerebral Circulation* 42 (2): 324–9.

151. Sinha, Rashmi, and Amanda J. Cross, et al. 2009. "Meat Intake and Mortality Prospective Study of Over Half a Million People." *Archives of Internal Medicine* 169 (6): 562–571.

152. Kontogianni, M. D., D. B. Panagiotakos, C. Pitsavos, C. Chrysohoou, et al. "Relationship Between Meat Intake and the Development of Acute Coronary Syndromes: The CARDIO2000 Case-Control Study." *European Journal of Clinical Nutrition* 62 (2):171–7.

153. Harvard Health Publications. "Red Meat and Colon Cancer (March 2008 Update)." www.health.harvard.edu. September 1, 2005.

154. Chao, A., and M. J. Thun, et al. 2005. "Meat Consumption and Risk of Colorectal Cancer." *JAMA* 293(2):172–82.

155. World Cancer Research Fund/American Institute for Cancer Research. 2011. "Continuous Update Project Report," May 23.

156. Ibid.

157. "The Assessment of Red Meat and Cancer Risk: A Summary of Findings from an Independent Research Assessment." National Cattlemen's Beef Association, May 22, 2011. Accessed May 10, 2016. http://www.beefnutrition.org/cmdocs /beefnutrition/theassessmentofredmeatandcancer.pdf.

158. The San Francisco Division of the Academic Senate. "Ballot on Tobacco Industry Funding Research." Accessed May 3, 2016. http://senate.ucsf.edu /townhallmeeting/index.html.

159. International Agency for Research on Cancer. 1978. "Monograph on the Evaluation of the Carcinogenic Risk of Chemicals to Humans: Some N-Nitroso Compounds." *IARC Monographs on the Evaluation of Carcinogenic Risks to Humans* 17:77–82.

160. Lijinsky, William. 1992. *Chemistry and Biology of N-Nitroso Compounds*. New York City, NY: Cambridge University Press.

161. Bingham, S. A., and B. Pignatelli, et al. 1996. "Does Increased Endogenous Formation of N-Nitroso Compounds in the Human Colon Explain the Association Between Red Meat and Colon Cancer?" *Carcinogenesis* 17 (3): 515-23.

162. Giovannucci, E., and E. Rimm, et al. 1994. "Intake of Fat, Meat, and Fibre in Relation to Risk of Colon Cancer in Men." *Cancer Research* 54: 2390–97.

163. Goldbohm, R. A, and P. van den Brandt, et al. 1994. "A Prospective Cohort Study on the Relation Between Meat Consumption and the Risk of Colon Cancer." *Cancer Research* 54: 718–723.

164. Samraj, Annie N. 2014. "A Red Meat-Derived Glycan Promotes Inflammation and Cancer Progression." *Proceedings of the National Academy of Sciences* 112 (2): 542–47. http://m.pnas.org/content/112/2/542.abstract.

165. Cummings, J.H. et al. 1979. "The Effect of Meat Protein on Colonic Function and Metabolism." *The American Journal of Clinical Nutrition* 32 (October): 2094-101.

166. Windey, K. et al. 2012. "Relevance of Protein Fermentation to Gut Health." *Molecular Nutriton and Food Research* 58:184–96.

167. Heinig, M., and R. J. Johnson. 2006. "Role of Uric Acid in Hypertension, Renal Disease, and Metabolic Syndrome." *Cleveland Clinic Journal of Medicine* 73 (12): 1059–64.

168. Dehghan, A., and M. van Hoek M, et al. 2008. "High Serum Uric Acid as a Novel Risk Factor for Type 2 Diabetes." *Diabetes Care* 31 (2): 361–2.

169. Norton, J. Renae. 2012. "Digesting Animal Protein." J Renae Norton. May 30. http://www.eatingdisorderpro.com/2012/05/30/digesting-animal-protein/.

170. Rattigan, Pat. 2003. *The Cancer Business.* The British AntiVivisection Association. Accessed May 10, 2016. http://www.checktheevidence.com/pdf/The%20 Cancer%20Business%20-%20Side%201.pdf.

171. Tsai, Chung-Jyi, Michael F Leitzmann, et al. 2007. "Heme And Non-Heme Iron Consumption and Risk of Gallstone Disease in Men." *American Journal of Clinical Nutrition* 85 (2): 518–22.

172. NY Times Health. 2013. "Acute Cholecystitis Surgery." NYTimes.com. August 26. Accessed May 3, 2016. http://www.nytimes.com/health/guides/disease /acute-cholecystitis-gallstones/surgery.html.

173. Pan A et al. 2011. "Red Meat Consumption and Risk of Type 2 Diabetes: 3 Cohorts of U.S. Adults and an Updated Meta-Analysis." *Am J Clin Nutr.,* August 10. ajcn.018978.

174. National Cattlemen's Beef Association news release. 2015. "Science Does Not Support International Agency Opinion on Red Meat and Cancer." National Cattlemans Beef Association, October 26. https://www.beefusa.org /newsreleases1.aspx?newsid=5418

175. Song, Y. et al. 2004. "A Prospective Study of Red Meat Consumption and Type 2 Diabetes in Middle-Aged and Elderly Women." *Diabetes Care* 27 (9): 2108–15.

176. van Dam, Rob M., et al. 2002. "Dietary Patterns and Risk for Type 2 Diabetes Mellitus in U.S. Men." *Annals of Internal Medicine* 136 (3): 201–09.

177. Goldstein, Myrna, and Mark A. Goldstein. 2002. *Controversies in Food and Nutrition* Westport, CT: Greenwood Press. p. 67.

178. Opposition to the Use of Hormone Growth Promoters in Beef and Dairy Cattle Production. American Public Health Association, November 10, 2009. Policy Number: 20098 https://www.apha.org/policies-and-advocacy /public-health-policy-statements/policy-database./

179. Holguin, Jaime. 2003. "Link Eyed Between Beef and Cancer." *CBS News,* May 20. Accessed May 10, 2106. http://www.cbsnews.com/news /link-eyed-between-beef-and-cancer/.

180. Mercola, Joseph. 2010. "The Alarming Reason Why More Girls Are Starting Puberty Early." Dr. Mercola, August 26. http://articles.mercola.com/sites/articles /archive/2010/08/26/why-are-more-girls-starting-puberty-early.aspx.

181. Wilkinson, Emma. 2010. "High Meat Diet Linked to Early Periods." BBC News, June 11.

182. Gandhi, R., and S. Snedeker. 2000. "Consumer Concerns about Hormones in Food. Fact Sheet #37, June 2000." Program on Breast Cancer and Environmental Risk Factors, Cornell University. http://envirocancer.cornell.edu /factsheet/diet/fs37.hormones.cfm. June 1. Retrieved July 20, 2011.

183. Hardin, Pete. 2007. "rbGH & Human Safety." *The Milkweed,* September. Accessed May 10, 2016. http://www.themilkweed.com/Feature_07_Sep.pdf.

184. Smith, Jeffery M. 2007. *Genetic Roulette: The Documented Health Risks of Genetically Engineered Foods.* Fairfield, IA: Yes Books. p. 157.

185. National Toxicology Program, Department of Health and Human Services. 2011. *National Toxicology Program, Department of Health and Human Services Report on Carcinogens, Twelfth Edition.*

186. Swan, S. H., and F. Liu, et al. 2007. "Semen Quality of Fertile U.S. Males in Relation to Their Mothers' Beef Consumption During Pregnancy." *Human Reproduction.* Advance Access published online March 28.

187. Holguin, Jaime. 2003. "Link Eyed Between Beef and Cancer." *CBS News*, May 20. Accessed May 10, 2106. http://www.cbsnews.com/news /link-eyed-between-beef-and-cancer/.

188. Raloff, Janet. 2002. "Hormones: Here's the Beef: Environmental Concerns Reemerge Over Steroids Given to Livestock." *Science News* 161(1): 10.

189. European Food Safety Authority. 2007. "Opinion of the Scientific Panel on Contaminants in the Food Chain on a Request from the European Commission Related to Hormone Residues in Bovine Meat and Meat Products." *The EFSA Journal*, June 12. Accessed May 10, 2016. http://www.efsa.europa.eu/en/scdocs /doc/510.pdf.

190. International Centre for Trade and Sustainable Development. 2003. "DSB: EC-US Disputes Top Agenda." *Bridges Weekly Trade News Digest* 7 (38). Accessed May 10, 2016. http://ictsd.org/i/news/bridgesweekly/7451/.

191. U.S. Congress Office of Technology Assessment. 1995. *Impacts of Antibiotic-Resistant Bacteria.* Washington, DC: U.S. Government Printing Office. Accessed May 10, 2016. www.fas.org/ota/reports/9503.pdf.

192. Levy, Stuart B. 2002. *The Antibiotic Paradox: How the Misuse of Antibiotics Destroys Their Curative Powers.* Cambridge, MA: Perseus Publishing.

193. Chiu, Cheng-Hsun, and Tsu-Lan Wu, et al. 2002. "The Emergence in Taiwan of Fluoroquinolone Resistance in Salmonella enterica Serotype Choleraesuis." *New England Journal of Medicine* 346:413–19.

194. Blezinger, Stephen B. "Debate Continues over Antibiotic Use in Cattle." CattleToday.com. Accessed May 3, 2016. http://www.cattletoday.com/ archive/2010/August/CT2302.php.

195. Couric, Katie. 2010. "Denmark's Case for Antibiotic-Free Animals." CBSNews. com, February 10. Accessed May 3, 2016. http://www.cbsnews.com /stories/2010/02/10/eveningnews/main6195054.shtml.

196. Mindfully.org. 1996. "Attorney General of the State of New York. Consumer Frauds and Protection Bureau. Environmental Protection Bureau. In the matter of Monsanto Company, respondent. Assurance of discontinuance pursuant to executive law § 63 (15). New York, NY, Nov." Accesssed May 10, 2106. http://www.mindfully.org/Pesticide/Monsanto-v-AGNYnov96.htm.

197. Benachour, Nora, and Gilles-Eric Séralini. 2008. "Glyphosate Formulations Induce Apoptosis and Necrosis in Human Umbilical, Embryonic, and Placental Cells." *Chemical Research in Toxicology* 22 (1): 97–105.

198. CBC News. 2009. "Complaints Halt Herbicide Spraying in Eastern Shore." *CBC News*, June 16. Accessed May 10, 2016.

199. "Tordon 101: picloram/2,4-D," Ontario Ministry of Agriculture Food & Rural Affairs, Reviewed January 21, 2008. http://www.omafra.gov.on.ca/english/crops/facts/notes/picloram2.htm.

200. Dinis-Oliveira, R. J., and F. Remião, et al. 2006. "Paraquat Exposure as an Etiological Factor of Parkinson's Disease." *NeuroToxicology* 27 (6):. 1110–22.

201. "Regulating Pesticides in Food." National Research Council, Board on Agriculture, Alternative Agriculture, 44; National Research Council, Board on Agriculture, October 1990, 78, Table 3, 20–22.

202. McCarthy, Colman. 1994. "Dioxin Burgers." *Washington Post*, September 24.

203. Institute of Food Technologists. "Food Technology." IFT.org. Accessed May 3, 2016. http://www.ift.org/food-technology.aspx.

204. Gardner, Amanda. 2011. "Well-Done Red Meat Linked to Aggressive Prostate Cancer." CNN.com., November 23. Accessed May 10, 2016. http://www.cnn.com/2011/11/23/health/well-done-red-meat-prostate-cancer/.

205. Douglass, William Campbell. 2010. "More Dangers from Overcooked Meat." HealthierTalk.com, March 26. Accessed May 3, 2016. www.healthiertalk.com/more-dangers-overcooked-meat-1621.

206. "Burden of Foodborne Illness: Findings" *Center for Disease Control and Prevention* July 15, 2016. https://www.cdc.gov/foodborneburden/2011-foodborne-estimates.html.

207. Woods, Jon B., and Clare K. Schmitt, et al. 2002. "Ferrets as a Model System for Renal Disease Secondary to Intestinal Infection with Escherichiacoli O157:H7 and Other Shiga Toxin-Producing *E. coli*." *The Journal of Infectious Diseases* 185 (4): 550–4.

208. Hill, Gaston J. S., and M. S. Lillicrap. 2003. "Arthritis Associated with Enteric Infection." *Best Practice & Research: Clinical Rheumatology* 17 (2): 219–39.

209. Department for Environment, Food, and Rural Affairs. 2007. "BSE: Disease Control & Eradication—Causes of BSE." The National Archives, March. Accessed May 10, 2016.

210. University of Michigan Health System. "L-Tryptophan." UofMHealth.org. Accessed May 3, 2016. http://www.uofmhealth.org/health-library/hn-10006312.

211. Science Daily. 2005. "Eating Chicken May Reduce Your Risk of Colon Cancer." ScienceDaily.com, December 21. Accessed May 3, 2016. http://www.sciencedaily.com/releases/2005/12/051221085444.htm.

212. Sears M.D., Bill. "Dietary Changes to Lower Cancer Risk" *Ask Dr. Sears*. 2013 http://www.askdrsears.com/topics/feeding-eating/family-nutrition/anticancer/12-dietary-changes-will-lower-your-cancer-risk.

213. Norat, Teresa et al. 2005. "The European Prospective Investigation into Cancer and Nutrition." *Journal of the National Cancer Institute* (2005) 97 (12): 906-916. www.mrc.ac.uk/consumption/groups/public/documents/content/mrc001870.pdf

214. Willett, W.C. et al. "Relation of meat, fat, and fiber intake to the risk of colon cancer in a prospective study among women." *New England Journal of Medicine* 1990: 323: 1664–72.

215. Russo, M. W., and S. C. Murray, et al. 1997. "Plasma Selenium Levels and the Risk of Colorectal Adenomas." *The Journal of Nutrition and Cancer* 28:125–9.

216. Patterson, B. H., and O. A. Levander. 1997. "Naturally Occurring Selenium Compounds in Cancer Chemoprevention Trials: A Workshop Summary." *Cancer Epidemiology and Biomarkers Prevention* 6:63–9.

217. Knekt, P., and J. Marniemi, et al. 1998. "Is Low Selenium Status a Risk Factor for Lung Cancer?" *American Journal of Epidemiology* 148:975–82.

218. Fleet, J. C. 1997. "Dietary Selenium Repletion May Reduce Cancer Incidence in People at High Risk Who Live in Areas with Low Soil Selenium." *Nutriton Review* 55:277–9.

219. Shamberger, R. J. 1985. "The Genotoxicity of Selenium." *Mutation Research* 154:29–48.

220. Young, K. L., and P. N. Lee. 1999. "Intervention Studies on Cancer." *European Journal of Cancer Prevention* 8:91–103.

221. Burguera, J. L., and M. Burguera. 1990. "Blood Serum Selenium in the Province of Merida, Venezuela, Related to Sex, Cancer Incidence and Soil Selenium Content." *Journal of Trace Elements and Electrolytes in Health and Disease* 4:73–7.

222. Combs Jr., G. F., and L. C. Clark, et al. 1997. "Reduction of Cancer Risk with an Oral Supplement of Selenium." *Journal of Biomedical and Environmental Sciences.* 10: 227–34.

223. Combs, G. F., and L. C. Clark, et al. 2001. "An Analysis of Cancer Prevention by Selenium." *BioFactors* 14: 153–9.

224. Rayman, M. P. 2000. "The Importance of Selenium to Human Health." *The Lancet* 356(9225): 233–41.

225. Nutritional Data of Food http://nutritiondata.self.com/facts /poultry-products/667/2.

226. Morris, M. C., and D.A. Evans, et al. 2004. "Dietary Niacin and the Risk of Incident Alzheimer's Disease and of Cognitive Decline." *Journal of Neurology, Psychiatry* 75:1093–1099.

227. University of California—Irvine. 2008. "Vitamin B3 Reduces Alzheimer's Symptoms, Lesions: Clinical Trial on Nicotinamide Effect in Alzheimer's Patients." *ScienceDaily*, November 5.

228. Wojcik, Oktawia P., and Karen L. Koenig, et al. 2013. "Serum Taurine and Risk of Coronary Heart Disease: A Prospective, Nested Case-Control Study." *European Journal of Nutrition* 52(1): 169–78.

229. Brown, W. V. 1995. "Niacin for Lipid Disorders." *Postgrad Med* 98:185–93.

230. Guyton, J. R. 1998. "Effect of Niacin on Atherosclerotic Cardiovascular Disease." *American Journal of Cardiology* 82(12A): 18U–23U.

231. Garg, R., and M. Malinow, et al. 1999. "Niacin Treatment Increases Plasma Homocyst(E)Ine Levels." *American Heart Journal* 138:1082–7.

232. Brattström, L., and D. E. Wilcken. 2000. "Homocysteine and Cardiovascular Disease: Cause or Effect?" *American Journal of Clinical Nutrition* 72 (2): 315–23.

233. FDA. "Letter to the Honorable John F. Kerry." February 22, 2011. Accessed May 3, 2016. http://desinfo411.files.wordpress.com/2011/04/page-1.jpg.

234. *Consumer Reports*. 2009. "*Consumer Reports*: Two-Thirds of Chickens Tested Harbor Dangerous Bacteria." ConsumerReports.org, November 30. Accessed May 3, 2016. http://pressroom.consumerreports.org/pressroom/2009/11 /cr-two-thirds-of-chickens-tested-harbor-dangerous-bacteria.html.

235. Ibid.

236. *Consumer Reports*. "Dangerous Contaminated Chicken: 97% of the Breasts Tested Harbored Bacteria That Could Make You Sick." ConsumerReports.org, January 7. http://www.consumerreports.org/cro/magazine/2014/02 /the-high-cost-of-cheap-chicken/index.htm.

237. "H.R. 965: Preservation of Antibiotics for Medical Treatment Act of 2011–2013." Accessed May 10, 2016. https://www.govtrack.us/congress/bills/112 /hr965/text.

238. Centers for Disease Control and Prevention. "Antimicrobial Resistance Threats in the United States, 2017." CDC.gov. Accessed February 3, 2017. http://www.cdc.gov/drugresistance/threat-report-2017/.

239. McKenna, Maryn. 2012. "How Your Chicken Dinner Is Creating a Drug-Resistant Superbug." TheAtlantic.com, July 11. Accessed May 3, 2016. http://www.theatlantic.com/health/archive/2012/07 /how-your-chicken-dinner-is-creating-a-drug-resistant-superbug/259700/.

240. The American Veterinary Medical Association (AVMA). http://www.avma.org /onlnews/javma/mar02/s031502h.asp.

241. "FDA Prohibits Nitrofuran Drug Use in Food-Producing Animals." 2002. *Journal of the American Veterinary Medical Association*. February 7. https://www.avma.org /News/JAVMANews/Pages/s031502h.aspx

242. Lewis, Betty. "Does Topic Flea Treatment Go into the Bloodstream?" *Pets*. http://pets.thenest.com/topical-flea-treatment-bloodstream-13025.html.

243. Food Safety and Inspection Service. "Nationwide Young Chicken Microbiological Baseline Data Collection Program." FSIS. USDA.gov. Accessed May 3, 2016. http://www.fsis.usda.gov/PDF/Baseline_Data_Young_Chicken.pdf.

244. Mach, Andrew. 2011. "Antibiotics in Livestock Fuel Debate Over Hazardous Meat and Poultry." Food Safety, October 2011. http://foodsafety.news21.com /2011/risks/antibiotics/.

245. Natural Resources Defense Council. 2012. "Court Orders FDA to Address Antibiotic Overuse in Livestock and Protect Effectiveness of Medicine for Humans: Group Wins Superbug Suit, Forcing FDA into Action After 35 Years of Delay." NRDC.org, March 23. Accessed May 3, 2016. http://www.nrdc.org /media/2012/120323.asp.

246. "FDA Seeks Public Input on Next Steps to Help Ensure Judicious Use of Antimicrobials in Animal Agriculture." 2016. FDA.gov, September 12. https://www.fda.gov/animalveterinary/newsevents/cvmupdates/ucm520110.htm

247. USDA. "Salmonella Questions and Answers." FSIS. USDA.org. Accessed May 6, 2016. http://www.fsis.usda.gov/wps/portal/fsis/topics/food-safety-education /get-answers/food-safety-fact-sheets/foodborne-illness-and-disease /salmonella-questions-and-answers/.

248. Centers for Disease Control (CDC). 2011. "CDC Estimates of Foodborne Illness in the United States, 2011." http://www.cdc.gov/foodborneburden /2011-foodborne-estimates.html.

249. Feodoroff, B., and A. Lauhio, et al. 2011. "A Nationwide Study of *Campylobacter jejuni* and *Campylobacter coli* Bacteremia in Finland Over a 10-Year Period, 1998–2007, With Special Reference to Clinical Characteristics and Antimicrobial Susceptibility." *Clinical Infectious Diseases* 53(8): e99–e106.

250. Foodborne Illness. "*Campylobacter*." FoodborneIllness.com. Accessed May 3, 2016. www.foodborneillness.com/campylobacter_food_poisoning/.

251. Centers for Disease Control and Prevention. 2009. Listeriosis. Available online: http://www.cdc.gov/nczved/divisions/dfbmd/diseases/listeriosis.

252. DeCuir, Lauren. 2015 "Finally! The FDA Admits That Nearly Over 70% of U.S. Chickens Contain Cancer-Causing Arsenic." MSN, January. http://www.msn.com /en-ca/foodanddrink/foodnews/finally-the-fda-admits-that-nearly-over-70percent- of-us-chickens-contain-cancer-causing-arsenic.

253. Hopey, Don. 2016. "Chicken Feed Additive May Pose Danger." *Pittsburgh Post- Gazette*, February 7. Accessed May 9, 2016.

254. Wallinga, David. 2006. "Playing Chicken: Avoiding Arsenic in Your Meat." The Institute for Agriculture and Trade Policy, April. Accessed May 9, 2016. http://www.iatp.org/files/421_2_80529.pdf.

255. Ibid.

256. The Nutrition and Food Web Archive. http://www.nafwa.org/general-nutrition /alternative-nutrition/31831-fda-finally-listened-and-removed-arsenic-from- chickens.html.

257. National Grain and Feed Association. 2011. "Pfizer Agrees to Suspend Sales of 3-Nitro (Roxarsone) after FDA Tests Detect Residues of Inorganic Arsenic in Chicken Livers." June 10. http://www.nytimes.com/2011/06/09/business/09arsenic. html.

258. *Burlington County Times*. 2011. "FDA: Some Chicken May Have Small Amount of Arsenic." June 8. Accessed May 3, 2016. http://www.burlingtoncountytimes.com /news/local/fda-some-chicken-may-have-small-amount-of-arsenic /article_252bf73c-a627-55c7-bc6f-8bc3aadc9ba8.html.

259. Agency for Toxic Substances and Disease Registry Division of Toxicology and Environmental Medicine. "Arsenic: Public Health Statement." Accessed May 3, 2016. http://www.atsdr.cdc.gov/toxprofiles/tp2-c1.pdf.

260. Environmental Health Association of Nova Scotia. "Arsenic Symptoms, Diagnosis and Treatment: Update Summer 2002." Accessed May 3, 2016. http://www.environmentalhealth.ca/summer02arsenic.html.

261. http://www.fda.gov/AnimalVeterinary/NewsEvents/CVMUpdates/ucm440668.htm

262. McDonalds Corporation. 2006. "McDonald's USA Ingredients Listing for Popular Menu Items." McDonalds.com, September 20. Accessed May 11, 2016.

263. U.S. Food and Drug Administration. 2011. "EAFUS: A Food Additive Database." FDA.gov, November. Accessed May 11, 2016.

264. Kobylewski Ph.D., Sarah, and Michael F. Jacobson, Ph.D. 2010. "Food Dyes: A Rainbow of Risks." Center for Science in the Public Interest, June 1. https://cspinet.org/resource/food-dyes-rainbow-risks.

265. Schlosser, Eric. 2002. *Fast Food Nation: The Dark Side of the All-American Meal.* New York City, NY: Perennial, pp. 126–7.

266. GRACE Communications Foundation. "Additives." SustainableTable.org. Accessed May 3, 2016. http://www.sustainabletable.org/issues/additives/#fn2.

267. Gharavi, N., and A. El-Kadi. 2005. "Tert-Butylhydroquinone Is a Novel Aryl Hydrocarbon Receptor Ligand." *Drug Metabolism & Disposition* 33 (3): 365–72.

268. Hirose, Masao, and Hideaki Yada, et al. "Modification of Carcinogenesis by A-Tocopherol, T-Butylhydro-Quinone, Propyl Gallate and Butylated Hydroxytoluene in a Rat Multi-Organ Carcinogenesis Model." *Carcinogenesis* (Oxford University Press) 14 (1): 2359–64.

269. The Law, Science & Public Health Law Site. "Circuit Court Allows Some Claims and Remands—Pelman V. McDonald's Corporation, 396 F.3d 508 (2d Cir. 2005)." Accessed May 3, 2016. http://biotech.law.lsu.edu/cases/food/pelman04.htm.

270. "The Chicken Which Should Be Banned." 2012. *Natural Healing News*, August 16. Environment, Food, Gen http://www.naturalhealingnews.com/the-chicken-which-should-be-banned/#.WOpceVPyvJM.

271. Sullivan, Kristie M., Michael A. Erickson, Chad B. Sandusky, and Neal D. Barnard. 2008. "Detection of PhIP in Grilled Chicken Entrées at Popular Chain Restaurants Throughout California." *Nutrition and Cancer* 60 (5).

272. Physicians Committee for Responsible Medicine. "KFC Grilled Chicken Products Contain Carcinogenic Chemicals: A Report from the Physicians Committee for Responsible Medicine May 2009." PRCM.org. Accessed May 2, 2016. http://www.pcrm.org/pdfs/health/KFCgrilledchickenPhIPreport-final.pdf.

273. Ibid.

274. Court of Appeal, Second District, Division 1, California. PHYSICIANS COMMITTEE FOR RESPONSIBLE MEDICINE, Plaintiff and Appellant, v. APPLEBEE'S INTERNATIONAL, INC., et al., Defendants and Respondents. February 27, 2014. http://caselaw.findlaw.com/ca-court-of-appeal/1658914.html.

275. Zheng, W., and S. Lee. 2009. "Well-Done Meat Intake, Heterocyclic Amine Exposure, and Cancer Risk." *Journal of Nutrition and Cancer* 61:437–446.

276. Greger M.D., Michael. 2013. "Avoiding Cooked Meat Carcinogens." Nutritionfacts.org. Accessed May 11, 2016. http://nutritionfacts.org/2013/07/04/avoiding-cooked-meat-carcinogens/.

277. Union of Concerned Scientists. "Industrial Agriculture: The Outdated, Unsustainable System That Dominates U.S. Food Production." UCSUSA.org. Accessed May 3, 2016. http://www.ucsusa.org/food_and_agriculture/science_and_impacts/impacts_industrial_agriculture/they-eat-what-the-reality-of.html.

278. Smith, Margaret, Mary Swalla, and Jim Ennis. "Literature Review of Consumer Research, Publications, and Marketing Communications Related to Pasture-Raised Animal Products and Production Systems." Iowa State University, Iowa InterFaith Ministries and Midwest Food Alliance. Accessed May 11, 2016.

279. Sustainable Agriculture Research and Education (SARE). 1999. "Pastured Poultry Products: Summary." SARE. https://projects.sare.org/sare_project/fne99-248/.

280. "Organic Certification" USA.gov. http://www.usda.gov/wps/portal/usda /usdahome?navid=ORGANIC_CERTIFICATION.

281. H. Katz, Solomon, and William Woys Weaver (eds). 2003. *Encyclopedia of Food and Culture, Volume 1.* New York City, NY: Charles Scribner's Sons, p. 558.

282. Maher, John. 2006. "Lutein and Zeaxanthin: Seeing into the Heart of the Matter." *Dynamic Chiropractic* 24, (21) October 12.

283. Inter-Society Commission for Heart Disease Resources: Prevention of Cardiovascular Disease. 1970. "Primary Prevention of the Atherosclerotic Diseases." *Circulation* 42: A55–A95.

284. American Heart Association. 1973. "Diet and Coronary Heart Disease." Dallas: American Heart Association.

285. Jiang, Yongzhi, and Sang K. Noh, et al. 2001. "Egg Phosphatidylcholine Decreases the Lymphatic Absorption of Cholesterol in Rats." *Journal of Nutrition* 131:2358–63.

286. Vandermark, Tracy. 2011. "What Are the Benefits of Egg Lecithin?" Livestrong. com, May 12.

287. Perkins, Cynthia. "Are Eggs Healthy or Do They Lead to an Early Death?" Holistichelp.net. Accessed May 10, 2106. http://www.holistichelp.net/blog /are-eggs-healthy-or-do-they-lead-to-an-early-death/. (Jamo8l:1387-94, Nut Metab Cas 2006; 9.8-12 Journal of Food Chemistry.).

288. *Daily Mail Reporter.* 2008. "Eating Two Eggs a Day Could Cut Your Cholesterol and Help You Lose Weight." DailyMail.co.uk. August 26. Accessed May 3, 2016. http://www.dailymail.co.uk/health/article-1049144/Eating-eggs-day-CUT-cholesterol-help-lose-weight.html.

289. Robbins, J. M., et al. 2014. Association of Egg Consumption and Calcified Atherosclerotic Plaque in the Coronary Arteries: The NHLBI Family Heart Study. *European e-Journal of Clinical Nutrition and Metabolism* 9 (3): e131–e135.

290. Reames, Elizabeth. 2010. "Make Fish, Seafood Part of Healthy Diet." LSU AgCenter News Release. November.

291. Harvard T. H. Chan School of Public Health. "Fish: Friend or Foe?" Accessed May 3, 2016. http://www.hsph.harvard.edu/nutritionsource /what-should-you-eat/fish/#1.

292. Boehnke, C., and U. Reuter, et al. 2004. "High-Dose Riboflavin Treatment Is Efficacious in Migraine Prophylaxis: An Open Study in a Tertiary Care Centre." *European Journal of Neurology* 11: 475–7.

293. Mitchell, Paul, and W. Smith, et al. 2003. "Nutritional Factors in the Development of Age-Related Eye Disease." *Asia Pacific Journal of Clinical Nutrition* 12 (Supp. 5).

294. Buydens-Branchey, L. and M. Branchey. 2008. "Long-Chain N-3 Polyunsaturated Fatty Acids Decrease Feelings of Anger in Substance Abusers." *Psychiatry Research* 157: 95–104.

295. Lawrence, Felicity. 2006. "Omega-3, Junk Food and the Link Between Violence and What We Eat." *The Guardian*, October 16. Accessed May 11, 2016. http://www.theguardian.com/politics/2006/oct/17/prisonsandprobation.ukcrime.

296. Park, Alice. 2011. "Brain Food: Eating Fish May Lower Your Risk of Alzheimer's." *Time*, December 1. Accessed May 3, 2016. www.healthland.time.com/2011/12/01 /brain-food-eating-fish-may-lower-your-risk-of-alzheimers/#ixzz1hlPPkzmO.

297. National Institutes of Mental Health. "Depression: What You Need to Know." NIMH. Accessed May 3, 2016. http://www.nimh.nih.gov/health/publications /depression/complete-index.shtml.

298. Tanskanen, Antti, et al. 2001. "Fish Consumption, Depression, and Suicidality in a General Population." *Archives of General Psychiatry* 58: 512–13.

299. Lalovic, Aleksandra, and Émile Levy, et al. 2007. "Fatty Acid Composition in Postmortem Brains of People Who Completed Suicide." *Journal of Psychiatry & Neuroscience* 32 (5): 363–70.

300. University of Maryland Medical Center. "Omega-3 Fatty Acids." UMM.edu. Accessed May 3, 2016. http://www.umm.edu/altmed/articles/omega-3-000316.htm.

301. Arthritis Foundation. "Best Fish for Arthritis." Arthritis.org. Accessed May 10, 2016. http://www.arthritis.org/living-with-arthritis/arthritis-diet/best-foods-for-arthritis /best-fish-for-arthritis.php.

302. Niu, K., et al. 2006. "Dietary Long-Chain N-3 Fatty Acids of Marine Origin and Serum C-Reactive Protein Concentrations Are Associated in a Population with a Diet Rich in Marine Products." *American Journal of Clinical Nutrition* 84:223–29.

303. Zampelas, A., et al. 2005. "Fish Consumption Among Healthy Adults Is Associated with Decreased Levels of Inflammatory Markers Related to Cardiovascular Disease: The ATTICA Study." *Journal of the American College of Cardiology* 46:120–24.

304. Tsitouras, P. D., et al. 2008. "Hormone and Metabolic Research; High Omega-3 Fat Intake Improves Insulin Sensitivity and Reduces CRP and IL6, But Does Not Affect Other Endocrine Axes in Healthy Older Adults." *Hormone and Metabolic Research* 40 (3): 199–205.

305. Van Bussell, B.C.T., et al. 2011. "Fish Consumption in Healthy Adults Is Associated with Decreased Circulating Biomarkers of Endothelial Dysfunction and Inflammation During a 6-Year Follow-up." *Journal of Nutrition* 141:1719–1725.

306. Crew, Bec. 2016. "The Ocean Is So Much Deeper Than You Think: Mount Everest Doesn't Even Come Close." *Science Alert*. Science Alert. http://www.sciencealert.com/the-ocean-is-so-much-deeper-than-you-think-it-is

307. Allen, Nick. 2010. "Microbe Eating Spilled Oil in Gulf of Mexico." *The Daily Telegraph*. August 25.

308. Lenntech Water Treatment Solutions. "Mercury—Hg." Lenntech.com. Accessed May 3, 2016. http://www.lenntech.com/periodic/elements/hg.htm.

309. Institute for Agriculture and Trade Policy, news release. 2009. "Much High Fructose Corn Syrup Contaminated With Mercury, New Study Finds." January 26.

310. Clifton, J. C. 2007. "Mercury Exposure and Public Health." *Pediatric Clinics of North America* 54 (2): 237–69, viii.

311. The International Academy of Oral Medicine and Toxicology (IAOMT). "The Scientific Case Against Amalgam." Accessed June 10, 2016. https://iaomt.org /wp-content/uploads/The-Case-Against-Amalgam.pdf.

312. Doheny, Kathleen. 2009. "FDA: Mercury Fillings Not Harmful." *WebMD Health News*. July 28. Accessed May 3, 2016. http://www.webmd.com/oral-health/news/20090728/fda-mercury-fillings-not-harmful.

313. Mercola, Joseph. 2011. "Are You Being Tricked into Having This Neurotoxin Placed Next to Your Brain?" Mercola.com, September 10. Accessed May 3, 2016. http://articles.mercola.com/sites/articles/archive/2011/09/10/americans-unaware-that-silver-fillings-are-50-percent-mercury.aspx

314. The International Academy of Oral Medicine and Toxicology (IAOMT). "The Scientific Case Against Amalgam." Accessed May 10, 2015. https://iaomt.org/wp-content/uploads/The-Case-Against-Amalgam.pdf.

315. Drasch, G., et al. 1998. "Mercury in Human Colostrum and Early Breast Milk: Its Dependence on Dental Amalgam and Other Factors." *Journal of Trace Elements in Medicine and Biology* 12 (1): 23–7.

316. DeNoon, Daniel. "FDA: Possible Risk From Dental Fillings To Settle Lawsuit, FDA Now Says Mercury From Fillings Might Pose Risk to Some." WebMD.com. Accessed May 10, 2016. http://www.webmd.com/oral-health/news/20080605/fda-dental-filling-risk-possible.

317. FDA. 2009. "FDA Issues Final Regulation on Dental Amalgam." FDA.gov., July 28. Accessed May 3, 2016. http://www.fda.gov/NewsEvents/Newsroom/PressAnnouncements/ucm173992.htm.

318. Tom Ricky. 1998. "Commercial Fish: Eat Up, Despite Low Levels of Mercury" Universisty of Rochester, August 26. http://www.rochester.edu/pr/releases/med/mercury.htm.

319. Barclay, Laurie. 2005. "Fish Consumption for Health: A Newsmaker Interview with Joshua Cohen, PhD." *Medscape Medical News*, October 19. http://www.medscape.com/viewarticle/515070.

320. Todd Datz. 2007. "Research Shows That the Benefits of Eating Seafood During Pregnancy Outweigh the Risks." *The Lancet* 369 (9561): 578–85.

321. Julvez, Jordi, et al. 2016. "Maternal Consumption of Seafood in Pregnancy and Child Neuropsychological Development: A Longitudinal Study Based on a Population with High Consumption Levels." *American Journal of Epidemiolgy* 183 (3): 169–82.

322. Daniels, Julie L., and Matthew P. Longnecker, et al. 2004. "Fish Intake During Pregnancy and Early Cognitive Development of Offspring." *Epidemiology* 15 (4): 394–402.

323. Lederman, Sally Ann, et al. 2008. "Relation Between Cord Blood Mercury Levels and Early Child Development in a World Trade Center Cohort." *Environmental Health Perspect.* 116 (8): 1085–91.

324. Grandjean, P., et al. 1997. "Cognitive Deficit in 7-Year-Old Children with Prenatal Exposure to Methylmercury." *Neurotoxicology and Teratology* 19 (6): 417–28.

325. Thomson, C.D., et al. 1980. "Selenium in Human Health and Disease with Emphasis on Those Aspects Peculiar to New Zealand." *American Journal of Clinical Nutrition.* 33 (2): 303–23.

326. Kaneko, J.J., et al. 2007. "Selenium and Mercury in Pelagic Fish in the Central North Pacific Near Hawaii." *Biological Trace Element* Research 119 (3): 242–54.

327. Longo, L. D. 1980. "Environmental Pollution and Pregnancy: Risks and Uncertainties for the Fetus and Infant." *American Journal of Obstetrics & Gynecology* 137 (2):162–73.

328. Harada, M. 1995. "Minamata Disease: Methylmercury Poisoning in Japan Caused by Environmental Pollution." *Critical Reveiws in Toxicology*. 25 (1): 1–24.

329. Ricky, Tom.1998. "Commercial Fish: Eat Up, Despite Low Levels Of Mercury." University of Rochester. http://www.rochester.edu/pr/releases/med/mercury.htm.

330. Kaplan, Melissa (compiler). 2014. "Common Sources of Ethylmercury." Melissa Kaplan's Chronic Neuroimmune Diseases. Accessed May 3, 2016. http://www.anapsid.org/cnd/diffdx/mercurysources.html.

331. Stratton, Kathleen, and Alicia Gable, et al. 2001. *Immunization Safety Review. Thimerosal-Containing Vaccines and Neurodevelopmental Disorders.* Washington, DC: The National Academies Press.

332. Minnesota Department of Health. "Frequently Asked Questions on Thimerosal." MDH. Accessed May 3, 2016. http://www.health.state.mn.us/divs/idepc/immunize /safety/faqthimerosal.html#6.

333. FDA. "Thimersoal in Vaccines." FDA.gov. Accessed May 3, 2016. http://www.fda.gov/cber/vaccine/thimerosal.htm#intro.

334. Bertrand, J., et al. 2001. "Prevalence of Autism in a United States Population: The Brick Township, New Jersey, Investigation." *Pediatrics* 108 (5): 1155–61. Accessed May 10, 2016. http://www.ncbi.nlm.nih.gov/pubmed/11694696.

335. Baillie-Hamilton, Paula. 2005. *Toxic Overload: A Doctor's Plan for Combating the Illnesses Caused by Chemicals in Our Foods, Our Homes, and Our Medicine Cabinets.* New York City, NY: Avery.

336. Immunization Safety Review Committee, Institute of Medicine. 2004. "Immunization Safety Review: Vaccines and Autism." National Academies Press, Accessed April 5, 2017.

337. Layton, Lyndsey. 2008. "FDA Draft Report Urges Consumption of Fish, Despite Mercury Contamination." *Washington Post*, December 12. Accessed May 3, 2016. http://www.washingtonpost.com/wp-dyn/content/article/2008/12/11 /AR2008121103394.html.

338. FDA and EPA. 2014. "Fish: What Pregnant Women and Parents Should Know." Draft Updated Advice by FDA and EPA. https://www.epa.gov/sites/production /files/2017-01/documents/draft-fish-advice-june-2014.pdf.

339. Barber, Richard T., and Patrick J. Whaling, et al. 1984. "Mercury in Recent and Century-Old Deep-Sea Fish." *Environmental Science & Technology* 18 (7): 552–5.

340. Mosbergen, Dominique. 2012. "Mercury in Fish More Dangerous Than Believed; Scientists Urge for Effective Treaty Ahead of UN Talks." (Report) *Huffington Post*: Healthy Living .http://www.huffingtonpost.com/2012/12/04 /mercury-in-fish-study-more-dangerous-treaty-un-talks_n_2238923.html.

341. Ibid.

342. First, Devra. 2008. "Catch of The Day?" *The Boston Globe*. July 2. Accessed May 3, 2016. http://archive.boston.com/lifestyle/food/articles/2008/07/02 /catch_of_the_day/.

343. Lohan, Tara. 2009. "How Farm-Raised Salmon Are Turning Our Oceans into Dangerous and Polluted Feedlots." Organic Consumers Association (OCA), September 2.

344. Jans, Nick. 2002. "Farmed Salmon Can't Beat Wild." *USA Today*, October 6. Accessed May 11, 2016.

345. UNEP Chemicals. 1999. *Guidelines for the Identification of PCBs and Materials Containing PCBs*. United Nations Environment Programme, p. 2.

346. "PCBs in Farm-Raised Salmon." *Environmental Working Group*. July 31, 2003. http://www.ewg.org/research/pcbs-farmed-salmon.

347. Knuth, Barbara A. "Health Risks and Health Benefits Associated with Eating Farmed and Wild Salmon." VIVO: Research & Expertise Across Cornell. Accessed May 3, 2016. http://vivo.cornell.edu/display/individual20834.

348. The Environmental Working Group. 2003. "PCBs in Farmed Salmon." EWG.org. Accessed May 3, 2016. http://www.ewg.org/reports/farmedpcbs.

349. Foran, J. A., and D. O. Carpenter. 2005. "Risk-Based Consumption Advice for Farmed Atlantic and Wild Pacific Salmon Contaminated with Dioxins and Dioxin-Like Compounds." *Environmental Health Perspectives* 113 (5): 552–6.

350. The Scotsman. 2003. "Food Colouring Causes Eye Problem." *The Scotsman*. Accessed May 3, 2016. http://www.scotsman.com/news/health /food_colouring_causes_eye_problem_1_638260.

351. Research News. 2011. "A Fish Test to Make Food Safer." Fraunhofer Press. Accessed May 11, 2016.

352. Foran, J. A., and D. O. Carpenter. 2005. "Risk-Based Consumption Advice for Farmed Atlantic and Wild Pacific Salmon Contaminated with Dioxins and Dioxin-Like Compounds." *Environmental Health Perspectives*113 (5): 552–6.

353. Roth, Myron. 2000. "The Availability and Use of Chemotherapeutic Sea Lice Control Products." *Contributions to Zoology* 69 (1/2).

354. Agency for Toxic Substances and Disease Registry (ATSDR). 1997. "Toxicological Profile for Dichlorvos." Public Health Service, U.S. Department of Health and Human Services, Atlanta, GA.

355. Organic Consumers Association. "Alaska Passes Law Requiring Mandatory Labeling of Genetically Engineered Fish." Accessed May 3, 2016. http://www.organicconsumers.org/ge/alaskabill051105.cfm.

356. Chatham Journal. 2006. "Consumer Reports Reveals That Farm-Raised Salmon Is Often Sold as 'Wild.'" Accessed May 3, 2016. http://www.chathamjournal.com/ weekly/living/food/cr-salmon-wild-60705.shtml.

357. Fish Watch U.S. Seafood Facts. Home page. NOAA's National Marine Fisheries Service. Accessed May 3, 2016. http://www.nmfs.noaa.gov/fishwatch/species /atl_salmon.htm.

358. Burros, Marian. 2005. "Salmon Gone Wild, or Is It Just Sold That Way?" *New York Times*. April 10. Accessed May 9, 2016.

359. *Consumer Reports* magazine. "Mystery Fish." December 2011. Accessed May 10, 2016. http://www.consumerreports.org/cro/magazine-archive/2011/december /food/fake-fish/overview/index.htm.

360. Ibid.

361. Warner, Kimberly, Patrick Mustain, Chris Carolin, et al. 2015."Oceana Reveals Mislabeling of America's Favorite Fish." http://usa.oceana.org/publications /reports/oceana-reveals-mislabeling-americas-favorite-fish-salmon#.

362. Council for Responsible Nutrition. 2010. "CRN Says There Are No Safety Issues with Fish Oil." Press Release. Accessed May 10, 2016. http://www.crnusa.org /CRNPR10CRNNoSafetyIssueswFishOil030210.html.

363. Kanner, J. 2007. "Dietary Advanced Lipid Oxidation Endproducts Are Risk Factors to Human Health." *Journal of Molecular and Nutrion Food Research* 51 (9): 1094–101.

364. Patton, Dominique. 2005. "Oxidised Fish Oils on Market May Harm Consumer, Warns Researcher." NutraIngredients.com. October 20. Accessed May 3, 2016. http://www.nutraingredients.com/Research/Oxidised-fish-oils-on-market-may-harm-consumer-warns-researcher.

365. Sears, Barry, interview with author. "Toxic Fat." *To Your Good Health Radio.*January 17, 2013 http://radiomd.com/show/to-your-good-health-radio /item/9486-toxic-fat.

366. Weil, Andrew. 2007. "Considering Krill Oil?" WEIL, July 3. Accessed May 3, 2016. http://www.drweil.com/drw/u/QAA400239/Consider-Krill-Oil.html.

367. Dharmananda, Subhuti. "Sea Buckthorn." Institute for Traditional Medicine, Portland, OR. Accessed May 3, 2016. http://www.itmonline.org/arts /seabuckthorn.htm.

368. Wood-Gush, D. G. M., and K. Vestergaard. 1991. "The Seeking of Novelty and Its Relation to Play." *Animal Behaviour* 42 (4): 599–606.

369. Hafez, E.S.E. (ed). 1975. *The Behaviour of Domestic Animals, 3rd Edition.* London, U.K.: Baillière Tindall, pp. 295–329.

370. Duchene, L. 2006. "Are Pigs Smarter Than Dogs?" Penn State News, May 8. www. rps.psu.edu/probing/pigs.html.

371. Helft, M. "Pig video arcades critique life in the pen." *Wired*, June 6, 1997. Accessed May 10, 2016. http://www.wired.com/1997/06 /pig-video-arcades-critique-life-in-the-pen/.

372. Watson, L. *The Whole Hog: Exploring the Extraordinary Potential of Pigs* Washington, DC: Smithsonian Books, 2004, p. 183.

373. Held, S., and M. Mendl, et al. 2001."Behaviour of Domestic Pigs in a Visual Perspective Taking Task." *Behaviour* 138: 1337–54.

374. Fuoco, Michael A. 1998. "Oinking for Help: Pot-Bellied Pig Saves Owner's Life by Lying in Front of a Car." *Pittsburgh Post-Gazette*, October 10.

375. Stolba, A., and D. G. M. Wood-Gush. 1989. "The Behaviour of Pigs in a Semi-Natural Environment." *Animal Production* 48 (2): 419–25.

376. Wood-Gush, D. G. M., and A. Stolba. 1982. "Behaviour of Pigs and the Design of a New Housing System." *Applied Animal Ethology* 8 (6): 583–4.

377. Stolba, A., and D. G. M. Wood-Gush. 1989. "The Behaviour of Pigs in a Semi-Natural Environment." *Animal Production* 48 (2): 419–25.

378. Fat Secret. "Sodium in Ham." FatSecret.com. Accessed May 3, 2016. http://www.fatsecret.com/calories-nutrition/food/ham/sodium.

379. Frame, Andy. 2012. "Cured Meat Is In, But Is it Safe?" *Food Safety News.* September 6.

380. EDinformatics. "Curing (Food Preservation)." Accessed May 3, 2016. http://www.edinformatics.com/math_science/science_of_cooking/curing_foods.htm.

381. Jakszyn, P., and C.A. Gonzalez. 2006. "Nitrosamine and Related Food Intake and Gastric and Oesophageal Cancer Risk: A Systematic Review of the Epidemiological Evidence." *World Journal of Gastroenterology* 12 (27): 4296–303.

382. Nordenberg, Tamar. 1998. "Heading Off Migraine Pain." *FDA Consumer Magazine.* U.S. Food and Drug Administration. Accessed May 10, 2016. http://permanent.access.gpo.gov/lps1609/www.fda.gov/fdac/features/1998/398_pain.html

383. Lijinsky, W., and S. Epstein. 1970. "Nitrosamines as Environmental Carcinogens." *Nature* 225 (5227): 2112.

384. BBC News Health. 2007. "Too Much Bacon 'Bad For Lungs.'" *BBC News*, April 17. Accessed May 3, 2016. http://news.bbc.co.uk/2/hi/health/6560121.stm.

385. Pogoda, J. M. 2001. "Maternal Cured Meat Consumption During Pregnancy and Risk of Paediatric Brain Tumour in Offspring: Potentially Harmful Levels of Intake." *Public Health Nutrition* 4 (2): 183–9.

386. Palk, David C., and David V. Saborio, et al. 2001. "The Epidemiological Enigma of Gastric Cancer Rates in the U.S.: Was Grandmother's Sausage the Cause?" *International Journal of Epidemiology* 30 (1): 181–82.

387. Mackerness, C. W., and S. A. Leach, et al. 1989. "The Inhibition of Bacterially Mediated N-Nitrosation by Vitamin C: Relevance to the Inhibition of Endogenous N-Nitrosation in the Achlorhydric Stomach." *Carcinogenesis* 10 (2): 397–9.

388. European Food Safety Authority. "Flavourings." EFSA. Accessed May 3, 2016. http://www.efsa.europa.eu/en/topics/topic/flavourings.htm.

389. BBC News Health. 2010. "'Smoked' Flavour Food Concerns." BBC News, January 8. Accessed May 3, 2016. http://news.bbc.co.uk/2/hi/health/8448184.stm.

390. Russel, Rex. 2006. *What the Bible Says About Healthy Living.* Revell, pp 147–50. Ada, MI.

391. Scholtissek, Christoph. 1992. "Cultivating a Killer Virus," *Natural History*, January.

392. "How Much Sodium Is in Bacon and in Link Sausage?" *Healthy Eating*, February 2014. http://healthyeating.sfgate.com/much-sodium-bacon-sausage-4706.html

393. Morton, Emma. 2009. "Bacon Is 'Danger' for Kids." *The Sun*, January 30. Accessed May 3, 2016. http://www.thesun.co.uk/sol/homepage/news/2192562/Bacon-is-danger-for-kids.html

394. Moisse, Katie. 2012. "A Link Between Sausage and Cancer?" ABC News, January 13. Accessed May 3, 2016. http://abcnews.go.com/blogs/health/2012/01/13/a-link-between-sausage-and-cancer/.

395. Duel, Diana. 2012. "Daily Doses of Bacon or Sausage Found to Increase Risk of Pancreatic Cancer." *The Examiner*, January 14.

396. Nöthlings, Ute, and Lynne R. Wilkens, et al. 2005. "Meat and Fat Intake as Risk Factors for Pancreatic Cancer: The Multiethnic Cohort Study." *Journal of the National Cancer Institute* 97 (19): 1458–65.

397. Datz, Todd. 2010. "Processed Meats Come with Increased Risk of Heart Disease, Diabetes." *Harvard School of Public Health*, May 17.

398. Hume, Tim, and Jen Christensen. 2014. "WHO: Imminent global cancer 'disaster' reflects aging, lifestyle factors." *CNN* February 4. http://www.cnn.com /2014/02/04/health/who-world-cancer-report/.

399. World Cancer Research Fund / American Institute for Cancer Research. *Food, Nutrition, Physical Activity, and the Prevention of Cancer: a Global Perspective.* Washington DC: American Institute for Cancer Research. 2007.

400. Baer, Arica A., et al. 2013. "Pathogens of Interest to the Pork Industry: A Review of Research on Interventions to Assure Food Safety." *Comprehensive Reviews in Food Science and Food Safety*, March 11.

401. Lawley, Richard. 2013. "Trichinella." Food and Safety Watch. January 1 http://www.foodsafetywatch.org/factsheets/trichinella/.

402. Medical FAQ. "How Long Can Tapeworms Grow?: Answers." Accessed May 3, 2016. http://www.medicalfaq.net/how_long_can_tapeworms_grow_/ta-134779.

403. Flisser, A. 1988. "Neurocysticercosis in Mexico." *Parasitology Today* 4 (5): 131–7.

404. Hirschmann, Jan V. 2001. "What Killed Mozart?" *Archives of Internal Medicine* 161:1381–9.

405. Richards, M. S., et al. 1993. "Investigation of a Staphylococcal Food Poisoning Outbreak in a Centralized School Lunch Program." *Public Health Reports* 108 (6): 765–71.

406. Voss, A., and F. Loeffen, et al. 2005. "Methicillin-Resistant Staphylococcus aureus in Pig Farming." *Emerging Infectious Disease* 11:1965–6.

407. Smith, Tara. 2009. "UI Study finds MRSA in Midwestern Swine, Workers." University of Iowa news release, January 23.

408. Science Daily Science News. 2011. "U.S. Meat and Poultry Is Widely Contaminated with Drug-Resistant Staph Bacteria, Study Finds." ScienceDaily. com, April 15. Accessed May 11, 2016.

409. O'Brien, Ashley M., and Blake M. Hanson, et al. 2012. "MRSA in Conventional and Alternative Retail Pork Products." *PLoS ONE* 7 (1): e30092 DOI: 10.1371 /journal.pone.0030092.

410. Ibid.

411. Bingham, Amy. 2011. "FDA: Hand Sanitizers Do Not Prevent MRSA Infection." ABC News, April 21. Accessed May 3, 2016. www.abcnews.go.com/US /fda-hand-sanitizers-make-false-claims-prevent-mrsa/story?id=13430582.

412. de Neeling, A. J., and M. J. van den Broek, et al. 2007. "High Prevalence of Methicillin Resistant *Staphylococcus aureus* in Pigs." *Vet Microbiology* 122: 366–72.

413. Mertens, P. L. 1999. "An Epidemic of *Salmonella typhimurium* Associated with Traditional Salted, Smoked, and Dried Ham," *Nederlands Tijdschrift voor Geneeskunde*, May 15.

414. Public Health Agency of Canada. "Notifiable Diseases On-Line." Accessed May 3, 2016. http://dsol-smed.phac-aspc.gc.ca/dsol-smed/ndis/index-eng.php.

415. Hald, T., and H. C. Wegener. 1999. "Quantitative Assessment of the Sources of Human Salmonellosis Attributable to Pork." *Proc 3rd International Symposium on Epidemiology and Control of Salmonella in Pork*, pp. 200–05.

416. Davies, R. H., and C. Wray. 1996. "Studies of Contamination of Three Broiler Breeder Houses with Salmonella Enteritidis Before and After Cleansing and Disinfection." *Avian Diseases* 40: 626–33. Duffy, E. A., and K. E. Belk, et al. 2000. "United States Retail Pork Microbiological Baseline." Proceedings. *Pork Quality and Safety Summit, National Pork Producers Council*, pp. 305–9.

417. Bayleyegn, Molla, et al. 2010. "Salmonella enterica in Commercial Swine Feed and Subsequent Isolation of Phenotypically and Genotypically Related Strains from Fecal Samples," *Applied Environmental Microbiology* 76:7188–7193. Science Daily. December 7, 2010. www.sciencedaily.com.

418. "Yersinia enterocolitica (Yersiniosis) Linked to Pork" Centers for Disease Control and Prevention. October 2016. https://www.cdc.gov/yersinia/.

419. Ryan, Kenneth J., and C. George Ray, et al. (eds.). 2004. *Sherris Medical Microbiology* (4th ed.). New York City, NY; McGraw Hill Professional.

420. Benvenga, S., and L. Santarpia, et al. 2006. "Human Thyroid Autoantigens and Proteins of *Yersinia* and *Borrelia* Share Amino Acid Sequence Homology That Includes Binding Motifs to HLA-DR Molecules and T-Cell Receptor." *Thyroid* 16 (3): 225–36.

421. Hoskins, Carolyn. 1986. "Pork Linked to Liver Cirrhosis." *Canadian Science News*, January.

422. Nanji, A. A., and S. W. French. 1985. "Relationship Between Pork Consumption and Cirrhosis." *Lancet* 1 (8430): 681–3.

423. Murphy, Karen J., et al. 2012. "Effects of Eating Fresh Lean Pork on Cardiometabolic Health Parameters." *Journal of Nutrients* 4 (7), 711–723.

424. Hortin, Audra E., and Peter J Bechtel, et al. 1991. "Efficacy of Pork Loin as a Source of Zinc and Effect of Added Cysteine on Zinc Bioavailability." *Journal of Food Science* 56 (6): 1505–7.

425. "Global Spending on Medicines from 2010 to 2021 (in Billion U.S. Dollars)." Statista. https://www.statista.com/statistics/280572/medicine-spending-worldwide/.

426. "Personal Care Products Manufacturing Report." *Research and Markets*, January 2017. ID #1052419 http://www.researchandmarkets.com/research/kxkcn7/personal_care Personal Care Products Council. Quarterly Update: November 28, 2011.

427. Kaiser Health. 2012. "Survey: Americans Spend More for Health Care Than People in Other Countries." *Kaiser Health News*, March 5. Accessed May 9, 2016. http://khn.org/morning-breakout/health-care-marketplace-surveys/.

428. U.S. Department of Health and Human Services. 1988. *The Surgeon General's Report on Nutrition and Health.* https://www.cambridge.org/core/journals/world-s-poultry-science-journal/article/div-classtitlestrategies-to-control-span-classitalicsalmonellaspan-in-the-broiler-production-chaindiv/F89BFBDD1CAF7302AB62EC4EB1A309AC.

429. Melina, Vesanto, and Brenda Davis. 2003. *Becoming Vegetarian: The Essential Guide to a Healthy Vegetarian Diet.* Volume 10. Healthy Living Publications.

430. Krikorian, Robert, and Marcelle D. Shidler, et. al. 2010. "Blueberry Supplementation Improves Memory in Older Adults." *Journal of Agricultural and Food Chemistry* 58 (7): 3996–4000.

431. Youdim, Kuresh A., et. al. 2000. "Short-Term Dietary Supplementation of Blueberry Polyphenolics: Beneficial Effects on Aging Brain Performance and Peripheral Tissue Function." *Nutritional Neuroscience* 3:383–97.

432. Drugs.com. "Aricept Side Effects." Accessed May 3, 2016. http://www.drugs.com /sfx/aricept-side-effects.html.

433. APUA. "Science of Resistance: Antibiotics in Agriculture." Alliance for the Prudent Use of Antibiotics (APUA). Accessed May 10, 2016. http://emerald.tufts.edu /med/apua/about_issue/antibiotic_agri.shtml.

434. Null, Gary, Carolyn Dean, Martin Feldman, Debora Rasio, and Dorothy Smith. 2004. "Death by Medicine." http://www.webdc.com/pdfs/deathbymedicine.pdf.

435. Bai, Yang, et al. 2015. "Sulforaphane Protects Against Cardiovascular Disease via Nrf2 Activation." *Oxidative Medicine* and *Cellular Longevity* 407580. Published online October 25, 2015. doi: 10.1155/2015/407580.

436. Farm Land Mineral Depletion. *1992 Earth Summit Report*. Medical Missionary Press. http://www.mmpress.info/id58.htm.

437. Hammel-Dupont, C. and S. Bessman 1970. "The Stimulation of Hemoglobin Synthesis By Porphyrins." *Biochemical Medicine* 4:55-60.

438. Linus Pauling Institute Micronutrient Information Center. "Chlorophyll and Chlorophyllin." Oregon State University. Accessed May 3, 2016. http://lpi. oregonstate.edu/infocenter/phytochemicals/chlorophylls/.

439. Hughes, J. H., and A. L. Latner. 1936. "Chlorophyll and Hemoglobin Regeneration after Hemmorhage." *Journal of Physiology* (University of Liverpool) 86 (4): 388–95.

440. Axe, Josh. 2013. "Chlorophyll Benefits: The Plant Pigment that Heals and Detoxes Better Than All Others." https://draxe.com/chlorophyll-benefits/

441. Morales, Lymari. 2010. "In U.S., Consumption of Fruits and Vegetables Trails Access." Gallup.com, September 22. Accessed May 9, 2016.

442. Willett, Walter C. 1991. "Health Professionals Follow-up Study (HPFS): Prospective Studies of Diet and Cancer in Men and Women." *Harvard School of Public Health*.

443. Zu, Era Ke, et al. 2014. "Dietary Lycopene, Angiogenesis, and Prostate Cancer: A Prospective Study in the Prostate-Specific Antigen." *National Cancer Institute* 106 (2): djt430.

444. Webb, Densie. 2014. "Anthocyanins." *Today's Dietitian* 16 (3): 20.

445. Subash, Selvaraju, et al. 2014. "Neuroprotective Effects of Berry Fruits on Neurodegenerative Diseases." *Journal of Neural Regeneration Research* 9 (16): 1557–66.

446. North Carolina Research Campus. Home page. Accessed May 3, 2016. www.ncresearchcampus.net.

447. David Murdock's feature "Living to Be 125" aired on *The Oprah Winfrey Show* on March 24, 2009. http://www.oprah.com/own-health/ david-murdocks-diet-and-fitness-routine-video.

448. Murdock, David H. 2009. "A Recipe for Longevity: 33 of the Healthiest Foods on Earth." *Huffington Post: Healthy Living*, June 20. Accessed May 3, 2016. www.huffingtonpost.com/david-h-murdock/a-recipe-for-longevity_b_205355.html.

449. Diamond, Harvey, interview with author. "Fit for Life with Harvey Diamond." *RadioMD*. Aired April 18, 2013. http://radiomd.com/show /to-your-good-health-radio/item/11271-fit-for-life-with-harvey-diamond.

450. "China-Cornell-Oxford Project," Cornell University. "Geographic Study of Mortality, Biochemistry, Diet and Lifestyle in Rural China," Clinical Trial Service Unit & Epidemiological Studies Unit, University of Oxford. 1989.

451. Campbell, T. Colin, interview with author. "Forks Over Knives." April 2, 2012. http://toyourgoodhealthradio.com/forks-over-knives/.

452. Ibid.

453. Dr. Oz. "Diet Changes to Lower Disease Risk, Pt 1." Video April 27, 2011. Accessed May 3, 2016. http://www.doctoroz.com/videos/diet-changes-lower-disease-risk-pt-1.

454. Esselstyn, C. B. 2001. "Resolving the Coronary Artery Disease Epidemic through Plant-Based Nutrition." *Preventive Cardiology* 4:171–177.

455. Luks, Joel. 2011. "Needless Heart Surgery? Houston Doctor Argues That a Plant-Based Diet Works Better Than a Bypass." *Vegging Out*, July 8.

456. O'Connor, Anahad. 2011. "Bill Clinton's Vegan Journey." *New York Times*, August 18. Accessed May 11, 2016. http://well.blogs.nytimes.com/tag /the-china-study/?_r=0.

457. Esselstyn Jr., Caldwell B. 2013. "Abolishing Heart Disease." T. Colin Campbell Center for Nutrition Studies, October 15. Accessed May 3, 2016. http://nutritionstudies.org/abolishing-heart-disease/.

458. Freston, Kathy. 2012. "Why Do Vegetarians Live Longer?" *Huffington Post*, October 28. Accessed May 11, 2016. http://www.huffingtonpost.com/kathy-freston /plant-based-diet_b_1981838.html.

459. Bortz, Walter. 1992. *We Live Too Short and Die Too Long: How to Achieve and Enjoy Your Natural 100-Year-Plus Life Span*. Bantam. New York.

460. LIFE Magazine. "161 Years Old and Growing Strong." *LIFE*, September 16, 1966: 121–27.

461. Leaf, Alexander. 1973. "Every Day Is a Gift When You Are Over 100." *National Geographic* 143 (1): 93–119.

462. Schinava, G. N., and N. N. Sachuk, et al. 1964. "On the Physical Condition of the Aged People of the Abkhasian ASSR." *Soviet Medicine* 5.

463. Robbins, John. 2006. *Healthy at 100: The Scientifically Proven Secrets of the World's Healthiest and Longest-Lived Peoples*. New York City, NY: Ballantine Books, 20.

464. Yuan, G. F., et al. 2009. "Effects of Different Cooking Methods on Health-Promoting Compounds of Broccoli." *Journal of Zheijang University SCIENCE B* 10 (8): 580–8.

465. Zeng, Chuli. 2013. "Effects of Different Cooking Methods on the Vitamin C Content of Selected Vegetables." *Nutrition & Food Science* 43 (5): 438–43.

466. Ibid.

467. Dewanto, Veronica, and Xianzhong Wu, et al. 2002. "Thermal Processing Enhances the Nutritional Value of Tomatoes by Increasing Total Antioxidant Activity." *Journal of Agriculture and Food Chemistry* 50 (10): 3010–4.

468. McDougall, John, interview with author. 2012. "Forks Over Knives" April 2. http://toyourgoodhealthradio.com/forks-over-knives/.

469. Marchione, Marilynn. 2009. "Ancient Mummies Show Signs of Heart Disease." *Associated Press*, November 18. http://www.ctvnews.ca/ancient-mummies-show-signs-of-heart-disease-1.455722.

470. Santos-Longhurst, Adrienne. 2017. "Type 2 Diabetes Statistics and Facts." *HealthLine*, February 27. http://www.healthline.com/health/type-2-diabetes/statistics.

471. Grady, Denise. "No Longer Just 'Adult-Onset.'" *New York Times*, May 7, 2012, p. A22. http://www.nytimes.com/2012/05/07/opinion/no-longer-just-adult-onset.html.

472. Barnard, Neal D., et al. 2005. "The Effect of a Low-Fat, Plant-Based Dietary Intervention on Body Weight, Metabolism, and Insulin Sensitivity." *American Journal of Medicine* 118: 991–97.

473. "Vegetarian Diet Improves Insulin Resistance and Oxidative Stress Markers More Than Conventional Diet in Subjects with Type 2 Diabetes." *Diabetic Medicine* 28: 549–559 (2011).

474. Barnard, Neal. 2008. *Dr. Neal Barnard's Program for Reversing Diabetes: The Scientifically Proven System for Reversing Diabetes without Drugs*. Rodale Books. New York.

475. Thomas, D. 2003. "A Study on the Mineral Depletion of the Foods Aailable to Us as a Nation Over the Period 1940 to 1991." *Journal of Nutrition and Health* 17 (2): 85–115.

476. Lindlahr, 1914; USDA: 1963 and 1997. "Average Mineral Content in Select Vegetables." p. 9. http://www.nutritionsecurity.org/PDF/Mineral%20Content%20in%20Vegetables.pdf.

477. LifeExtension. 2001."Vegetables Without Vitamins." *LE Magazine*. Accessed May 3, 2016. http://www.lifeextension.com/Magazine/2001/3/report_vegetables/Page-01.

478. Glass, Anthony. 2003. "Nitrogen Use Efficiency of Crop Plants: Physiological Constraints upon Nitrogen Absorption." *Critical Reviews in Plant Sciences* 22 (5): 453.

479. Ward, Mary. 2009. "Too Much of a Good Thing? Nitrate from Nitrogen Fertilizers and Cancer." *Reviews on Environmental Health* 24 (4): 357–63.

480. Ecological Society of America. 1997. "Human Alteration of the Global Nitrogen Cycle: Causes and Consequences." *Issues in Ecology*, Ecological Society of America.

481. The National Academies of Science, Engineering, and Medicine. Home page. Accessed May 3, 2016. Www.nationalacademies.org.

482. Braun, Heder, et al. 2016. "Soil Science and Plant Nutrition: Carbohydrates Concentration in Leaves of Potato Plants Affected by Nitrogen Fertilization Rates." *The Journal Revista Ceres* 63 (2): 241–248.

483. "Ammonium Nitrate (Alias of Varioform I): CAS RN:6484-52-2." U.S. National Library of Medicine. https://www.nlm.nih.gov/.

484. EPA Chemical Safety Alert. EPA/ATF/OSHA Chemical Advisory: Safe Storage, Handling, and Management of Ammonium Nitrate (Aug. 2013). https://www.osha.gov/chemicalexecutiveorder/an_guidelines_IAFC-IME-NSSGA-ISEE.pdf.

485. University of California. "Organic Production." Vegetable Research & Information Center. Accessed May 3, 2016. http://vric.ucdavis.edu/veg_info_topic/organic_production.htm.

486. Mercola, Joseph. 2014. "Glyphosate May Be Worse Than DDT, Which Has Now Been Linked to Alzheimer's Disease, Decades after Exposure." Dr. Mercola, February 13. http://articles.mercola.com/sites/articles/archive/2014/02/13/glyphosate-ddt-alzheimers.aspx.

487. Mercola, Joseph. 2016. "Worse Than DDT: When You Eat This, It Ends Up Lingering in Your Gut." Dr. Mercola, January 15. Accessed May 3, 2016. http://articles.mercola.com/sites/articles/archive/2012/01/15/dr-don-huber-interview-part-2.aspx.

488. Goldstein, D. A., and J. F. Acquavella, et al. 2002. "An Analysis of Glyphosate Data from the California Environmental Protection Agency Pesticide Illness Surveillance Program." *Journal of Toxicology. Clinical Toxicology* 40 (7): 885–92.

489. U.S. EPA Communications and Public Affairs 1991 Press Advisory. "EPA Lists Crops Associated with Pesticides for Which Residue and Environmental Fate Studies Were Allegedly Manipulated." San Francisco Estuary, Invasive Spartina Project, Spartina Control Program. Volume 2 March 29.

490. U.S. Environmental Protection Agency. 1983. *Summary of the IBT Review Program: Office of Pesticide Programs.* Washington D.C.; Office of Pesticides and Toxic Substances.

491. Schneider, K. 1983. "Faking It: The Case Against Industrial Bio-Test Laboratories." *The Amicus Journal* Spring: 14–26.

492. U.S. Dept. of Justice. United States Attorney. Western District of Texas 1992. "Texas Laboratory, Its President, 3 Employees Indicted on 20 Felony Counts in Connection with Pesticide Testing." Austin, TX, September 29, 1992.

493. Environmental Protection Agency R.E.D. FACTS "Glyphosate." September 1993. https://archive.epa.gov/pesticides/reregistration/web/pdf/0178fact.pdf.

494. Ji, Sayer. 2011. "Are You Eating, Drinking and Breathing Monsanto's New Agent Orange?" Salem-News.com, December 16. Accessed May 10, 2016.

495. American Academy of Environmental Medicine. "Genetically Modified Foods." July 2013. Accessed May 10, 2016. https://www.aaemonline.org/gmo.php.

496. "About Genetically Engineered Foods." *Center for Food Safety.* 2013. http://www.centerforfoodsafety.org/issues/311/ge-foods/about-ge-foods#.

497. Wechsler, Seth J. 2016. "Recent Trends in GE Adoption" *USDA*, November 3. https://www.ers.usda.gov/data-products/adoption-of-genetically-engineered-crops-in-the-us/recent-trends-in-ge-adoption.aspx.

498. Smith, Jeffrey M. 2013. "Genetically Engineered Foods May Be Far More Harmful Than We Thought." *Western Price Foundation.* October 23. https://www.westonaprice.org/health-topics/modern-foods/genetically-engineered-foods-may-be-far-more-harmful-than-we-thought/.

499. Smith, Jeffrey M. "Lyme/Autism Group Blasts Genetically Modified Foods as Dangerous." Institute for Responsible Technology. Accessed May 3, 2016. http://responsibletechnology.org/lymeautism-group-blasts-genetically-modified-foods-as-dangerous/.

500. "How Far Does Your Food Travel to Get to Your Plate?" Center for Urban Education about Sustainable Agriculture. 2014. http://www.cuesa.org/learn/how-far-does-your-food-travel-get-your-plate

501. Hamburg, Margaret A. 2013. "Food Safety Modernization Act: Putting the Focus on Prevention." Food Safety.gov. https://www.foodsafety.gov/news/fsma.html

502. Charles, Dan. 2014. "Are Organic Vegetables More Nutritious?" *National Public Radio News*, July 11. http://www.npr.org/sections/thesalt/2014/07/11/330760923/are-organic-vegetables-more-nutritious-after-all.

503. Foucard, T., and Malmheden Yman I. 1999. "A Study on Severe Food Reactions in Sweden: Is Soy Protein an Underestimated Cause of Food Anaphylaxis?" *Allergy* 54 (3): 261–65.

504. Bilello, Stanley. 2016. *21ˢᵗ Century Homestead: Nitrogen-Fixing Crops.* p 119. Lulu Press, Inc. Morrisville, NC.

505. Henry Ford Organization. https://www.thehenryford.org/collections-and-research/digital-resources/popular-topics/soy-bean-car/.

506. "What's So Bad about Tofu?" Dr. Mercola interview with Dr. Kaayla T. Daniel, author of *The Whole Soy Story: The Dark Side of America's Favorite Health Food* (New Trends, March 2005). September 16, 2008. http://articles.mercola.com/sites/articles/archive/2008/09/16/what-s-so-bad-about-tofu.aspx.

507. Setchell, K. D., et al. "Isoflavone Content of Infant Formulas and the Metabolic Fate of These Early Phytoestrogens in Early Life." *American Journal of Clinical Nutrition*, December 1998 Supplement, 1453S–1461S.

508. Ross, R. K., et al. 1983. "Effect of In-Utero Exposure to Diethylstilbestrol on Age at Onset of Puberty and on Post-Pubertal Hormone Levels in Boys." *Canadian Medical Association Journal* 128 (10): 1197–8.

509. Setchel, K. D., and L. Zimmer-Nechemias, et al. 1997. "Exposure in Infants to Phyto-Oestrogens From Soy-Based Infant Formula." *Lancet* 350 (9070): 23–27.

510. Fallon, Sally, and Mary G. Enig. 2000. "Tragedy and Hype: The Third International Soy Symposium—Part II." The Weston A. Price Foundation, March 26. Accessed May 10, 2016. http://www.tldp.com/issue/11_00/soy.htm.

511. Shomon, Mary J. 2005. *Living Well With Hypothyroidism* (2nd ed.). New York City, NY; HarperCollins/HarperResource.

512. Divi, R. L., and H. C. Chang, et al. 1997. "Anti-Thyroid Isoflavones from Soybean: Isolation, Characterization, and Mechanisms of Action." *Biochem Pharmacol* 54 (10): 1087–96.

513. Steven Reinberg. 2008. "Soy Linked to Low Sperm Count." *Washington Post.* July 24. http://www.washingtonpost.com/wp-dyn/content/article/2008/07/23/AR2008072303151.html.

514. Sutardi and K. A. Buckle. 2006. "Reduction in Phytic Acid Levels in Soybeans During Tempeh Production, Storage and Frying." *Journal of Food Science* 50 (1): 260–63.

515. Van Rensburg, S.J., et al. 1983. "Nutritional Status of African Populations Predisposed to Esophageal Cancer." *Nutrition and Cancer* 4: 206–16. Moser, P. B. et al. 1988. "Copper, Iron, Zinc and Selenium Dietary Intake and Status Of Nepalese Lactating Women and Their Breastfed Infants." *American Journal of Clinical Nutrition* 47: 729–734. Harland, B. F. et al. 1988. "Nutritional Status and Phytate: Zinc And Phytate X Calcium: Zinc Dietary Molar Ratios of Lacto-Ovovegetarian Trappist Monks: 10 Years Later." *Journal of the American Dietetic Association* 88:1562–66.

516. Prasad, A. S. 1983. "Zinc Deficiency in Human Subjects." *Progress in Clinical and Biological Research* 129:1–33.

517. Prasad, A. S. 1991. "Discovery of Human Zinc Deficiency and Studies in an Experimental Human Model." *American Journal of Clinical Nutrition* 53 (2): 403–12.

518. Rackis, J. J., and M. R. Gumbmann. 1981. "Protease Inhibitors: Physiological Properties and Nutritional Significance." *Antinutrients and Natural Toxicants in Foods*. Westport, CT, USA: Food and Nutrition Press. http://naldc.nal.usda.gov /naldc/download.xhtml?id=26115&content=PDF.

519. Heathcock, J. N. 1991. "Residue Trypsin Inhibitor: Data Needs for Risk Assessment." *Advances in Experimental Medicine and Biology* 289:273–79.

520. Somoza, Veronika, and Elisabeth Wenzel, et al. 2006. "Dose-Dependent Utilisation of Casein-Linked Lysinoalanine, N(Epsilon)-Fructoselysine and N(Epsilon)-Carboxymethyllysine in Rats." *Molecular Nutrition & Food Research* 50 (9): 833–41.

521. Scanlan, Richard A. 2000. "Nitrosamines and Cancer." *The Linus Pauling Institute*. http://margotbworldnews.com/News/Apr/Apr22/nitrosamines.html Accessed May 10, 2016.

522. Jakszyn, P., and C. A. Gonzalez. 2006. "Nitrosamine and Related Food Intake and Gastric and Oesophageal Cancer Risk: A Systematic Review of the Epidemiological Evidence." *World Journal of Gastroenterology* 12 (27): 4296–303.

523. Doerge, D. R., and D. M. Sheehan. 2002. "Goitrogenic and Estrogenic Activity of Soy Isoflavones." *Environmental Health Perspectives* 110(Suppl 3): 349–53. http:// www.ncbi.nlm.nih.gov/pmc/articles/PMC1241182/.

524. Fallon, Sally, and Mary G. Enig. 2000. "Soy Products: Tragedy and Hype." *Nexus Magazine* 7 (3).

525. Health News. 2008. "Eating Soy Linked to Memory Loss." United Press International, July 5. Accessed May 10, 2016.

526. White, L. R., et al. 2000. "Brain Aging and Midlife Tofu Consumption." *Journal American College of Nutrition* 19:242.

527. Goddard, et al. 2003. "Soy-Induced Brain Atrophy?" *Journal of Anti Aging Medicine* 6 (4): 335–6.

528. Hartley, et al. 2003. "Soya Phytoestrogens Change Cortical and Hippocampal Expression of BDNF Mrna in Male Rats." *Neuroscience Letters* 338 (2): 135–8.

529. FDA Poisonous Plant Database CFSAN/Office of Plant and Dairy Foods. United States Food and Drug Administration. February 2004; March 2006 Update. https://www.accessdata.fda.gov/scripts/plantox/.

530. Sheehan, Daniel M., and Daniel R. Doerge. Letter to FDA regarding Docket # 98P-0683.

531. Ocean Health. "Chemistry of Seawater: Ocean Salt Composition and Concentration Is in 'Steady State.'" Accessed April 15, 2017. oceanplasma.org/documents/chemistry. html#Steady_State.

532. Dagnelie, Pieter C. 1997. "Comments on the Paper by Rauma et al. (1995)." *Journal of Nutrition* 127 (2): 379.

533. Rauma, Anna-Liisa, and Riitta Törrönen, et al. 1995. "Vitamin B-12 Status of Long-Term Adherents of a Strict Uncooked Vegan Diet ('Living Food Diet') Is Compromised." *Journal of Nutrition* 125 (10): 2511.

534. Richter, Brian. 2012. "Walking Water: H20 and the Human Body." The Nature Conservancy and University of Virginia. *National Geographic*. March 6, 2012.

535. PubMed. "Apoptosis Fucoidan Search Result." Accessed May 3, 2016. www.ncbi. nlm.nih.gov/pubmed?term=apoptosis%20fucoidan.

536. Paul, T. M., and S. C. Skoryna, et al. 1966. "Studies on Inhibition of Intestinal Absorption of Radioactive Strontium." *Canadian Medical Association Journal* 95 (19): 957–60.

537. Skoryna, S.C., et al., 1964. "Intestinal Absorption of Radioactive Strontium." *Canadian Medical Association Journal* 191.

538. Tanaka,Y. et al. 1968. "Studies on Inhibition of Intestinal Absorption of Radioactive Strontium." *Canadian Medical Association Journal* July 27; 99(4): 169–75.

539. Drum, Ryan. "Botanicals for Thyroid Function and Dysfunction." Medicines From the Earth: Official Proceedings, 3–5, June 2000.

540. *Physicians' Desk Reference 1996* (50th ed. Issn 0093-4461) Hardcover–Page 1542. Published by Medical Economics. North Olmsted, OH.

541. Integrated Biomolecule. "Welcome to IBC." Accessed May 3, 2016. www.integratedbiomolecule.com.

542. Yochum, Terry R., and Lindsay J. Rowe. 2004. *Essentials of Skeletal Radiology* (2 Vol. Set). 3rd edition. Philadelphia, PA: LWW.

543. MLA style: "Physiology or Medicine for 1999—Press Release." *Nobelprize.org*. Nobel Media AB 2014. Web. 15 April 2017. <http://www.nobelprize.org/nobel_ prizes/medicine/laureates/1999/press.html>.

544. LeBoeuf-Little, Nicole. "Vitamin Isolates & Liver Problems." January 18, 2011 |. www.livestrong.com.

545. Lee, Royal. "How and Why Synthetic Poisons Are Being Sold as Imitations of Natural Foods and Drugs." Lee Foundation for Nutritional Research. August 7, 2013. https://price-pottenger.org/diet-nutrition-research/how-and-why-synthetic-poisons-are-being-sold-imitations-natural-foods-and.

546. Thiel, Robert. "The Truth about Vitamins in Nutritional Supplements." Doctors' Research. Accessed May 3, 2016. http://www.doctorsresearch.com/articles4.html.

547. "The Truth About Nutritional Supplements." Hipprocraties Institute. https://www. organicconsumers.org/news/nutri-con-truth-about-vitamins-supplements.

548. FDA. "Dietary Supplements." FDA.gov. Accessed May 3, 2016. http://www.fda.gov /food/dietarysupplements/default.htm.

549. Dateline: "The Hansen Files": Supplements, Part 2, Season 2012: Episode 0319. March 19, 2012.

550. Ibid.

551. Brody, Jane E. 1998. "Taking Too Much Vitamin C Can Be Dangerous." *New York Times*, April 9. Accessed May 10, 2016.

552. Olabisi, Avodele O. 2005. "The Chemistry of L-Ascorbic Acid Derivatives in the Asymmetric Synthesis of C2- and C3- Substituted Aldono-γ-lactones." *Wichita State University*, August.

553. Davies, M. B. 1991. "Vitamin C: Its Chemistry & Biochemistry." *CRC Press*; 1st edition, September 13.

554. Dykes, M. H., and P. Meier. 1975. "Ascorbic Acid and the Common Cold. Evaluation of Its Efficacy and Toxicity." *JAMA* 231:1073–9.

555. Taft, G., and P. Fieldhouse. 1978. "Vitamin C and the Common Cold." *Public Health* 92:19–25.

556. Truswell, A. S. 1986. "Ascorbic Acid (Letter)." *New England Journal of Medicine* 315:709. Walker, G. H., et al. 1967. "Trial of Ascorbic Acid in Prevention of Colds." *British Medical Journal* 1:603–06.

557. Pauling, L. 1982. "Speech at Natural Foods Exposition, March 29, 1982." *Natural Foods Merchandiser* June: 65.

558. Schwartz, A. R., and R.B. Hornick, et al. 1973. "Evaluation of the Efficacy of Ascorbic Acid in Prophylaxis of Induced Rhinovirus 44 Infection in Man." *Journal of Infectious Diseases* 128: 500–05.

559. Ibid.

560. Facts and Statistics. *International Osteoporsosis Foundation*. 2012. https://www.iofbonehealth.org/facts-statistics.

561. Theil, R. J. 2003. "The Truth about Vitamin Supplements." *ANMA Monitor* 6 (2): 6–14.

562. Ross, Edward A., and Nancy J. Szabo, et al. 2000. "Lead Content of Calcium Supplements." *JAMA* 284 (11): 1425–29.

563. Schorr, Melissa. 2000. "Lead Found in Calcium Supplements." *ABC News*, September 19. Accessed May 10, 2016. http://abcnews.go.com/Health/story?id=117953

564. Adluri, R. S., and L. Zhan, et al. 2010. "Comparative Effects of a Novel Plant-Based Calcium Supplement with Two Common Calcium Salts on Proliferation and Mineralization in Human Osteoblast Cells." *Molecular and Cellular Biochemistry* 340 (1-2): 73–80. Epub March 7, 2010.

565. Kaats, G. R., and H. G. Preuss, et al. 2011. "A Comparative Effectiveness Study of Bone Density Changes in Women Over 40 Following Three Bone Health Plans Containing Variations of the Same Novel Plant-sourced Calcium." *International Journal of Medicine and Science* 8 (3): 180–91.

566. Mayo Clinic Proceedings: Vitamin D Deficiency, December 9, 2003. The Vitamin D Council Press Release. http://www.cholecalciferol-council.com.

567. Tovey, A., and Cannell, J. J. 2016. "Are We Currently Amid a Vitamin D Deficiency Pandemic?" *The Vitamin D Council Blog & Newsletter*. https://www.vitamindcouncil.org/are-we-currently-amid-a-vitamin-d-deficiency-pandemic/.

568. NIH Office of Dietary Supplements. "Vitamin D: Fact Sheet for Consumers." Accessed May 13, 2016. https://ods.od.nih.gov/factsheets/VitaminD-Consumer/.

569. Thiel, R. 2003. "Vitamin D, Rickets, and Mainstream Experts." *International Journal of Naturopathy* 2 (1).

570. Holick, M. F. 1999. *Modern Nutrition in Health and Disease* (9th ed.). Baltimore, MD: Wolters Kluwer Health, pp. 329–45.

571. Zittermann, A., and J. F. Gummert, et al. 2009. "Vitamin D Deficiency and Mortality." *Current Opinion in Clinical Nutrition and Metabolic Care* 12 (6): 634–9.

572. Palacios, Cristina. 2014. "Is Vitamin D Deficiency a Major Global Public Health Problem?" *Journal of Steroid Biochemistry* and *Molecular Biology* 144PA: 138–45.

573. Holick, Michael F. 2004. "Sunlight and Vitamin D For Bone Health and Prevention of Autoimmune Diseases, Cancers, and Cardiovascular Disease." *American Journal of Clinical Nutrition* December 80 (6): 1678S–1688S.

574. Edwards, Kim. 2007. "Study Shines More Light on Benefit of Vitamin D in Fighting Cancer: 600,000 Cases a Year of Breast and Colorectal Cancer Could Be Prevented Each Year by Adequate Intake of Vitamin D, According to Researcher." UC San Diego, August 21. Accessed May 10, 2016. http://ucsdnews.ucsd.edu/archive/newsrel/health/08-07VitaminDKE-.asp.

575. Ibid.

576. Westerdahl, J., and C. Ingvar, et al. 2000. "Sunscreen Use and Malignant Melanoma." *International Journal of Cancer* 87 (1): 145–50.

577. Weinstock, M. A. 1999. "Do Sunscreens Increase or Decrease Melanoma Risk: An Epidemiologic Evaluation." *Journal of Investigative Dermatology Symposium Proceedings* 4 (1): 97–100.

578. Vainio, H., and F. Bianchini. 2000. "Cancer-Preventive Effects of Sunscreens Are Uncertain." *Scandinavian Journal of Work Environment and Health* 26: 529–31.

579. "Sunscreens Exposed: Nine Surprising Truths." EWG's Skin Deep. August 1, 2012. Accessed May 10, 2016. http://beforeitsnews.com/health/2012/08/sunscreens-exposed-nine-surprising-truths-2444536.html.

580. Hope, Jenny. 2014. "Skin Cancer Rates Rising Fastest in Older Men: Cases of Melanoma Have Risen 12% Each Year In Males Over 60." DailyMail.com, August 29. Accessed May 10, 2016. http://www.dailymail.co.uk/health/article-2738152/Skin-cancer-rates-rising-fastest-older-men-Cases-melanoma-risen-12-year-males-60.html.

581. Newton-Bishop, Julia A., and Yu-Mei Chang, et al. 2011. "Relationship Between Sun Exposure and Melanoma Risk for Tumours in Different Body Sites in a Large Case-Control Study in a Temperate Climate." *European Journal of Cancer* 47 (5): 732–41.

582. "Sunscreens Exposed: Nine Surprising Truths." EWG's Skin Deep. August 1, 2012. Accessed May 10, 2016. http://beforeitsnews.com/health/2012/08/sunscreens-exposed-nine-surprising-truths-2444536.html.

583. Mearini, L., and A. Zucchi, et al. 2013. "Low Serum Testosterone Levels Are Predictive of Prostate Cancer." *World Journal of Urology* 31 (2): 247–52.

584. Dellorto, Danielle. 2012. "Avoid Sunscreens with Potentially Harmful Ingredients, Group Warns." *CNN Health*, May 16. http://www.cnn.com /2012/05/16/health/sunscreen-report/.

585. "Is your sunscreen more dangerous than the sun?" *PRN Newswire*. August 2, 2007, http://www.prnewswire.com/news-releases/is-your-sunscreen-more-dangerous-than-the-sun-57784587.html.

586. Dellorto, Danielle. 2012. "Avoid Sunscreens with Potentially Harmful Ingredients, Group Warns." *CNN Health*, May 16. Accessed May 11, 2016.

587. Gray, Richard. 2010. "Weekend Sunshine 'Can Protect Against Skin Cancer.'" *The Telegraph*, December 5. Accessed May 11, 2016. http://www.telegraph.co.uk/ news/newstopics/howaboutthat/8181447/Weekend-sunshine-can-protect-against-skin-cancer.html.

588. Shils, M., et al. (eds). 1999. *Modern Nutrition in Health & Disease*, 9th ed. Baltimore, MD: Williams & Wilkins.

589. Traber, M. G., et al. 1998. "Synthetic as Compared with Natural Vitamin E Is Preferentially Excreted as A-CEHC in Human Urine: Studies Using Deuterated A-Tocopheryl Acetate." *FEBS Letters* 437: 145–8.

590. Acuff, R. V., and R. G. Dunworth, et al. 1998. "Transport of Deuterium-Labeled Tocopherols During Pregnancy." *American Journal of Clinical Nutrition* 67 (3): 459–64.

591. Grimes, Melanie. 2010. "Vitamin E Grows Hair." *Natural News*, January 29. Accessed May 11, 2016. http://www.naturalnews.com/028050_vitamin_E_hair.html.

592. Wittman, Leigh. 2011. "What Are the Health Benefits of Taking Vitamin E?" Livestrong.com, June 14. Accessed May 11, 2016.

593. Klein, Eric A., and Ian M. Thompson, et al. 2011. "Vitamin E and the Risk of Prostate Cancer: The Selenium and Vitamin E Cancer Prevention Trial." *JAMA* 306 (14): 1549–56. doi:10.1001/jama.2011.1437.

594. "Study Shows High-Dose Vitamin E Supplements May Increase Risk of Dying." Johns Hopkins Medicine. November 10, 2004. Accessed May 3, 2016. http://www.hopkinsmedicine.org/Press_releases/2004/11_10_04.html.

595. Ibid.

596. Sesso, H. D., and J. E. Buring, et al. 2008. "Vitamins E and C in the Prevention of Cardiovascular Disease in Men: The Physicians' Health Study II Randomized Controlled Trial." *JAMA: The Journal of the American Medical Association* 300 (18): 2123–33.

597. New York Daily News. 2012. "Osteoporosis Linked to Vitamin E Intake." NYDailyNews.com, March 5. Accessed May 11, 2016.

598. Gilbère, Gloria. 2007. "The Science Behind Wheatgrass Juice and Health." *The Environmental Illness Resource*, May 21. Accessed April 18, 2017. http://www.ei-resource.org/expert-columns/dr-gloria-gilberes-column /the-science-behind-wheatgrass-juice-and-health-dr-gloria-gilbere/.

599. Bircher-Benner, Maximillian. 1928. *Food Science for All: New Sunlight Theory of Nutrition*. Health Research Press. Champaign, IL.

600. Meyerowitz, S. 1999. *Wheat Grass: Nature's Finest Medicine*. Summertown, TN: Book Publishing Co.

601. Ben-Arye, E., and E. Goldin, et al. 2002. "Wheat Grass Juice in the Treatment of Active Distal Ulcerative Colitis: A Randomized Double-Blind Placebo-Controlled Trial." *Scandinavian Journal of Gastroenterology* 37 (4): 444–9.

602. Hotta, Y. "Stimulation of DNA Repair-synthesis by P4-D I." 1984 Lecture in Honolulu, Hawaii.

603. Kubota, K., et al. "Isolation of Potent Anti-Inflammatory Protein from Barley Leaves." Dept. of Pharmaceutical Sciences, Science University of Tokyo (Ichigaya-funagawara-machi, Shinjuku-ku), 162, Japan.

604. Hagiwara, Yoshihide. Tokyo, Japan: Association of Green and Health Distributors, 1981. "The Wheatgrass Book: How to Grow and Use Wheatgrass to Maximize Your Health and Vitality." New York: Avery.

605. "Home Remedies for Tooth Decay and Cavities." *The Healthy Archive.* July 2014. http://www.thehealthyarchive.info/2014/11/home-remedies-for-tooth-decay-and.html

606. Martin, Kristina. 2015. "FDA Cracks Down Walmart, GNC, Other Companies Selling Supplements That Do Not Contain the Herbs on the Label." Natural News. February 5. www.naturalnews.com/048514_supplement_scam_big_business_FDA.html

607. Altman, Lawrence K. 1984. "James Fixx: The Enigma of Heart Disease." *New York Times*, July 24. Accessed May 9, 2016. http://www.nytimes.com/1984/07/24/science/the-doctor-s-world-james-fixx-the-enigma-of-heart-disease.html?pagewanted=all

608. Robbins, John. 2011. "What Should We Learn from The Deaths of Fitness Icons?" *Huffington Post*, January 31. Accessed May 9, 2016. http://www.huffingtonpost.com/john-robbins/what-should-we-learn-from_b_815943.html.

609. Smith, David B. 2005. "Running Yourself to Death." *The Voice of Prophecy*, January 25. Accessed May 9, 2016. http://www.institutefornaturalhealing.com/2011/11/running-yourself-to-death/.

610. Shelton, Herbert M. 1999. "Hygienic System Vol. II – Orthotrophy." *Health Research Books*, February, p. 229. .

611. Innes, Emma. 2014. "People Who Live in the Northern Hemisphere Are Fatter 'Because of the Cold Climate.'" *Dailymail*, February. http://www.dailymail.co.uk/health/article-2556969/Britain-fattest-nation-Europe-cold-climate.html#ixzz4edk9oqrE

612. Sachs, Andrea. 2011. "Weight Watchers Dieters Can Have a Free Lunch?" *Time* magazine, Saturday, February 19. http://content.time.com/time/magazine/article/0,9171,2042344,00.html

613. Wedick, Nicole M., et al. 2012. "Dietary flavonoid intakes and risk of type 2 diabetes in US men and women." *American Journal of Clinical Nutrition.* February 22. http://ajcn.nutrition.org/content/early/2012/02/20/ajcn.111.028894.abstract

614. Ibid.

615. Church, T. S., and C. K. Martin, et al. 2009. "Changes in Weight, Waist Circumference and Compensatory Responses with Different Doses of Exercise among Sedentary, Overweight Postmenopausal Women." *PLoS ONE* 4 (2): e4515. doi:10.1371/journal.pone.0004515

616. Wang, Z., et al. 2001. "Resting Energy Expenditure: Systematic Organization and Critique of Prediction Methods." *Obesity Research* 9 (5): 331–6.

617. Forbes, Alice G. 2012. "How Much Sugar Are Americans Eating?" *Forbes*, August 30.

618. Lapid, Nancy. "How Common Is Celiac Disease?" *Very Well*. June 21, 2017. https://www.verywell.com/how-common-is-celiac-disease-562738.

619. Zhang, Yu Jie, et al. 2015. "Impacts of Gut Bacteria on Human Health and Diseases." *International Journal of Molecular Sciences* April, 16 (4): 7493–519.

620. Anantharaj, Preethi G., et al. 2016. "An Overview on the Role of Dietary Phenolics for the Treatment of Cancers." *Nutrition Journal* September: 15:99.

621. de Munter, J. S., et al. "Whole Grain, Bran, and Germ Intake and Risk of Type 2 Diabetes: a Prospective Cohort Study and Systematic Review." *PLoS Medicine* 2007, 4: e261.

622. Isaksson, Hanna, et al. 2011. "Rye Kernel Breakfast Increases Satiety in the Afternoon—an Effect of Food Structure." *Journal of Nutrition* April 11, 10: 31.

623. Sandberg, J. C., I. M. E. Björek, and A. C. Nilsson. 2016. "Rye-Based Evening Meals Favorably Affected Glucose Regulation and Appetite Variables at the Following Breakfast; A Randomized Controlled Study in Healthy Subjects." *PLoS ONE* 11 (3): e0151985.

624. Benjamin Lebwohl, et al. 2017. "Long Term Gluten Consumption in Adults without Celiac Disease and Risk of Coronary Heart Disease: Prospective Cohort Study." *British Medical Journal* April 3, 357: j1892.

625. *Science Daily*. "Whole grains decrease colorectal cancer risk, processed meats increase the risk." September 7, 2017. www.sciencedaily.com/releases/2017/09/170907093623.htm.

626. Sifferlin, Alexandra. "Many Probiotics Contain Traces of Gluten." *Time Magazine*. May 15, 2015. http://time.com/3860361/probiotics-gluten.

627. Delzenne, N. M., et al. 2005. "Impact of Inulin and Oligofructose on Gastrointestinal Peptides." *British Journal of Nutriton* 93 (Suppl 1): S157–61.

628. Genta, S., et al. 2009. "Yacon Syrup: Beneficial Effects On Obesity And Insulin Resistance In Humans." *Journal of Clinical Nutrition* 28 (2):182–7.

629. Patel, S.R., et al. 2006. "Association Between Reduced Sleep and Weight Gain in Women." *American Journal of Epidemiology* 164 (10): 947–54.

630. Knutson, Kristen L. 2012. "Does Inadequate Sleep Play a Role in Vulnerability to Obesity?" *American Journal of Human Biology* 24 (3): 361–71.

631. Jaslow, Ryan. 2012. "Study Confirms Not Enough Sleep Raises Diabetes, Obesity Risks." *CBS News*, April 12. Accessed May 10, 2016. http://www.cbsnews.com/news/study-confirms-not-enough-sleep-raises-diabetes-obesity-risks/.

632. Ogden, Cynthia, and Margaret Carroll. 2010. "Obesity Rates Among All Children in the United States." *NCH Data Brief 82*, Hyattsville, MD: National Center for Health Statistics, Division of Health and Nutrition Examination Surveys.

633. Dr. Michael Breus, interview with author, "Sleep Your Pounds Away." May 22, 2015. *Health Radio Network* http://toyourgoodhealthradio.com/to-your-good-health-radio-pocasts/.

634. WebMD. "Fatty Liver Disease." WebMD.com. Accessed May 11, 2016. http://www.webmd.com/hepatitis/fatty-liver-disease.

635. Molitch, M. E., and D. R. Clemmons, et al. 2006. "Evaluation and Treatment of Adult Growth Hormone Deficiency: An Endocrine Society Clinical Practice Guideline." *Journal of Clinical Endocrinology and Metabolism* 91 (5): 1621–34.

636. Lauderdale, D. S., and K. L. Knutson, et al. 2006. "Objectively Measured Sleep Characteristics Among Early-Middle-Aged Adults: The CARDIA Study." *American Journal of Epidemiology* 164 (1): 5–16.

637. Ferrie, J. E., and M. J. Shipley, et al. 2007. "A Prospective Study of Change in Sleep Duration: Associations with Mortality in the Whitehall II Cohort." *Sleep* 30 (12): 1659–66.

638. N. Vgontzas, Alexandros, and Duanping Liao, et al. 2010. "Insomnia with Short Sleep Duration and Mortality: The Penn State Cohort." *SLEEP* 33(9).

639. Valcavi, R., and M. Zini, et al. 1993. "Melatonin Stimulates Growth Hormone Secretion Through Pathways Other Than the Growth Hormone-Releasing Hormone." *Clinical Endocrinology* (Oxf). 39 (2): 193–9.

640. Aydin, Mehmet, and Sinan Canpolat, et al. 2008. "Effects of Pinealectomy and Exogenous Melatonin on Ghrelin and Peptide YY in Gastrointestinal System and Neuropeptide Y in Hypothalamic Arcuate Nucleus: Immunohistochemical Studies in Male Rats." *Regulatory Peptides* 146 (1–3): 197–203.

641. James, Francine O., and Nicolas Cermakian, et al. 2007. "Circadian Rhythms of Melatonin, Cortisol, and Clock Gene Expression During Simulated Night Shift Work." *SLEEP* 30 (11): 1427–36.

642. Park, Alice. "Why Shift Work and Sleeplessness Lead to Weight Gain and Diabetes." *Time*. April 12, 2012. Accessed May 10, 2016.

643. Ostrow, Nicole. "Lack of Sleep May Lead to Obesity, Harvard Study Suggests." *Bloomberg*. April 11, 2012. Accessed May 10, 2016. http://www.bloomberg.com /news/articles/2012-04-11/lack-of-sleep-may-lead-to-obesity-harvard-study-suggests.

644. Björntorp, P. 1997. "Body Fat Distribution, Insulin Resistance, and Metabolic Diseases." *Nutrition* 13 (9): 795–803.

645. "Chemicals in Food Can Make You Fat." *CBS News*. February 11, 2010 http://www.cbsnews.com/news/chemicals-in-food-can-make-you-fat/.

646. Stanhope, K. L. 2012. "Role of Fructose-Containing Sugars in the Epidemics of Obesity and Metabolic Syndrome." *Annual Review of Medicine* 63: 329–43.

647. Teff, Karen L., et al. 2004. "Dietary Fructose Reduces Circulating Insulin and Leptin, Attenuates Postprandial Suppression of Ghrelin, and Increases Triglycerides in Women." *Journal of Clinical Endocrinology & Metabolism* June. 89 (6): 2963-2972.

648. Stanhope, Kimber L., et al. 2009. "Consuming Fructose-Sweetened, Not Glucose-Sweetened, Beverages Increases Visceral Adiposity and Lipids and Decreases Insulin Sensitivity in Overweight/Obese Humans." *Journal of Clinical Investigation* 119 (5): 1322–34. doi: 10.1172/JCI37385. Epub 2009 Apr 20.

649. Raloff, Janet. 2009. "Concerned about BPA: Check Your Receipts." *Science News*, October 7. Accessed May 10, 2016.

650. Tavernise, Sabrina. 2012. "F.D.A. Makes It Official: BPA Can't Be Used in Baby Bottles and Cups." *New York Times*, July 17.

651. Liao, C., and K. Kannan. 2011. "High Levels of Bisphenol A in Paper Currencies From Several Countries, and Implications for Dermal Exposure." *Environmental Science & Technology* 45 (16): 6761–8.

652. Vom Saal, F. S., and S. C. Nagel, et al. 2012. "The Estrogenic Endocrine Disrupting Chemical Bisphenol A (BPA) and Obesity." *Molecular and Cellular Endocrinology* 354 (1-2): 74–84.

653. Thayer, K. A., and J. J. Heindel, et al. 2012. "Role of Environmental Chemicals in Diabetes and Obesity: A National Toxicology Program Workshop Report." *Environmental Health Perspectives* 120 (6): 779–89.

654. National Heart, Lung, and Blood Institute, United States National Institutes of Health. 1998. "Clinical Guidelines on the Identification, Evaluation, and Treatment of Overweight and Obesity in Adults—The Evidence Report. National Institutes of Health" *Obesity Research* 6 (Suppl 2): 51S–209S.

655. Blumberg, Bruce. 2012. "Chemicals That Make You Fat." *Living On Earth:* PRI's Environmental News Magazine, June 1. Accessed May 11, 2016. http://www.loe.org /shows/shows.html?programID=12-P13-00022#feature2.

656. Shankar, A., and J. Xiao J, et al. 2011. "Perfluoroalkyl Chemicals and Elevated Serum Uric Acid in U.S. Adults." *Clinical Epidemiology* 3: 251–8.

657. Holtcamp, Wendee. 2012. "An Environmental Link to Obesity." *Environmental Health Perspectives* 120:a62–a68.

658. Wang, Y., et al. 2009. "Meat Consumption Is Associated with Obesity and Central Obesity Among U.S. Adults." *International Journal of Obesity (Lond)*. 33 (6): 621–28. Accessed May 10, 2016. http://www.nature.com/ijo/index.html.

659. Today Health & Wellness. 2013. "U.S. Obesity Mystery: We're Eating Fewer Calories, Getting Fatter." *TodayHealth*, March 7. http://www.today.com/health /us-obesity-mystery-were-eating-fewer-calories-getting-fatter-1C8747683.

660. Mortelmans, M. J., and M. Van Loo, et al. 2008. "Seizures and Hyponatremia After Excessive Intake of Diet Coke." *European Journal of Emergency Medicine* 15 (1): 51.

661. Evangelista, Arthur M. 2010. "Aspartame: The History Of A Killer—The Whole Story." Rense.com, March. http://www.rense.com/general50/killer.htm.

662. Thomas, Pat. 2005. "Aspartame—The Shocking Story of the World's Bestselling Sweetener." *The Ecologist*. September; 35–51.

663. Hull, Janet Starr. "Aspartame's FDA Approval Process Shows Significant Flaws." Accessed May 3, 2016. www.sweetpoison.com.

664. Reported Aspartame Toxicity Effects. Aspartame Toxicity Information Center. Accessed May 13, 2016. http://www.fda.gov/ohrms/dockets/dailys/03 /jan03/012203/02p-0317_emc-000199.txt.

665. Mercola, Joseph. 2014. "Supporting Evidence for Aspartame-Alzheimer's Link Emerges." Dr. Mercola, June 26. http://articles.mercola.com/sites/articles /archive/2014/06/26/aspartame-methanol-alzheimers.aspx

666. Bowen, James, and Arthur M. Evangelista. 2002. "Brain Cell Damage from Amino Acid Isolates: A Primary Concern From Aspartame-Based Products and Artificial Sweetening Agents." Quality Systems, GMP, and Regulatory Site, May 6. Accessed May 3, 2016. http://qualityassurance.synthasite.com /public-health-information-research.php.

667. Gold, Mark. "The Bitter Truth About Artificial Sweeteners." *Nexus*, 2 (28) (Oct– Nov '95) and 3 (1) (Dec '95 –Jan '96). Accessed May 3, 2016. https://www. nexusmagazine.com/products/downloads/individual-articles-downloads /volume-2-article-downloads/vol-2-no-28-downloads/bitter-truth-on-artificial- sweeteners-part-1-2-detail.

668. Gold, Mark. 2003. "Letter to FDA. Docket # 02P-0317 Recall Aspartame as a Neurotoxic Drug: File #6: Aspartame and Parkinson's Disease." FDA.gov, January 12. Accessed May 3, 2016. http://www.fda.gov/ohrms/dockets /dailys/03/Jan03/012203/02P-0317_emc-000201.txt.

669. U.S. Environmental Protection Agency. "Benzene." EPA. Accessed May 3, 2016. http://www.epa.gov/ttnatw01/hlthef/benzene.html.

670. Splenda International Patent A23L001-236 and PEP Review #90-1-4 (July 1991). "How Splenda is Made." April 18, 2003. Janet Hull, Ph.D., CN. *Healthy News* http://www.janethull.com/healthynews/blog/2013/04 /how-splenda-is-made-hidden-chemicals-you-dont-know-about/.

671. Mercola, Joseph. 2011. "Avoiding Artificial Sweeteners? This Study Will Surprise You . . ." Dr. Mercola, September 20. Accessed May 3, 2016. http://articles.mercola.com/sites/articles/archive/2011/09/20/why-are-millions-of- americans-getting-this-synthetic-sweetener-in-their-drinking-water.aspx.

672. Conis, Elena. "Saccharin's mostly sweet following." *Los Angeles Times*. December 27, 2010 http://www.latimes.com/health/la-he-nutrition-lab-saccharin-20101227- story.html

673. Center for Science in the Public Interest. 1977. "Saccharin Still Poses Cancer Risk, Scientists Tell Federal Agency." CSPI Press Release, October 28. Accessed May 3, 2016. www.cspinet.org/new/saccharn.htm.

674. Ibid.

675. "Everything You Need to Know about Monk Fruit Sweeteners." *Food Insight* August 24, 2016. http://www.foodinsight.org/blogs/ everything-you-need-know-about-monk-fruit-sweeteners.

676. Kim, M., and H. K. Shin. 1996. "The Water-Soluble Extract of Chicory Reduces Glucose Uptake from the Perfused Jejunum in Rats." *Journal of Nutrition* 126 (9): 2236–42.

677. UT Health Center San Antonio Press Release, "New Analysis Suggests 'Diet Soda Paradox'—Less Sugar, More Weight," June 14, 2005. https://news.uthscsa.edu /new-analysis-suggests-diet-soda-paradox-less-sugar-more-weight/.

678. Zerbe, Leah. "Diet Soda = Diabetes Soda." Rodale News. Accessed May 10, 2016. http://www.rodalesorganiclife.com/food/diet-soda-and-diabetes.

679. Mann, Denise. 2011. "Can You Get Hooked on Diet Soda?" CNN Health.com, March 2. Accessed May 9, 2016. http://www.cnn.com/2011/HEALTH/03/01 /diet.soda.health/.

680. National Institutes of Health. The Heart Truth. "Media Kit." Accessed May 10, 2016. http://www.nhlbi.nih.gov/health/educational/hearttruth/media-room /sponsor-dietcoke.htm.

681. Carroll, Linda. 2011. "Daily Diet Soda Tied to Higher Risk for Stroke, Heart Attack." *MSNBC*, February 10. http://www.nbcnews.com/id/41479869/ns /health-diet_and_nutrition/t/daily-diet-soda-tied-higher-risk-stroke-heart-attack/#.Wc7MjNQrLs0.

682. Nettleton, Jennifer A., and Pamela L. Lutsey, et al. 2009. "Diet Soda Intake and Risk of Incident Metabolic Syndrome and Type 2 Diabetes in the Multi-Ethnic Study of Atherosclerosis (MESA)." *Diabetes Care* 32 (4): 688–94.

683. U.S. Dept of Health and Human Services. 2009. "Inspections, Compliance, Enforcement, and Criminal Investigations. General Mills, Inc." FDA.gov, May 5. Accessed May 10, 2106. http://www.fda.gov/ICECI/EnforcementActions /WarningLetters/ucm162943.htm.

684. Marturano, Janice L. 2009. "Re: Initial Response to Warning Letter of May 5, 2009." FDA.gov, May 14. Accessed May 3, 2016. http://www.fda.gov/downloads /AboutFDA/CentersOffices/ORA/ORAElectronicReadingRoom/UCM167463.pdf.

685. Society for Science-Based Medicine. 1994. "General Nutrition Inc. Agrees to Pay $2.4 Million Civil Penalty to Settle Charges It Violated Two Previous FTC Orders." FTC News Release. April 28. Accessed May 11, 2016.

686. "General Nutrition Corp. To Pay $600,000 to Settle Charges It Made False and Misleading Advertising Claims about Food Supplements." Consent Agreement Settles 1984 Charges About Healthy Greens and Additional Charges about Six Other Food Supplements. June 13, 1988. https://www.casewatch.org/ftc/news /1988/gncconsent.shtml.

687. Federal Trade Commission. 2009. "QVC to Pay $7.5 Million to Settle Charges That It Aired Deceptive Claims." FTC.gov, March 19. Accessed May 3, 2016. https://www.ftc.gov/news-events/press-releases/2009/03/qvc-pay-75-million-settle-charges-it-aired-deceptive-claims.

688. Kendall, Brent. 2015. "Pom Wonderful's Ads Were Deceptive, Appeals Court Agrees With FTC." *Wall Street Journal*, January 30 https://www.wsj.com/articles /appeals-court-upholds-ftcs-deception-findings-on-pom-wonderful-1422633948

689. Federal Trade Commission. 2008. "Makers of Airborne Settle FTC Charges of Deceptive Advertising; Agreement Brings Total Settlement Funds to $30 Million." FTC.gov, August 14. Accessed May 3, 2016. https://www.ftc.gov/news-events /press-releases/2008/08/makers-airborne-settle-ftc-charges-deceptive-advertising.

690. McMullen, Troy. 2010. "Dannon to Pay $45M to Settle Yogurt Lawsuit." ABC News, February 26. http://abcnews.go.com/Business/dannon-settles-lawsuit /story?id=9950269.

691. Federal Trade Commission. 2005. "FTC Puts the Squeeze on Tropicana's Orange Juice Claims: Tropicana Settles FTC Charges It Lacked Evidence to Support Heart and Stroke-Related Claims Made for Its 'Healthy Heart' Juice." FTC.gov, June 2. Accessed May 11, 2016.

692. Federal Trade Commisssion. 1997. "Nu Skin to Pay $1.5 Million Penalty to Resolve FTC Charges Over Fat-Loss Claims for Supplements." FTC.gov, August 6. Accessed May 11, 2016.

693. Society for Science-Based Medicine. 1993. "Revlon, Inc. To Settle Charges of Unsubstantiated Ad Claims for 'Anti-Cellulite.'" FTC News Release, August 24. Accessed May 11, 2016.

694. PR Newswire. 2011. "FDA Seizes Elderberry Juice Concentrate at Kansas Company." PRNewswire.com, June 3. Accessed May 11, 2016.

695. Armstrong, David. 2006. "How the *New England Journal* Missed Warning Signs on Vioxx." Wall Street Journal, May 15. Accessed May 11, 2016. http://www.wsj.com /articles/SB114765430315252591.

696. Doheny, Kathleen. 2011. "The Real Dangers of Weight-Loss Drugs." *Consumers Digest*, May.

697. Harvey-Berino, Jean. 2005. "The Impact of Calcium and Dairy Product Consumption on Weight Loss." *Journal of Obesity Research* 13 (10): 1720–6.

698. Chen, M., A. Pan, V. S. Malik, F. B. Hu. 2012. "Effects of Dairy Intake on Body Weight and Fat: A Meta-Analysis of Randomized Controlled Trials." *American Journal of Clinical Nutrition* 96: 735–47.

699. Berkey, Catherine S. et al. 2005. "Milk, Dairy Fat, Dietary Calcium, and Weight Gain: A Longitudinal Study of Adolescents." *Archives of Pediatrics and Adolescent Medicine* 159 (6): 543–50.

700. Steenhuysen, Julie. 2007. "Mother Nature Still a Rich Source of New Drugs" *Reuters*, March 19. http://www.reuters.com/article/environment-drugs-nature-dc-idUSN1624228920070320.

701. Shurtleff, W., and A. Aoyagi. 2012. *History of Koji—Grains and/or SoyBeans Enrobed with a Mold Culture (300 BCE to 2012).* Lafayette, California: Soyinfo Center.

702. Lin, C. C., et al. 2005. "Efficacy and Safety of Monascus Purpureus Went Rice in Subjects with Hyperlipidemia." *European Journal of Endocrinology*. November.

703. Endo, A. 2004. "The Origin of the Statins." *Atherosclerosis Supplements* 5 (3): 125–30.

704. FDA News Release. 2007. "FDA Warns Consumers to Avoid Red Yeast Rice Products Promoted on Internet as Treatments for High Cholesterol: Products Found to Contain Unauthorized Drug." August 9.

705. Wolfe, Sidney, and Steven Galson, et al. "How Independent is the FDA?: Interview with Sidney Wolfe MD." *Frontline PBS*. Accessed May 3, 2016. http://www.pbs. org/wgbh/pages/frontline/shows/prescription/hazard/independent.html

706. Feuer, Elaine. 1996. *Innocent Casualties: The FDA's War Against Humanity.* Pittsburgh: Dorrance Pub Co.

707. Fassa, Paul. 2013. "Medical Authority's System Kills: FDA-Approved Drugs Kill Over 100,000 People Annually." *Natural Society*, July 23. Accessed May 3, 2016. http://naturalsociety.com/medical-system-fda-approved-drugs-kill-100000-annually/#ixzz45B0uqjJW.

708. Anderson, Chris. 2003. "What Is Your Body Worth?" *Wired*, August 16. www.soundmedicine.iu.edu/archive/2003.

709. Koop, C. Everett. 1988. "The Surgeon General's Report on Nutrition and Health." U.S. Department of Health and Human Services. DHHS (PHS) Publication No. 88-50210.

710. Roizen, Michael, interview with the author. 2014. "YOU having a baby." *To Your Good Health Radio*. Health Radio Network. http://toyourgoodhealthradio.com /celebrity-interviews/.

711. McDougall, John, interview with the author. 2012. "Forks Over Knives" *To Your Good Health Radio*, April 4. http://toyourgoodhealthradio.com/forks-over-knives/.

712. United States Press International. 2011. "Why You Can't Eat Just One Potato Chip." UPI.com, July 5. Accessed May 11, 2016. http://www.upi.com /Health_News/2011/07/05Why-you-cant-eat-just-one-potato-chip/14221309839490/.

713. "Water." *The Honor Society Magazine*. July 15, 2016. https://www.honorsociety.org /articles/water.

714. Kallio, P., and M. Kolehmainen, et al. 2007. "Dietary Carbohydrate Modification Induces Alterations in Gene Expression in Abdominal Subcutaneous Adipose Tissue in Persons with the Metabolic Syndrome: The FUNGENUT Study." *American Journal of Clinical Nutrition* 85(5): 1417–27.

INDEX

Acidic *versus* alkaline pH, 13

Additives, food, 76–77, 121, 131. *See also* Artificial sweeteners

Aging, 67. *See also* Elderly
achieving healthy longevity, 149–151
biological age *versus* real age, 256–257
milk, accelerated by, 25
sleep deprivation and, 221

Airborne Health, Inc., 246, 248

AlgaeCal, 189–190

Alkaline *versus* acidic pH, 13

Allergies. *See* Food allergies

Almond milk, 39

Aluminum, 168

Alzheimer's disease, 67, 90, 169, 231

American Dairy Association and Dairy Council, Inc. (ADADC), 22–23

Anatomy. *See* Human biology and anatomy

Antibiotic-resistant pathogens, 56, 70–71, 126–127

Antibiotics, 136
in chicken, 69, 70–72, 79, 227
in cow's milk, 33
in fish, 106, 108–109, 227
obesity, linked to, 227
in red meat, 55–56, 62

Appendicitis, 1

Arsenic, 73–76

Artificial additives and flavorings, 76–77, 121, 131

Artificial sweeteners, 165, 228–237

Ascorbic acid. *See* Vitamin C

Aspartame, 165, 228–232

Aspirin, 252

Athletes and bodybuilders, 43–44, 82–84

Atkins diet, 3–4, 5

Autism, 30, 104–105, 163

Babies, 120. *See also* Children and infants
breastfeeding *versus* cow's milk, xxi, 20–22, 24–25, 37
calcium/magnesium required for, 24–25
cow's milk, health risks of, 20, 21, 31, 36–37
soy-based formulas, 167

Bacon, 120, 123–124, 130, 132

Bacteria, 13, 137
in chicken, 69–73
in pork, 126–127
in red meat, 11, 56, 57–59

Barnard, Neal, xiii, 60, 78, 243–244

Beef. *See* Red meat

Beef industry, 48–49, 51–52, 69

Belly (visceral) fat, 220, 221, 225

Biological age *versus* real age, 256–257

Biology. *See* Human biology and anatomy

Bison, 61

Bisphenol-A (BPA), 225–226

Blood pressure, high, 31, 82–83, 136, 148, 152–155

Blood sugar levels, 222–223
diet soft drinks and, 235–236
fruit, sugar content in, 208–209
insulin resistance, 154
rye bread and, 215
sleep deprivation and, 219, 220
"white foods," 212, 216

Bodybuilders, 43–44, 82–84

Bone health
calcium supplements and, xvii–xviii, 188–190

317